T0381805

A Social History of Wet Nursing in America: From Breast to Bottle examines the intersection of medical science, social theory, and cultural practices as they shaped relations among wet nurses, physicians, and families from the colonial period through the twentieth century. It explores how Americans used wet nursing to solve infant-feeding problems in the eighteenth century, shows why wet nursing became controversial in the nineteenth century as motherhood slowly became medicalized, and elaborates how the development of scientific infant feeding eliminated wet nursing by the beginning of the twentieth century.

Setting these changes in the context of women's history and the history of medicine, the book makes a significant contribution to our understanding of the cultural authority of medical science, the role of physicians in shaping child-rearing practices, the social construction of motherhood, and the profound dilemmas of class and culture that played out in the private space of the nursery.

A social history of wet nursing in America

Cambridge History of Medicine

Edited by

CHARLES ROSENBERG, Professor of History and Sociology of Science, University of Pennsylvania

Other titles in the Series:

Health, medicine and morality in the sixteenth century EDITED BY
CHARLES WEBSTER
The Renaissance notion of woman: A study in the fortunes of scholasticism and medical science in European intellectual life IAN MACLEAN
Mystical Bedlam: Madness, anxiety and healing in sixteenth-century England
MICHAEL MACDONALD
From medical chemistry to biochemistry: The making of a biomedical discipline
ROBERT E. KOHLER
Joan Baptista Van Helmont: Reformer of science and medicine
WALTER PAGEL
A generous confidence: Thomas Story Kirkbride and the art of asylum-keeping, 1840–1883 NANCY TOMES
The cultural meaning of popular science: Phrenology and the organization of consent in nineteenth-century Britain ROGER COOTER
Madness, morality and medicine: A study of the York Retreat, 1796–1914
ANNE DIGBY
Patients and practitioners: Lay perceptions of medicine in pre-industrial society
EDITED BY ROY PORTER
Hospital life in Enlightenment Scotland: Care and teaching at the Royal Infirmary of Edinburgh GUENTER B. RISSE
Plague and the poor in Renaissance Florence ANNE G. CARMICHAEL
Victorian lunacy: Richard M. Bucke and the practice of late nineteenth-century psychiatry S. E. D. SHORTT
Medicine and society in Wakefield and Huddersfield, 1780–1870
HILARY MARLAND
Ordered to care: The dilemma of American nursing, 1850–1945
SUSAN M. REVERBY
Morbid appearances: The anatomy of pathology in the early nineteenth century
RUSSELL C. MAULITZ
Professional and popular medicine in France, 1770–1830: The social world of medical practice MATTHEW RAMSEY
Abortion, doctors and the law: Some aspects of the legal regulation of abortion in England, 1884–1984 DONALD DENOON
Health, race and German politics between national unification and Nazism, 1870–1945 PAUL WEINDLING
The physician-legislators of France: Medicine and politics in the Early Third Republic, 1870–1914 JACK D. ELLIS

Continued on page following the Index

A social history of wet nursing in America

From breast to bottle

JANET GOLDEN
Rutgers University, Camden

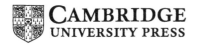
CAMBRIDGE
UNIVERSITY PRESS

CAMBRIDGE
UNIVERSITY PRESS

32 Avenue of the Americas, New York NY 10013-2473, USA

Cambridge University Press is part of the University of Cambridge.

It furthers the University's mission by disseminating knowledge in the pursuit of education, learning and research at the highest international levels of excellence.

www.cambridge.org
Information on this title: www.cambridge.org/9780521495448

© Cambridge University Press 1996

First published 1996

A catalogue record for this publication is available from the British Library

Library of Congress Cataloguing in Publication data
Golden, Janet Lynne
A social history of wet nursing in America : from breast to bottle
/ Janet Golden.
p.   cm. – (Cambridge history of medicine)
Includes index.
ISBN 0-52 1-49544-X (hc)
1. Wet-nurses – United States – History.   2. Motherhood – United
States – History.   3. Infants – United States – Nutrition – History.
4. Breast feeding – United States –History.   5. Physician and patient –
United States – History.
I. Title.   II. Series.
RJ216.063   1996
649′.33′0973 – dc20   95-22149
                                                                    CIP

ISBN 978-0-521-49544-8 Hardback

CONTENTS

List of tables	*page* vi	
Acknowledgments	ix	
List of abbreviations	xii	
Introduction	1	
1	Public discourse and private relations: Wet nursing in colonial America	11
2	The new motherhood and the new view of wet nurses, 1780–1865	38
3	Finding "just the right kind of woman": The urban wet nurse marketplace, 1830–1900	64
4	"Victims of distressing circumstances": The wet nurse labor force and the offspring of wet nurses, 1860–1910	97
5	Medical oversight and medical dilemmas: The physician and the wet nurse, 1870–1910	128
6	"Obliged to have wet nurses": Relations in the private household, 1870–1925	156
7	"Therapeutic merchandise": Human milk in the twentieth century	179
	Epilogue: From commodity to gift	201
	Index	207

TABLES

3.1 Advertisements in the *Philadelphia Public Ledger*,
1837–1897 *page* 68
3.2 Sample of advertisements in the *Boston Evening Transcript*,
1861–1896 69
3.3 Advertisements in the *Baltimore Sun*, 1875 71
3.4 Placement of wet nurses discharged from the Boston City
Temporary Home, 1862–1864 79
3.5 Wages earned by wet nurses discharged from the Boston
City Temporary Home, 1862–1864 81
3.6 Requests regarding wet nurses at the Protestant Home,
1882–1887 85
3.7 Wet nurses placed by the Nursery and Child's Hospital,
1857–1871 93
4.1 Marital status of Boston City Temporary Home registrants
by occupational choice 100
4.2 Infant status of Boston City Temporary Home registrants by
occupational choice 101
4.3 Age of wet nurses in the Massachusetts Infant Asylum 103
4.4 Age of private-duty wet nurses discharged from the
Massachusetts Infant Asylum, the Boston Lying-In Hospital,
and the New England Hospital for Women and Children 104
4.5 Occupation of fathers of wet nurses' babies, Massachusetts
Infant Asylum, 1868–1907 105
4.6 Marital status of wet nurses at the Massachusetts Infant
Asylum, 1868–1907 106
4.7 Marital status of women discharged as wet nurses from the
Boston City Temporary Home, 1862–1864 106
4.8 Marital status of wet nurses from Boston's private
institutions, 1868–1907 107
4.9 Birthplace of wet nurses entering the Nursery and Child's
Hospital, 1859–1860 108

4.10 Birthplace of wet nurses discharged from the Boston City Temporary Home, 1862–1864   109

4.11 Birthplace of private-duty wet nurses in Boston, 1868–1907   109

4.12 Birthplace of wet nurses in the Massachusetts Infant Asylum, 1868–1907   110

4.13 Previous occupations of wet nurses from Boston's private institutions, 1868–1907   111

4.14 Previous occupations of wet nurses employed at the Massachusetts Infant Asylum   111

4.15 Infant mortality rates for institutionalized infants suckled by their mothers   122

4.16 Outcome of wet nurses' infants placed in the Massachusetts Infant Asylum, 1868–1911   123

4.17 Outcome of wet nurses' infants placed at the Philadelphia Home for Infants, 1873–1899   124

4.18 Age of wet nurses' infants at the Philadelphia Home for Infants by outcome   125

4.19 Age of wet nurses' infants at the Nursery and Child's Hospital, 1859–1860   125

4.20 Age of wet nurses' infants at the Charles Street Temporary Home, 1862–1864   126

ACKNOWLEDGMENTS

This book took a long time to write. In the process, I built up a lot of intellectual debts that I am pleased to acknowledge. I must begin with my graduate school professors: Sol Levine, Diana Long, Roslyn Feldberg, and Sam Bass Warner, Jr. Each of them encouraged my interests and pushed me to work harder. Diana Long, my thesis advisor, supplied me with friendship, support, and a critical eye. While in graduate school I benefited from the advice and support of members of the Boston Women's Social History Group: Charlotte Borst, Barbara Hobson, Ellen Holzman, Diana Long, Margaret Thompson, Susan Reverby, and Kathleen Scharf. Two special friends, Joan Zoref and Ron Sanfield, helped me by sharing meals and good conversations that had nothing to do with history.

Over the years many librarians and archivists provided me with the materials I needed for my work. I want to acknowledge Christine Ruggere, Jean Carr, and Tom Horrocks of the College of Physicians of Philadelphia, Carol Pine and Richard Wolfe of the Countway Medical Library, Fred Miller and David Weinberg of the Temple Urban Archives, Adele Lerner of the New York Hospital Cornell Medical Center Archives, Sister Elaine Wheeler of the Daughters of Charity Northeast Province Archives, and Karl Kabelac of the University of Rochester Library. I also want to thank the staffs of the American Antiquarian Society, the Hagley Museum and Library, the Historical Society of Pennsylvania, the Massachusetts Historical Society, the New-York Historical Society, the Philadelphia City Archives, and the Schlesinger Library. Charles Rosenberg graciously allowed me access to his private library.

Support for my research came from a Beveridge Grant from the American Historical Association and from Research Grant 1 RO1 LMO5150–01, awarded by the National Library of Medicine of the National Institutes of Health. Parts of the book appeared in "From Wet Nurse Directory to Milk Bank: The Delivery of Human Milk in Boston, 1909–1927," *Bulletin of the History of Medicine* 62 (1988), and in "Trouble in the Nursery: Physicians, Families and Wet Nurses at the End of the Nineteenth Century," in Carol

Groneman and Mary Beth Norton, eds., *"To Toil the Livelong Day":
America's Women at Work, 1780–1980* (Ithaca: Cornell University Press,
1987), and I thank the journal and the press for granting permission for
their use.

References to wet nurses are hard to find and so I am grateful to the
many individuals who sent me citations by what is now known as snail
mail: Janet Carlisle Bogdan, Faye Dudden, Sally Dwyer-McNulty, Sonya
Michel, Randall Miller, Susan Porter, and Lynn Weiner. I benefited from
the research assistance provided at key points by two scholars, Sarah Tracey and Virginia Montijo. I appreciate the help given to me by the late
Clement A. Smith who shared his personal papers and the late Samuel X.
Radbill who supplied me with several references.

Over more years than I care to recount the members of the Chester
Avenue Seminar – David Allmendinger, Len Braitman, George Dowdall,
Svend Holsoe, Emma Lapsansky, Adele Lindenmyer, Cindy Little, Ran-
dall Miller, and Marion Roydhouse – read and commented on chapters,
giving generous, detailed criticism that improved this work enormously.
Other colleagues who read chapters or the papers from which they evolved
include Rima Apple, Gretchen Condran, Lori Ginzburg, Brian Gratton,
Joel Howell, Ed Morman, Rosemary Stevens, Janet Tighe, and Lynn
Weiner. Each of them offered insights that have worked their way into
many parts of the book. Barbara Bates, Susan Porter, Morris Vogel, and
Charles Rosenberg read the entire manuscript, generously taking time
from their own work. I benefited greatly from their wisdom and their vast
knowledge of the history of medicine and women's history. I hope that
they will see how the manuscript developed under their kind encouragement. As I prepared the final manuscript my colleague Laurie Bernstein
pushed me to sharpen my writing and clarify my ideas so that the book
would be accessible to a wide range of readers. She also helped me keep up
my sense of humor and my momentum.

In the final stage of finishing the book, I received help from several
others. The anonymous readers for Cambridge University Press took great
care in commenting on the manuscript, doing exactly what we expect of
our peers when we place a manuscript in their hands. Loretta Carlisle
suggested the title for the book and helped me prepare the manuscript in its
final form. Susan Greenberg provided skillful copyediting. Helen Wheeler,
production editor, was enormously helpful. My editor, Alex Holzman,
helped me make some important decisions, including placing the book in
the Cambridge History of Medicine Series. Most deserving of thanks is my
family. My parents, Arthur and Doris Golden, my brother, Richard
Golden, and my late mother-in-law, Gunde Joucken Schneider, always
supported my academic interests and promoted my inquisitiveness. Saman-
tha Bristow, Ruth Hotger, Beate Ittenbach, and Anita Nitsch contributed

significantly to my work by helping to care for my children and by being my friends. My children, Alex Schneider and Ben Schneider, made me think in new ways about the experiences of the mothers I write about. I thank them for this and for always tempting me to leave the confines of my study to play. My greatest debt is to Eric Schneider. He did all he could do to see that this book was written: reading every draft, taking over chores, being a single parent of two young children during my research trips, and inspiring me always with his dedication to his own scholarship. More important than all this, however, is the life we live together, and it is for this reason that I have dedicated the book to him with love.

ABBREVIATIONS

Manuscript Collections

AAS	American Antiquarian Society Worcester, Massachusetts
CCP	College of Physicians of Philadelphia Historical Collections Philadelphia, Pennsylvania
DCA	Daughters of Charity of St. Vincent de Paul Northeast Province Archives Albany, New York
FACLM	Francis A. Countway Library of Medicine Harvard Medical School Boston, Massachusetts
HLUMB	Healy Library, University of Massachusetts, Boston Boston, Massachusetts
HML	Hagley Museum and Library Wilmington, Delaware
HSP	Historical Society of Pennsylvania Philadelphia, Pennsylvania
MHS	Massachusetts Historical Society Boston, Massachusetts
NYHCMC	New York Hospital Cornell Medical Center Archives New York, New York
NYHS	New-York Historical Society New York, New York
PCA	Philadelphia City Archives Philadelphia, Pennsylvania

SLRC	Schlesinger Library, Radcliffe College Cambridge, Massachusetts
TUA	Urban Archives, Temple University Philadelphia, Pennsylvania
URL	University of Rochester Library Rochester, New York

INTRODUCTION

In her autobiography, *Blackberry Winter* (1972), Margaret Mead recalled the impending birth of her first child. Clearly influenced by her field work in regions where neither bottles nor formulas were available, the eminent anthropologist wrote of how she promised herself that she would hire a wet nurse if she could not breast-feed her child.[1]

Mead would have been hard pressed to hire a wet nurse in 1939, the year of her daughter's birth. Although hospitals sometimes kept women on call to provide breast milk to premature infants, wet nursing as a form of domestic service was fast becoming extinct. Women who could not or would not breast-feed their babies typically provided them with an artificial formula composed of modified cow's milk.[2] Indeed, by the middle of the twentieth century, many American families routinely chose bottle-feeding over breast-feeding, perceiving the former to be the modern, scientific way to rear children. Mead thus was far out of step with her contemporaries.[3] Her field work in less developed regions had taught her something most Americans preferred to forget: that human infants are most likely to survive and flourish when fed human milk.[4]

There are only three ways to nourish an infant: with its own mother's milk, with an artificial food, or with the milk of a woman who is not its mother – a wet nurse. An obvious question is why Americans rejected wet nursing, assuming that what "science" produced was superior to what "nature" provided. This book sets out to answer that question by chroni-

1 Margaret Mead, *Blackberry Winter: My Earlier Years* (New York: William Morrow, 1972), pp. 265–82. In 1975 Mead helped found the Human Lactation Center, a nonprofit organization to promote and research breast-feeding. See Dana Raphael and Flora Davis, *Only Mothers Know: Patterns of Infant Feeding in Traditional Cultures* (Westport: Greenwood Press, 1985), p. 9.
2 On the history of artificial feeding, see Rima D. Apple, *Mothers and Medicine: A Social History of Infant Feeding, 1890–1950* (Madison: University of Wisconsin Press, 1987).
3 On rates of bottle-feeding, see Apple, *Mothers and Medicine*, pp. 152–5.
4 See, for example, Margaret Mead, *Coming of Age in Samoa: A Psychological Study of Primitive Youth for Western Civilisation* (New York: William Morrow, 1928), p. 21.

cling the history of wet nursing in the United States, from the colonial period through the early twentieth century. By examining how Americans used wet nursing to solve infant-feeding problems in the eighteenth century, why wet nursing became particularly problematic in the nineteenth century, and how the development of scientific infant feeding eliminated wet nursing by the beginning of the twentieth century, it makes clear why Margaret Mead could not have easily found a wet nurse.

In rejecting scientific, technological, and economic determinism, I seek to place the end of wet nursing in a broader interpretive framework. I begin with two assumptions. The first is that wet nursing did not "lose" a competition with artificial feeding because the latter was less expensive or was more convenient. I believe its "defeat" evidenced instead the growing social class divisions between the women who were employed as wet nurses and the families in which they worked, the changing cultural perceptions of motherhood and infancy that were linked to the rise of America's middle class, the growing authority of medical science, the expanding role of physicians in shaping child-rearing practices, and the profound ethical dilemmas raised by the practice of wet nursing in the nineteenth century.

My second assumption is that infant feeding is a significant subject. Feeding decisions materially influence infant mortality rates and thus the demographic and economic structure of a society as well as its long-term viability. Additionally, the ways in which infants are fed and cared for reflects and in turn helps determine how a society is organized in terms of individual, family, and state responsibilities. In the United States, infant-feeding customs have played a critical role in defining the practice of mothering, the cultural meaning of motherhood, and thus the experiences of a majority of women.[5]

Although wet nursing offers a critical window into the historical construction of motherhood, it is a subject that has not been studied very much in the American context. Whereas historians have written a variety of books about women and children in the United States, they have largely ignored the subject of wet nursing. Most discuss the topic incidentally and anecdotally, obscuring it within their broader investigations of childbearing or of child-rearing practices, of the medical care of infants, or of family history.[6] By contrast, historians have made numerous studies of wet nurs-

5 Vanessa Maher, ed., *The Anthropology of Breast-Feeding: Natural Law or Social Construct* (Oxford: Berg, 1992); and Valerie Fildes, *Wet Nursing: A History from Antiquity to the Present* (Oxford: Basil Blackwell, 1988).
6 See, for example, Apple, *Mothers and Medicine*; Richard A. Meckel, *"Save the Babies": American Public Health Reform and the Prevention of Infant Mortality, 1850–1929* (Baltimore: Johns Hopkins University Press, 1990); Judith Walzer Leavitt, *Brought to Bed: Childbearing in America, 1750 to 1950* (New York: Oxford University Press, 1986); Sylvia D. Hoffert, *Private Matters: American Attitudes toward Childbearing and Infant Nurture in the Urban North, 1800–1860* (Urbana: University of Illinois Press, 1989); Sally G. McMillen, *Motherhood in*

ing in Europe, from the medieval period through the early twentieth century.[7]

There are good reasons for the absence of attention to the American experience. To begin with, the evidence is elusive. We do not know precisely how many infants were wet nursed, or for how long they were suckled, or whether they were fed in their own homes or in the homes of their wet nurses, or whether the wet-nursed babies lived or died. A related concern is our inability to determine the number of women who acted as wet nurses. How many women fed a neighbor's child once or twice? How many remained on the job for weeks or months? How many were paid? How many made wet nursing a career? These are valid questions, and none is answerable with precision. Instead of gathering exact counts of wet nurses, we must take snapshots of the wet-nursing population and trace its growth or decline in particular eras and regions. Instead of painting the vast panorama of wet-nursing experiences, we must sketch a series of tableaux, relying on the testimony of eyewitnesses at different points in time. The sources of information on American wet nursing are significantly fewer than the sources available to historians of other nations. European scholars can turn to the archives of the church and of the state, as each institution was deeply involved in caring for infants and placing them with wet nurses. The relative absence of American religious and secular authorities from the oversight of wet nursing has set social historians of America on a different path; nevertheless, the paucity of data linked to official organizations is in itself a vital clue about the American situation.

Another reason American historians have not fully explored the history of wet nursing is a perception that the subject is outside traditional disciplinary boundaries. It perches on the edge of two specialties – the history of medicine and women's history – and it challenges some of the central tenets of each. Recent histories of American medicine have, for example, paid close attention to the growth of medical prestige and dominance and to the development of institutions such as hospitals and academic medical schools that have supported and enhanced that growth, as well as to the changes in therapeutic practice and knowledge, particularly the germ theory of disease, that have accounted for and helped shape professional development.[8] Wet nursing was peripheral to each of these phenomena. It

the *Old South: Pregnancy, Childbirth, and Infant Rearing* (Baton Rouge: Louisiana State University Press, 1990); and Paula J. Treckel, "Breastfeeding and Maternal Sexuality in Colonial America," *Journal of Interdisciplinary History* 20 (1989): 25–51.

7 For a select bibliography on wet nursing in Western societies, see Fildes, *Wet Nursing*, pp. 281–90; and idem, *Breasts, Bottles, and Babies: A History of Infant Feeding* (Edinburgh: Edinburgh University Press, 1986).

8 See, for example, Charles E. Rosenberg, *The Care of Strangers: The Rise of America's Hospital System* (New York: Basic Books, 1987); Paul Starr, *The Social Transformation of American Medicine* (New York: Basic Books, 1982); John Harley Warner, *The Therapeutic Perspective: Medical Practice, Knowledge, and Identity in America, 1820–1885* (Cambridge, Harvard University Press, 1986); Rosemary Stevens, *In Sickness and in Wealth: American Hospitals in the*

was based in the home, not the hospital, and it was a traditional practice that was ultimately replaced by one defined as scientific. Most importantly, the job of managing wet nurses was perceived by physicians to be antithetical to their quest for professional authority. Yet, for all their reluctance to employ wet nurses, physicians still wrote about them and still had to supervise those working in private homes in the eighteenth and nineteenth centuries and in hospitals in the twentieth century. The history of wet nursing, therefore, illuminates the practice of medicine in private as well as in institutional settings and helps link the development of professional authority in each sphere.

Similarly, the history of wet nursing is identified with many currents in women's history, including studies of the intertwined worlds of home and work, the expression of gender ideology in institutions of public welfare, and the substitution of professional authority for traditional patriarchal control of the family.[9] An examination of wet nursing contributes to each inquiry by helping clarify how new mothers contributed to the family economy, how the meaning of motherhood changed over time, and how public and private authorities regulated unwed motherhood.[10] In sum, the historical evolution of wet nursing presents in microcosm the interactions of families, physicians, social arbiters, and civic authorities. Several critical themes emerge from studying the beliefs and experiences that guided these historical actors.

The first theme involves the ways in which women and physicians negotiated professional authority. The history of wet nursing displays the sometimes paradoxical relationship between the cultural and the scientific authority of medicine. Families turned to doctors because physicians supplied "scientific" answers, but the questions the families posed were social as well as medical. Was the wet nurse medically necessary? Would she

Twentieth Century (New York: Basic Books, 1989); and Kenneth M. Ludmerer, *Learning to Heal: The Development of American Medical Education* (New York: Basic Books, 1985).

9 See, for example, Jeanne Boydston, *Home and Work; Housework, Wages, and the Ideology of Labor in the Early Republic* (New York: Oxford University Press, 1990); Linda Gordon, ed., *Women, the State, and Welfare* (Madison: University of Wisconsin Press, 1990); and Robyn Muncy, *Creating a Female Dominion in American Reform, 1890–1935* (New York: Oxford University Press, 1991).

10 See, for example, Alice Kessler-Harris, *Out to Work: A History of Wage-Earning Women in the United States* (New York: Oxford University Press, 1982); Carol Groneman and Mary Beth Norton, eds., *"To Toil the Livelong Day": America's Women at Work* (Ithaca: Cornell University Press, 1987); Sheila M. Rothman, *Woman's Proper Place: A History of Changing Ideals and Practices, 1870 to the Present* (New York: Basic Books, 1978); Marian J. Morton, *And Sin No More: Social Policy and Unwed Mothers in Cleveland, 1855–1990* (Columbus: Ohio State University Press, 1993); Peggy Pascoe, *Relations of Rescue: The Search for Female Moral Authority in the American West, 1874–1939* (New York: Oxford University Press, 1990); Rickie Solinger, *Wake Up Little Susie: Single Pregnancy and Race Before Roe v. Wade* (New York: Routledge: 1992); and Regina G. Kunzel, *Fallen Women, Problem Girls: Unmarried Mothers and the Professionalization of Social Work, 1890–1945* (New Haven: Yale University Press, 1993).

disrupt the household? Doctors answered with the knowledge that what was best for the baby had to be weighed against the family's other concerns. When physicians began promoting infant formulas, assuring families that they were superior to the milk of wet nurses, a similar kind of cultural and scientific accounting occurred. Doctors knew that many families were averse to hiring wet nurses because the women's personal characteristics made them unwelcome in middle- and upper-class homes. Furthermore, buying formula proved cheaper than paying a wet nurse and was often easier to use. Physicians also understood that in discouraging the use of wet nurses and championing "scientific infant feeding" they were bolstering their own status. In these instances, scientific certainty – the knowledge that breast milk was best for babies – was traded for social authority – the use of medical knowledge to shape private behavior. Whereas professionalization rests on acquisition of skills and development of formal institutions, its critical achievement is the attainment of autonomy from lay evaluation and control. Historically this involves a process of negotiation and exchange with the client group and thus physicians made alliances with women over the issue of infant care.[11]

The changing meaning of motherhood is a second theme. Mothering is an activity gendered by a culture just as it is defined by political, legal, economic, social, intellectual, emotional, and medical paradigms.[12] Its definition is neither fixed by biology nor universally applied; instead it changes over time and varies according to social class, race, age, and marital status. Wet nursing links the biological necessity of feeding an infant with the social meaning of motherhood and infancy, and thus casts light on these shifts and variations. To oversimplify, we see the eighteenth-century condemnation of the "woman of leisure" who hired a wet nurse superseded first by the nineteenth-century outcry against women who permitted "moral lepers" into their nurseries and finally by the twentieth-century celebration of "scientific mothers." In each period, the religious, domestic, and medical literature offered a construction of motherhood based on implicit and explicit comparisons between women of different social classes, as represented by the wet nurse and her employer. Over time, we can see the growing power of the medical discourse, as it infused both popular accounts and private writings and as it shaped behavior in the nursery. Historians have called for the "decoding" of public language in

---

11 For the classic formulation of professionalization in medicine, see Eliot Freidson, *Profession of Medicine: A Study of the Sociology of Applied Knowledge* (New York: Harper & Row, 1970).
12 The history of emotions is a relatively new field of study. A critical work on the development of mother love is Jan Lewis, " 'Mother's Love': The Construction of an Emotion in Nineteenth-Century America," in Andrew E. Barnes and Peter N. Stearns, eds., *Social History and Issues in Human Consciousness: Some Interdisciplinary Connections* (New York: New York University Press, 1989), pp. 209–29.

order to understand the underlying emotional realities. The task is much the same for those studying private language. Women's private, emotional writings about their infants and their wet nurses reveal the influence of shifting and often publicly formulated ideas regarding medical science, social welfare, and the proper responsibilities of women.[13] These private writings reveal, in particular, the gradual medicalization of motherhood that began in the nineteenth century.

A third and related theme is the way in which class conflict came to be expressed in the private domain. In the nineteenth century, wet nursing evolved into an occupation for single mothers, and it became linked to the development of new social-welfare institutions, such as homes for unwed mothers, and to new medical facilities, such as lying-in hospitals. The consequences of these changes were many. Wet nurses, like other poor women, experienced increased regulation and increased stigmatization. They became more differentiated from other women in the domestic labor force, marked by out-of-wedlock births and by their passage through the social-welfare system. By the middle of the nineteenth century, wet nursing embodied essential class, ethnic, and religious conflicts, demonstrating that the clash of cultures that characterized the American experience could be found in the nursery as well as on the shop floor.

The role of the marketplace in the organization of wet nursing is the fourth theme. In a fundamental sense, wet nursing was a way for women to earn a living by selling what they produced. Certainly, in some cases wet nursing was an informal relationship governed by rules of community exchange in which the expectation of reciprocity rather than of cash was typical. In many instances, however, it was a form of paid labor – a service. The marketplace rules of supply and demand governed wet nursing in the nineteenth century just as much as did the moral guidelines preached by ministers and the medical rules offered by physicians. In the twentieth century the role of the marketplace became even more explicit as wet nursing became largely extinct and breast milk was transformed into a commodity and divorced from the physical presence of its now autonomous producer.

In tracing the historical experience of wet nursing, I have listened to both the evolving discourse and the individual voices of participants. One can generalize that the seventeenth- and eighteenth-century discourse centered around religious views of motherhood, although it became increasingly secularized as physicians and family advisors joined the chorus. In the nineteenth century, the discourse about motherhood continued, but it

---

13 Carroll Smith-Rosenberg, "Hearing Women's Word's: A Feminist Reconstruction of History," in Carroll Smith-Rosenberg, *Disorderly Conduct: Visions of Gender in Victorian America* (New York: Knopf, 1985), pp. 11–52.

incorporated new themes – heredity, morality, and science – and was increasingly articulated by physicians.

Beyond the matter of discourse lies that of experience. Wet nursing, though publicly discussed, occurred in private. The task of seeing wet nursing as a historical phenomenon requires that we peel back its many layers and explain how each stratum of experience contoured public discourse. At its core, wet nursing involves the almost untraceable interactions of a woman and two infants: the woman's own child and the baby she has been hired to feed. Women became wet nurses for many reasons – primarily to earn money – and, in the nineteenth century, to escape from welfare institutions. In addition, wet nursing was for some women a means of rejecting responsibility for their infants while capitalizing on the most valuable commodity yielded by childbirth: human milk. Unfortunately, the words of wet nurses, like those of so many other poor working people, are lost to historians. To understand their lives we are forced to turn to those who chronicled their existence and who, because of their own positions, must be presumed to have left a biased and incomplete account.

Employers, their relatives, and their friends wrote about their encounters with wet nurses, describing feelings that ranged from hostility to gratitude and experiences that concluded with the death of an infant or its restoration to health. Although modeled on relations between domestic servants and their employers, relations that arose between wet nurses and the families they served could be far more emotionally charged precisely because the life of a baby sometimes hung in the balance. At this level of analysis – one that probes family relations – we can trace how perceptions of wet nursing were shaped by changing cultural values regarding science and motherhood and equally, and perhaps more powerfully, by individual experiences.

The next stratum is comprised of the discourse created by those who observed but did not participate directly in the wet nursing relationship. The individuals who watched and wrote about wet nursing included religious authorities, household advisors, and medical experts, whose social roles gave them particular perspectives from which to assess the arrangement as well as various motives for offering advice. Typically, their counsel was in harmony, but the voices of some grew louder as others faded. Physicians were, of course, those who ultimately sang the loudest and whose words were most clearly articulated. The rhetoric and rationale of science slowly infused the discussion of wet nursing, whereas the domestic and religious discourse remained steady but, ultimately, became less resonant.

Cultural values and social structures comprise the outermost layers of this study. We can trace the process by which wet nurses, their employers, and medical professionals responded to the changing ideology of motherhood even as they helped to construct it and give it practical meaning. To achieve this dual vision, it becomes critical to understand the private family nursery as a place in which larger social forces – an expanding labor market, immigration, urbanization, and class conflict – were apparent and, ideally, managed. Studying the everyday task of feeding a baby, the most vital act of social survival, permits us to see elements that have, historically, mattered to Americans.

Other societies also coped with the need to insure the survival of their youngest and most vulnerable members, and studies of wet nursing in other cultures provide important points of comparison. Most significantly, the experience in European nations and regions offers a means of seeing how particular social structures, cultural values, and family economies influenced the understanding and use of wet nurses. The contrast, for example, between France, which instituted state regulation of its extensive wet nursing system in the nineteenth century, and England, in which wet nursing had become far less popular and therefore far less regulated, points to differences of religion, government, and family economy.[14] Where appropriate, I have made comparisons between American and European wet nursing or have demonstrated the influence of European thinking and practices.

A Social History of Wet Nursing in America is divided into three parts and an epilogue. The first section explores wet nursing in antebellum America. Chapter 1 begins with an overview of colonial wet nursing. Describing infant-feeding practices in the seventeenth and eighteenth centuries, it also investigates the overlapping religious and medical discourse on motherhood as it related to the question of wet nurses. Chapter 2 interprets how the emergence of a new view of motherhood in the nineteenth century changed medical and popular perceptions of wet nurses. In the context of changing family demographics and an emerging urban middle-class culture, a new calculus of risk appeared. This reflected both that wet nurses began to be drawn from the ranks of the urban lower classes and that middle-class mothers were given new responsibilities for shaping the character of their children.

The second section of the book describes wet nursing in the post–Civil

14 On France, see Louise A. Tilly and Joan W. Scott, *Women, Work, and Family* (New York: Holt, Rinehart & Winston, 1978); George D. Sussman, *Selling Mothers' Milk: The Wet-Nursing Business in France, 1715–1914* (Urbana: University of Illinois Press, 1982); and Rachel Ginnis Fuchs, *Abandoned Children: Foundlings and Child Welfare in Nineteenth-Century France* (Albany: State University of New York Press, 1984). On England, see Lawrence Stone, *Family, Sex, and Marriage in England, 1500–1800* (New York: Harper & Row, 1977); Ann Roberts, "Mothers and Babies: The Wet Nurse and Her Employer in Mid-Nineteenth Century England," *Women's Studies* 3 (1976): 279–93; and Valerie Fildes, "The English Wet Nurse and Her Role in Infant Care, 1538–1800," *Medical History* 32 (1988): 142–73.

War years. Chapter 3 explicates the modernization of the urban wet nurse marketplace, examining the sources for wet nurses and how, over time, the marketplace was both rationalized and segmented. Chapter 4 describes the wet nurse labor force and attempts to answer two questions: Who were the wet nurses who came to live in urban middle- and upper-class homes, and what were the consequences of their employment? Both chapters incorporate material from the case records of hospitals and welfare agencies. In all cases, the names of the wet nurses and other significant identifying characteristics have been changed.

The third section of the book looks at relations among all the participants in the wet nursing business during the period from about 1870 to about 1910. Chapter 5 focuses on the emergence of pediatrics as a medical specialty inextricably linked to the development of a science of infant feeding. It then analyzes the relationship between wet nurses and doctors in the late nineteenth and early twentieth centuries. Chapter 6 provides a parallel examination of the relationship between wet nurses and their employers. It aims to show the penetration of medical authority into the private nursery and also to explicate the sometimes contrasting experiences and opinions of medical professionals and private families. Together, Chapters 5 and 6 also explain why artificial infant feeding became the most favored alternative to maternal nursing and why wet nursing declined in popularity. Chapter 7 traces the end of wet nursing in the twentieth century. It demonstrates how the medical, social, and cultural changes that began in the late nineteenth century rapidly gained momentum, leading to the demise of the occupation. It also describes the wet nurse's replacement: the woman who sold bottled breast milk. The brief epilogue that follows describes the late twentieth-century transformation of bottled breast milk from a commodity to a gift.

I have employed terms that may be unfamiliar to modern readers accustomed to referring to infant foods by their brand names. "Hand-feeding" refers to the provision of food in a bottle or "pap boat" (a feeding vessel with a long spout used for feeding liquids and soft foods to infants and children).[15] As bottles became the more common device, the term most often used became "bottle-feeding." The substances delivered by bottle or pap boat were "artificial foods" – a reference to the fact that they were not human milk. Most consisted of animal milks (typically cow's or goat's milk), sometimes mixed with water or grain. The modern term for these mixtures is "formula." Formulas produced by manufacturers are referred to as "proprietary infant foods". In the nineteenth and early twentieth centuries, formulas mixed by mothers following medical instructions were commonly termed "scientific infant foods." The term, of course, implied

15 Thomas E. Cone, Jr., *History of American Pediatrics* (Boston: Little, Brown, 1979), pp. 63–4.

that the physician's scientific expertise allowed for the prescription of an artificial infant food that was best for the baby – better, perhaps, than what a woman herself produced.

Although there are many ways of describing artificial feeding, there are no synonyms for "wet nurse." Instead, we must track the descriptions of the women engaged in the occupation. In the eighteenth century, we find wet nurses described as poor mothers earning a living; in the nineteenth century, they become "moral monsters"; and, by the twentieth century, they are "manufacturers of milk." As these words suggest, the language of wet nursing communicated a complex and changing reality.

1

Public discourse and private relations: Wet nursing in colonial America

Women who refuse to suckle their infants are "dead while they live," wrote Cotton Mather in 1710.[1] The celebrated Puritan minister's sentiments foreshadowed generations of "family advisers," who praised mothers for breast-feeding and excoriated those who hired wet nurses. Yet social observers, including Mather, understood that families sometimes needed wet nurses – women who played a vital, indeed life-giving, role in the nursery. Mather himself retained a wet nurse for at least one of his fifteen children, and he kept his own former wet nurse on his charity list.[2]

The breach between cultural prescription and biological need marked Mather's writings as well as his life. In the former, he articulated both the religious objections to wet nurses and the practical reasons for using them. *Elizabeth in Her Holy Retirement* (1710), written to "Prepare a Pious Woman for Her Lying In," instructed mothers to suckle their own infants when possible and chided those who refused to do so: "be not such an ostrich as to decline it." However, for those who tried and failed he had words of solace: "entertain it with submission to the will of God."[3] More pragmatic advice appeared in *The Angel of Bethesda* (1722), in which Mather summarized his knowledge of medicine, including the treatment of common illnesses and the promotion of health. In this volume, Mather suggested ways to increase the milk of either a wet nurse or a mother through the use

---

1 Cotton Mather, *Elizabeth in Her Holy Retirement; An Essay to Prepare a Pious Woman for Her Lying In . . .* (Boston: Printed for B. Green, 1710), p. 35.
2 Ralph Boas and Louise Boas, *Cotton Mather, Keeper of the Puritan Conscience* (Hamden, Conn.: Archon Books, 1964), p. 7. It is difficult to determine how many of the Mather children were wet nursed. Catherine Scholten argues that wet nurses were "routinely" employed by the Mathers. Catherine M. Scholten, *Childbearing in American Society, 1650–1850* (New York: New York University Press, 1987), p. 62. In 1695 Mather recorded in his diary the death of his daughter Mehetable, attributing it to her having been overlaid (accidentally smothered in her sleep) by her wet nurse. See Cotton Mather, *The Diary of Cotton Mather, 1681–1724* (Boston: Massachusetts Historical Society, 1911–12), pp. 185–6.
3 Mather, *Elizabeth in Her Holy Retirement*, p. 35.

of drugs and diet.[4] Like other colonial Americans, Mather believed that God would judge women who deliberately neglected their children. For the virtuous few who could not meet their maternal obligations, Mather and others offered useful advice about hand-feeding and wet nursing.

Colonial Americans knew of three kinds of wet nursing: informal wet nursing, which occurred unrecorded in communities throughout the colonies; commercial wet nursing, in which women were paid to suckle the offspring of others; and rhetorical wet nursing, the discussion of wet nurses (and their employers) within an analysis of female domesticity. Ironically, the historical record of the rhetorical wet nurse is the most extensive. Religious, social, and medical writers painted vivid portraits of these household workers, although the images are heavily encrusted with moral analysis.

Ministers used the rhetorical wet nurse and the issue of infant feeding largely as a trope to analyze women's obligations to their offspring, to their husbands, and ultimately, to God. Minister and Harvard president Benjamin Wadsworth, like Cotton Mather, spoke harshly of mothers who refused to nurse their babies, calling them "criminal and blame-worthy." Wadsworth knew that the "crime" occurred, recalling in his treatise *The Well-Ordered Family; Or, Relative Duties* (1719) the women who "seem[ed] to dislike and reject that method of nourishing their children which God's wise bountiful Providence has provided as most suitable."[5] The politics of class inevitably emerged in these homilies, as authors criticized idle, upper-class women who sought pleasure not in the fulfillment of their maternal responsibilities but in a whirlwind of social activity and a life of luxury. In the epistolary novel *Memoirs of the Bloomsgrove Family* (1790), the Congregationalist minister Enos Hitchcock censured women who, "from a love of ease, or a fancied superiority to the drudgery of giving sustenance to their helpless offspring," put their children out to nurse.[6] The collective voice of the clergy rose not to condemn wet nurses, nor even to condemn those families who had a good reason to employ them, but to warn against following the example of an upper class that shunned a domestic and religious obligation.

---

4 Cotton Mather, *The Angel of Bethesda,* . . . ed. and with intro. and notes by Gordon W. Jones (Barre, Mass.: American Antiquarian Society, 1972), p. 248. For an analysis of Mather's and other ministers' views of mothers see Laurel Thatcher Ulrich, "Vertuous Women Found: New England Ministerial Literature, 1668–1735," *American Quarterly* 28 (1976): 20–40; and Martha Saxton, "Being Good: Moral Standards for Puritan Women, Boston: 1630–1730" (Ph.D. diss., Columbia University, 1989), pp. 271–320.
5 Benjamin Wadsworth, *The Well-Ordered Family; Or, Relative Duties* . . . (Boston: Printed by B. Green, 1712), p. 46.
6 Enos Hitchcock, *Memoirs of the Bloomsgrove Family: In a Series of Letters to Respectable Citizens of Philadelphia* . . . (Boston: Printed at Thomas and Andrews, 1790), p. 81.

Although clergymen framed their sermons in biblical terms, the core of their argument encompassed many of the same Enlightenment ideas influencing European secular theorists. Across Europe, eighteenth-century writers celebrated domesticity and the womanly duty of breast-feeding, espousing a new bourgeois ideology that embraced the private realm and the mother's role as ruler of this separate kingdom. The best-known account came from Jean-Jacques Rousseau who, after abandoning five of his own children to a foundling hospital, passionately denounced wet nursing and lauded maternal responsibility in *Emile* (1762).[7] His work proved to be popular but not particularly influential in terms of infant-feeding practices. Wealthy French families persisted in the use of wet nurses.[8] In Germany as well, medical and moral authorities opposed wet nurses, but the well-to-do continued to hire them.[9]

Only the English bourgeoisie turned from the employment of wet nurses in the middle of the eighteenth century, propelled by changes in family culture. Thus the doctors who promoted maternal nursing in this period were not making converts so much as they were preaching to believers.[10] The public culture of the English bourgeoisie helped to silence wet nursing's aristocratic defenders. In one telling example, Countess Elizabeth Clinton, English author of *The Countesse of Lincolnes Nursery* (1752), carefully detailed the reasons why women should suckle their own children. Like Rousseau, however, she herself had sent all of her children – eighteen of them – to wet nurses, in her case at the urging of her husband.[11]

The physicians and social philosophers who made eloquent arguments on behalf of female domesticity and maternal nursing often overlooked the fact that infant feeding was not a woman's choice, but a family's decision. The need for a woman's participation in the family economy sometimes dictated that an infant be sent to a wet nurse so that its mother could earn a living. The proscription against sexual relations during nursing also led couples to hire wet nurses and may have accounted for Countess Clinton's actions. And, finally, the desire for a male heir could result in the dispatching of infant daughters to wet nurses so that women could quickly

---

7 For a discussion of the French literature on infant feeding, see Nancy Senior, "Aspects of Infant Feeding in Eighteenth-Century France," *Eighteenth Century Studies* 16 (1983): 367–88.
8 George D. Sussman, *Selling Mothers' Milk: The Wet-Nursing Business in France, 1715–1914* (Urbana: University of Illinois Press, 1982), pp. 19–32.
9 Mary Lindemann, "Love for Hire: The Regulation of the Wet-Nursing Business in Eighteenth-Century Hamburg," *Journal of Family History* 6 (1981): 379–95.
10 Lawrence Stone, *The Family, Sex, and Marriage in England, 1500–1800* (New York: Harper & Row, 1977), pp. 429–32.
11 Ernest Caulfield, "The Countesse of Lincolnes Nurserie," *American Journal of Diseases of Children* 43 (1932): 151–62.

become pregnant again.[12] The reasons and the choices both necessitated and helped to maintain an entrenched wet nursing system. Furthermore, the developing custom of sending babies to the countryside may have served to discourage maternal nursing among some social groups by making it seem an unnatural choice. As the historical record makes clear, whatever the precise reasons for its longevity, wet nursing outlived its critics.

If the religious and secular observers appear shortsighted about the complex economic, social, and cultural foundations of wet nursing, they can be credited with an astute understanding of its consequences. Nearly every European commentator knew that wet nursing increased infant mortality. Wet-nursed infants were more likely to die than were infants suckled by their mothers, and the wet nursing system itself contributed to infant mortality by inducing poor women to abandon their own offspring in order to find employment suckling the children of others. The problem was made visible not by the private wet nursing arrangements of the upper classes, but in the systems of foundling care that developed in many European nations. Foundling hospitals, which employed large numbers of poor wet nurses to suckle abandoned babies, failed miserably in preventing the infants' deaths. Many who witnessed this wholesale tragedy quickly become advocates for maternal nursing. Benjamin Franklin, while resident in Paris, examined the statistics of the local Foundling Hospital – which had an infant mortality rate in excess of 85 percent in the first half of 1781 – and remarked in his plainspoken style: "there is no nurse like a mother."[13] Physicians, many of whom were familiar with the consequences of wet nursing, were more candid. Their writings on wet nursing wove together a discourse on righteousness with a discourse on risk. The former commented on the decisions of wealthy families, the latter on the consequences of the wet nursing system for poor mothers and babies.

Although American colonists lived in a world far different from that described by urban European physicians, they too worried about the health of their own infants, and they too were confronted with the problem of caring for abandoned infants. Thus, European medical books on child rearing found a market across the Atlantic, bringing the insights gleaned from their authors' observations of foundling homes and upper-class nurseries to the colonial American audience.[14] Readers of the *South Carolina*

---

12 Jan Lewis and Kenneth A. Lockridge, " 'Sally has been Sick': Pregnancy and Family Limitation among Virginia Gentry Women, 1780–1830," *Journal of Social History* 22 (1988): 12; and Linda Pollock, comp., *A Lasting Relationship: Parents and Children over Three Centuries* (Hanover, N.H.: University Press of New England, 1987), p. 53.

13 Franklin is cited in Samuel X. Radbill, "Centuries of Child Welfare in Philadelphia: Part II, Benjamin Franklin and Pediatrics," *Philadelphia Medicine* 71 (1975): 320. For the mortality rate at the Paris foundling asylum in 1781, see Sussman, *Selling Mothers' Milk*, p. 67.

14 On the domestic and imported pediatric literature in the seventeenth and eighteenth centuries, see William M. Schmidt, "Health and Welfare of Colonial American Children,"

Gazette in 1749 found in their newspaper excerpts from William Cadogan's *An Essay upon Nursing, and the Management of Children* only a year after its publication in England.[15] Copies of this popular and highly regarded child-rearing manual could be purchased in the colonies soon thereafter.[16]

A physician to the London Foundling Hospital and therefore a seasoned observer of infants, Cadogan, like his religious contemporaries, exalted women who suckled their offspring and reproached the "leisured ladies" who shirked their God-given responsibility. His work in the foundling asylum had taught him that mother's milk was, unequivocally, the best food for babies. Yet, Cadogan was obliged to provide more than moral instruction. Despite his misgivings about wet nurses, he had to advise mothers who could not for medical reasons suckle their babies. Weakened by childbirth, stricken with illness, or unable to produce a sufficient supply of milk, some women required instructions for hiring wet nurses or hand-feeding babies.[17]

Physicians debated the risks of nourishing an infant by artificial means against the hazards of using sick or ill-tempered wet nurses, and they also considered the likelihood of convincing well-to-do women to take their maternal responsibilities seriously. George Armstrong, for example, favored hand-feeding and was attacked for this opinion by a fellow practitioner, Michael Underwood.[18] Another influential English physician with an American audience, Hugh Smith, shared with Cadogan the belief that all mothers should nurse their infants. Smith recalled those mothers who had "ruined their health by not suckling their children."[19] Unlike Cadogan,

American Journal of Diseases of Children 130 (1976): 694–701; Joseph I. Waring, "American Pediatric Writings of the Eighteenth Century," *American Journal of Diseases of Children* 130 (1976): 741–6; and Ian G. Wickes, "A History of Infant Feeding, Part II: Seventeenth and Eighteenth Centuries," *Archives of Diseases of Childhood* 28 (1953): 232–40; and idem, "A History of Infant Feeding, Part III: Eighteenth and Nineteenth Century Writers," *Archives of Diseases of Childhood* 28 (1953): 332–40.

15 Joseph Ioor Waring, *A History of Medicine in South Carolina, 1670–1825* (Columbia: South Carolina Medical Association, 1964), pp. 67–8.

16 Within twenty nine editions had appeared, making it one of the most popular books on child rearing. Ernest Caulfield, "Infant Feeding in Colonial America," *Journal of Pediatrics* 41 (1952): 677; and John Ruhrah, ed. and comp., *Pediatrics of the Past: An Anthology* (New York: Paul B. Hoeber, 1925), p. 384.

17 William Cadogan, *An Essay Upon Nursing, and the Management of Children From Their Birth to Three Years of Age: In a Letter to One of the Governors of the Foundling Hospital* (London: J. Roberts, 1748). See also Thomas E. Cone, Jr., *History of American Pediatrics* (Boston: Little, Brown, 1979) p. 58; and Morwenna Rendle-Short and John Rendle-Short, *The Father of Child Care: Life of William Cadogan* (Bristol: Wright, 1966).

18 George Armstrong, *An Essay on the Diseases Most Fatal to Infants* . . . (London: T. Cadell, 1767), pp. 99, 101; Michael Underwood, *A Treatise on the Diseases of Children: With General Directions for the Management of Infants from the Birth* . . . , new ed., rev. and enlgd. (Philadelphia: T. Dobson, 1793), pp. 329–30. On Armstrong, see Evan Charney, "George Armstrong: An Early Activist," *American Journal of Diseases of Children* 128 (1974): 824–6.

19 Hugh Smith, *The Female Monitor: Consisting of a Series of Letters to Married Women on Nursing and the Management of Children*, 1st Am. ed. from the 6th London (Philadelphia: Matthew Carey, 1792), p. 84.

however, Smith preferred bottle-feeding to wet nursing. Wet nurses, Smith believed, carried disease. He was also critical because of their willingness to abandon their own babies in order to find work.[20] Colonial citizens read excerpts from Smith's *Letters to Married Women on the Nursing and Management of Children* (1772) in their local newspapers and purchased imported volumes of the book until an American edition appeared in 1792.

America's most illustrious physician, Benjamin Rush, issued his own opinions on the subject of infant feeding and the relative merits of wet nurses and artificial foods. He defended wet nurses with faint praise, instructing his students that these women were a necessary evil, to be employed when mothers had weak constitutions or when they were exhausted by "enervating pleasures." Rush recommended that in these circumstances a woman "snatch her offspring from her own breast and send it to repair the weakness of its stamina with the milk of a ruddy cottager."[21] His remarks stand in stark contrast to those of his British counterparts, not in his belief in the value of maternal nursing, but in his profound optimism that healthy farm women with wholesome milk could in fact be hired. Foreign writers were nearly unanimous in thinking that wet nurses generally lacked both health and morals.

The allegations differed among the various tracts. Some doctors feared that wet nurses were "given to drinking and other vices."[22] Others labeled them mercenaries and accused them of thoughtlessly casting aside their own babies in order to obtain a comfortable and well-paying position. Only a few professional men understood the sacrifice made by "poor women who suckle other people's children."[23] With suspicions running high, advice on detecting and avoiding immoral women became part of the stock-in-trade of medical writers.[24] Look for a healthy woman, wrote William Buchan, one with an abundant supply of milk, healthy children, clean habits, and a sound temperament.[25] Buchan, a Scottish physician who had worked at the Foundling Hospital in Ackworth, Yorkshire, was the author of two best-selling books, *Domestic Medicine* (1769) and *Advice to Mothers* (1803), that found a vast audience in the United States as well

20 Smith, *Female Monitor*, p. 61. On Smith's American audience, see Cone, *History of American Pediatrics*, p. 61.
21 Quoted in Samuel X. Radbill, "The Pediatrics of Benjamin Rush," *Transactions and Studies of the College of Physicians of Philadelphia*, series IX, 40 (1973): 154; and idem, "Centuries of Child Welfare, Part III: Pediatrics of the First Medical Teachers," *Philadelphia Medicine* 71 (1975): 361.
22 Armstrong, *Essay on the Diseases Most Fatal to Infants*, p. 104.
23 Underwood, *Treatise on the Diseases of Children*, p. 333.
24 See, for example, George Armstrong, *An Account of the Diseases Most Incident to Children* . . . , new ed. (London: T. Cadell and W. Davies, 1808); Smith, *Female Monitor*; and Alexander Hamilton, *A Treatise of Midwifery* . . . (Edinburgh: J. Dickson, W. Creech, and C. Elliot, 1781).
25 William Buchan, *Advice to Mothers, on the Subject of their own Health; and of the Means of Promoting the Health, Strength, and Beauty of Their Offspring* (Boston: Printed for Joseph Bumstead, 1809), p. 68.

as throughout Britain.[26] His mixture of warnings and recommendations resounded with the flamboyance of the pulpit, but he addressed an audience demanding practical advice. Buchan and other physicians understood that readers consulted home medical guides not to learn lessons of morality, but to resolve a crisis in the nursery.

Infant-feeding problems arose quickly following the death or sudden illness of a mother and left families with two choices: artificial feeding or the wet nurse. Artificial feeding met numerous obstacles. It was difficult for infants to suck the proper amount from the feeding utensils generally available: spoons, pap boats (often made of soft pewter and thus having a high lead content), or imported bottles. More critically, artificial foods, typically consisting of animal milk or a pap of flour, water, and milk, were neither as nutritious as human milk nor as easy to digest. Often the feeding implements and the food itself became contaminated with harmful bacteria. Contemporaries understood the problems of artificial feeding not in terms of neonatal sucking and swallowing reflexes, toxicology, nutrition, or bacteriology, but from observation: artificial feeding proved far less successful than wet nursing or breast-feeding at keeping babies alive.[27] For this reason, families used artificial feeding as a last resort, when a wet nurse could not be found.

The death of a mother often instigated a quest for a wet nurse. Seventeenth-century court records from Charles County, Maryland, reveal the efforts of Arthur Turner to find a woman to suckle his motherless child. His odyssey, which began at the home of one woman who was unable to wet nurse, led him to a Mrs. Ashbrooke, whom he observed in the act of nursing her own child before requesting Mr. Ashbrooke's permission to hire her.[28] The negotiation illustrates both that breast-feeding was a public act and that a woman's earnings as a wet nurse belonged, under the law, to her husband.[29]

How many men found themselves in Turner's position is difficult to

26 William Buchan, *Domestic Medicine, or, a Treatise on the Prevention and Cure of Diseases by Regimen and Simple Medicines* [Adapted to the Climate and Diseases of America by Isaac Cathrall] (Philadelphia: 1797); and idem, *Advice to Mothers*. On Buchan see Cone, *History of American Pediatrics*, p. 46, and Charles E. Rosenberg, "Medical Text and Social Context: Explaining William Buchan's *Domestic Medicine*," *Bulletin of the History of Medicine* 57 (1983): 22–42. On Cadogan's influence on Buchan, see Rendle-Short and Rendle-Short, *Father of Child Care*, pp. 18–20.

27 Cone, *History of American Pediatrics*, pp. 58–63.

28 Lorena S. Walsh, " 'Till Death Us Do Part': Marriage and Family in Seventeenth-Century Maryland," in Thad W. Tate and David L. Ammerman, eds., *The Chesapeake in the Seventeenth Century: Essays on Anglo-American Society* (Chapel Hill: Published for the Institute of Early American History and Culture by the University of North Carolina Press, 1979), pp. 141–2.

29 On public suckling of babies, see Laurel Thatcher Ulrich, *Good Wives: Image and Reality in the Lives of Women in Northern New England, 1650–1750* (New York: Knopf, 1982), pp. 138–9.

determine. The death rate of colonial mothers remains an elusive figure, clearly varying by locale, over time, and according to environmental conditions and economic circumstances. In the Chesapeake region, where Arthur Turner lived, and in the Southern colonies as a whole, maternal mortality rates were high and linked to endemic malaria, which, during pregnancy, nullified immunity and led to a build-up of parasites causing health problems in both mother and fetus.[30] In New England, maternal mortality rates appear to have been lower than in the South, but women of childbearing age still faced considerable risk of death.[31] One study estimated that between 3 and 10 percent of women who married between 1630 and 1670 died following childbirth.[32]

Reports of maternal deaths in the eighteenth century are likewise limited and often anecdotal, but they too reveal a population at risk. In Newport, Rhode Island, the Reverend Ezra Stiles recorded ten childbed deaths over the course of 1,600 deliveries for 900 women that occurred between 1760 and 1764. Maine midwife Martha Ballard, who delivered 998 babies between 1777 and 1812, recorded five maternal deaths.[33] On the island of Nantucket, calculations of maternal mortality for three birth cohorts of

30 David Patterson, "Disease Environments of the Antebellum South," in Ronald L. Numbers and Todd L. Savitt, eds., *Science and Medicine in the Old South* (Baton Rouge: Louisiana State University Press, 1989), p. 154; and Darrett B. Rutman and Anita H. Rutman, "Of Agues and Fevers: Malaria in the Early Chesapeake," *William and Mary Quarterly*, 3d ser., 33 (1976): 31–60. See also Lois Green Carr and Lorena S. Walsh, "The Planter's Wife: The Experience of White Women in Seventeenth-Century Maryland, *William and Mary Quarterly*, 3d ser., 34 (1977): 542–71; Russell R. Menard, "Immigrants and Their Increase: The Process of Population Growth in Early Colonial Maryland," in Aubrey C. Land, Lois Green Carr, and Edward C. Papenfuse, eds., *Law, Society, and Politics in Early Maryland. Proceedings of the First Conference on Maryland History* (Baltimore: Johns Hopkins University Press, 1977), p. 95; Darrett B. Rutman and Anita H. Rutman, " 'Now-Wives and Sons-in-Law': Parental Death in a Seventeenth-Century Virginia County," in Tate and Ammerman, *The Chesapeake in the Seventeenth Century*, pp. 153–82; and Walsh, " 'Till Death Us Do Part,' " pp 126–52.
31 Maris A. Vinovskis, "Mortality Rates and Trends in Massachusetts Before 1860," *Journal of Economic History* 32 (1972): 201.
32 Richard Archer, "New England Mosaic: A Demographic Analysis for the Seventeenth Century," *William and Mary Quarterly*, 3d ser., 47 (1990): 494. Archer sampled records of emigrants to New England. Most other estimates of maternal mortality come from studies of individual communities. See, for example, John Demos, *A Little Commonwealth: Family Life in Plymouth Colony* (New York: Oxford University Press, 1970), pp. 60, 131–44; and Philip J. Greven, Jr., *Four Generations: Population, Land, and Family in Colonial Andover Massachusetts* (Ithaca: Cornell University Press, 1970), pp. 28–9. For a review of maternal mortality and comparative European statistics, see Irvine Loudon, *Death in Childbirth: An International Study of Maternal Care and Maternal Mortality, 1800–1950* (Oxford: Clarendon Press, 1992).
33 Richard W. Wertz and Dorothy C. Wertz, *Lying-In: A History of Childbirth in America* (New York: Free Press, 1977), p. 134; Laurel Thatcher Ulrich, *A Midwife's Tale* (New York: Knopf, 1990), p. 373, n. 7. See also Laurel Thatcher Ulrich, " 'The Living Mother of Living Child': Midwifery and Mortality in Post-Revolutionary New England," *William and Mary Quarterly*, 3d ser., 41 (1989): 27–48.

women from 1660 to 1799 yield rates ranging from a high of 16.3 per 1,000 births to a low of 12.8 in the later decades of the eighteenth century.[34] The lack of substantive demographic data makes it impossible to determine whether maternal mortality rates generally were rising, falling, or holding steady over the course of the eighteenth century.[35] Nevertheless, it is safe to assume that maternal mortality rates ranged from a low of 6 per 1,000 births to a high of perhaps 20 per 1,000 in regions of endemic malaria. Some of the deaths undoubtedly resulted from stillbirths and undelivered pregnancies, but in other instances, the mother alone perished and the surviving infant needed a wet nurse.[36]

Maternal morbidity as well as mortality created a demand for wet nurses, as colonial women suffered from anatomical, physical, and mental conditions that limited their ability to breast-feed their infants. Severe physical illnesses prevented women from taking an infant to the breast, whereas mental disorders and other conditions resulting in fatigue probably interfered with the psychophysiological phenomenon known as the "let-down reflex" – the ability to excrete milk. Understood to be the single most important factor in the success of breast-feeding, and the most complex, the let-down reflex is influenced by hormones as well as by the psyche. Conditions such as pain, stress, and mental anguish interfere in some cases with the ability to suckle. Additional limits on maternal nursing result from nipple malformations, breast abnormalities, and a failure to make milk, a condition referred to in contemporary medical terminology as primary or secondary hypoprolactinemia.[37] A modern estimate of the number of women physically incapable of lactation places the figure at 5

34 Barbara J. Logue, "In Pursuit of Prosperity: Disease and Death in a Massachusetts Commercial Port, 1660–1850," *Journal of Social History* 25 (1991): 320–2.
35 Logue sees maternal mortality declining in the eighteenth century; Norton finds it rising in Ipswich. Logue, "In Pursuit of Prosperity," p. 322; and Susan L. Norton, "Population Growth in Colonial America: A Study of Ipswich, Massachusetts," *Population Studies* 25 (1971): 440. In the Chesapeake, female survival rates increased between 1650 and 1775. See Allan Kulikoff, *Tobacco and Slaves: The Development of Southern Cultures in the Chesapeake, 1680–1800* (Chapel Hill: Published for the Institute of Early American History and Culture by the University of North Carolina Press, 1986), pp. 60–3. For an overview of mortality rates, see Stephen J. Kunitz, "Mortality Change in America, 1620–1920," *Human Biology* 56 (1984): 559–82.
36 The estimations are in line with comparative data from European populations. For a discussion of maternal mortality and the problem of counting deaths in cases of stillbirths and in instances when the mother died in the weeks following pregnancy see Roger Schofield, "Did the Mothers Really Die? Three Centuries of Mortality in 'The World We Have Lost,' " in Lloyd Bonfield, Richard M. Smith, and Keith Wrightson, eds., *The World We Have Gained: Histories of Population and Social Structure* (Oxford: Basil Blackwell, 1986), pp. 231–60.
37 On lactation see Derrick B. Jelliffe and E. F. Patrice Jelliffe, *Human Milk in the Modern World: Psychosocial, Nutritional, and Economic Significance* (Oxford: Oxford University Press, 1978); and Ruth A. Lawrence, *Breastfeeding; A Guide for the Medical Profession*, 3d ed. (St. Louis: Mosby, 1989).

percent.[38] Another 2.5 percent suffer from mastitis, a painful breast infection that may lead a woman to cease nursing.[39] Other women no doubt suffered from such physical and mental ailments as postpartum weakness, fevers, and other short- and long-term physical and mental difficulties, which led them as well to relinquish the suckling of their babies.[40]

The correspondence between an individual mother's illness and the likelihood of her family obtaining a substitute is indeterminate. Illness could be an excuse as well as a reason for not nursing, and, conversely, women sometimes ignored enormous physical and mental discomfort in order to breast-feed. Furthermore, maternal nursing and wet nursing or artificial feeding were not mutually exclusive; in some instances, women recovered from an illness and began or resumed suckling their babies. One Philadelphia woman, Betsy Rhoads Fisher, had breast problems that kept her from nursing her baby – a situation she deeply regretted and, according to her husband, found "a greater trial of her fortitude than her own bodily pains."[41] Had she recovered quickly, Fisher might have tried to nurse the child herself. Martha Ballard wrote in her diary in 1789 of two neighbors who nursed a newborn child while the mother was ill with a postpartum fever. All parties presumed that the mother would eventually resume suckling her baby.[42] Similarly, Hannah Parkman, the second wife of Massachusetts minister Ebenezer Parkman, experienced sore breasts after the birth of each of her children and relied on friends to suckle her babies until she recovered.[43] Unlike the wealthy women described in the religious and medical literature, who allegedly used the slightest case of fatigue as an excuse for hiring a substitute, many mothers hoped to nurse their babies and were not easily deterred by illness.

Just as the prescriptive literature presumed that rich women eschewed maternal nursing, it also concluded that wet nursing was a paid arrangement. However, the experiences of Hannah Parkman and of Martha Ballard's patient suggest that women sometimes relied on the kindness of neighbors rather than on hired strangers. In a society with a high birth rate and probably frequent instances of postpartum ailments, brief, informal assistance was part of a patchwork of reciprocal relations that knit commu-

38 Dana Raphael, The Tender Gift: Breastfeeding (Englewood Cliffs, N.J.: Prentice-Hall, 1973), p. 67.
39 Lawrence, Breastfeeding, p. 209.
40 Examples from the eighteenth century are cited in Daniel Blake Smith, Inside the Great House: Planter Family Life in Eighteenth-Century Chesapeake Society (Ithaca: Cornell University Press, 1980), pp. 35–7.
41 Cited in Mary Beth Norton, Liberty's Daughters: The Revolutionary Experience of American Women, 1750–1800 (Boston: Little, Brown, 1980), p. 90.
42 Ulrich, A Midwife's Tale, p. 196. For a Southern example see Smith, Inside the Great House, p. 36.
43 Rose Lockwood, "Birth, Illness and Death in 18th-Century New England," Journal of Social History 12 (1978): 121–2.

nities together. Its casual and often spontaneous nature rendered it largely invisible; woven into the fabric of everyday life, it remained beyond the gaze of critics, ministers, and doctors. The importance of communal wet nursing lay in the lives of the infants saved and in the fact that these collective instances of informal assistance made wet nursing an accepted and acceptable part of daily living.[44]

Of course, not all temporary wet nursing involved informal arrangements. Some families hired women to suckle infants until the mother's milk "came in" – a period that could last approximately five days for a woman giving birth the first time and two or three days for subsequent births. Boston merchant Samuel Sewall recorded in his diary in 1677 that Bridget Davenport fed his son John until he was six days old and his mother could begin to suckle him.[45] The next thirteen children Hannah Sewall bore over a twenty-five-year period she apparently suckled without the assistance of a temporary wet nurse. However, following the birth of the last Sewall child, Judith, a wet nurse once again entered the Sewall home, for reasons left unstated. She was not a temporary assistant like Bridget Davenport. "Nurse Randal" lived with the Sewalls for over fourteen months, until she fell ill with "Ague in her Brest." At that point, Samuel Sewall wrote in his diary, "my wife begins to wean Judith though it be a few days before we intended."[46] The reference to his wife's weaning apparently refers to her overseeing the process, rather than to the act itself.

44 Lyle Koehler suggests that wet nursing was mostly temporary, short-term employment and often unremunerated and that wet nurses may not have thought of themselves as being employed. Although he makes an important point about the probable "undercounts" of short-term arrangements and those that involved no monetary exchange, I believe he understates the extent to which wet nurses were also employed on a long-term basis and the number of families who placed their infants out. There is insufficient evidence to determine under what circumstances wet nurses viewed themselves as workers. Lyle Koehler, *A Search for Power: The "Weaker Sex" in Seventeenth-Century New England* (Urbana: University of Illinois Press, 1980), p. 114.

45 Samuel Sewall, *The Diary of Samuel Sewall, 1674–1729*, M. Halsey Thomas, ed. (New York: Farrar, Straus & Giroux, 1973), vol. 1, pp. 41–2. Sewall uses the term "nurse" when he is speaking of women who took care of the sick as well as when he is referring to the women who suckled his children. I have discussed only those instances when Sewall refers to his children's being suckled. Lockwood discusses a similar utilization of interim wet nurses by Hannah Parkman, wife of Ebenezer Parkman, a minister in Westborough, Massachusetts, in the early eighteenth century. Lockwood, "Birth, Illness and Death," p. 122. The custom of giving infants purgatives followed by milk from a wet nurse persisted until the middle of the eighteenth century. The Glasgow physician John Burns, for example, reported that it was "customary to give some food before the child be applied to the breast." John Burns, *Principles of Midwifery, Including the Diseases of Women and Children* (New York: Printed by I. Riley, 1810), p. 380. Underwood favored the use of castor oil and took issue with Buchan who opposed this measure. Underwood, *Treatise on the Diseases of Children*, pp. 357–8; and Buchan, *Advice to Mothers*, p. 163. Fildes argues that publication of Cadogan's *Essay upon Nursing* in 1748 marked a turning point in ideas and practices. Valerie A. Fildes, *Breasts, Bottles, and Babies: A History of Infant Feeding* (Edinburgh: Edinburgh University Press, 1986), pp. 81–91.

46 Sewall, *Diary*, vol. 1, pp. 460, 482–3.

The Sewalls, a wealthy family, could have easily afforded wet nurses for all of their offspring, and thus it seems clear that for them breast-feeding was a deliberate choice. English Puritans eschewed wet nursing for religious reasons and in reaction to the prevailing upper-class custom of sending children out to nurse, and the Sewalls, as Puritans, may have been influenced by this custom.[47] However, women in all regions of colonial America breast-fed their children, making it difficult to conclude that Hannah Sewall was demonstrating her Puritan values by suckling her babies. Cultural convention rather than religious doctrine may have been a stronger argument among members of the Sewall family. One reason for suspecting this is that the fashion appears to have shifted over generations.

Rural wet nurses cared for several Sewall grandchildren. In 1704 Samuel Sewall wrote in his diary that his granddaughter, Mary Hirst, had a nurse from Salem, Massachusetts. Mary Sewall, another granddaughter, died in 1712 while in the care of a wet nurse. Eight years later, in the summer of 1720, Sewall wrote that he had gone to visit his four-month-old grandson Henry while the boy was "at Nurse."[48] The custom of sending children out to wet nurse became popular among other Bostonians. Some urban families assumed that the city was an unhealthy environment, rife with both epidemic and endemic diseases. The countryside, many believed, provided a more salubrious setting, especially in the early months of life. Evidence gathered by historians would later prove them correct.[49]

The use of rural wet nurses as prophylaxis cost money, and thus health concerns and status seeking converged when families sent their infants to the country. According to one scholar, wet nursing evolved into a cottage industry in some rural communities. Newspaper advertisements placed by women looking for babies to wet nurse often reported their distance from the city. The coastal towns outside of Boston, where the Sewall grandchil-

---

47 Fildes, *Breasts, Bottles, and Babies*, pp. 98–9. Fildes points out that Roman Catholic theologians supported wet nursing as a solution to the incompatibility of breast-feeding and conjugal relations (p. 105). For other discussions of the beliefs of English Puritans regarding wet nursing see Stone, *Family, Sex, and Marriage*, p. 263; and R. V. Schnucker, "The English Puritans and Pregnancy, Delivery and Breast Feeding," *History of Childhood Quarterly* 1 (1974): 648; and Joseph E. Illick, "Child-Rearing in Seventeenth-Century England and America," in Lloyd deMause, ed., *The History of Childhood* (New York: Harper & Row, 1975), p. 325. Illick argues that New England Puritans may have been more likely to breast-feed than their English counterparts not because of deeper religious feeling, but because their background was less aristocratic. However, he provides no evidence to support this assertion nor does he have any information about the extent of wet nursing among English and New England Puritans.

48 Sewall, *Diary*, vol. 1, pp. 496–7, and vol. 2 (New York: Farrar, Straus & Giroux, 1973), pp. 696–7, 953. Caulfield concludes that Mary Sewall was placed at a wet nurse to treat her for convulsions. The entries in Sewall's diaries refer only to his visiting the child in Brookline and to her death there. Caulfield, "Infant Feeding in Colonial America," p. 676.

49 Gerald F. Moran and Maris A. Vinovskis, "The Puritan Family and Religion: A Critical Reappraisal," *William and Mary Quarterly*, 3d ser., 39 (1982): 50.

dren presumably were sent, developed a reputation for having healthy wet nurses. Ironically, the best evidence of these New England wet nursing enclaves comes from the town death records for the "nurse children."[50]

As Samuel Sewall's remarks about his children and grandchildren suggest, responsibility for child rearing rested on all family members, although mothers shouldered the primary burden of care.[51] Husbands, fathers, and other male relatives concerned themselves with the health of family members and, therefore, with choices regarding infant feeding. Some, like Sewall, recorded their wives' and daughters' struggles to breast-feed or to hire wet nurses.

One man, Dr. Richard Hill, took up the question of his grandchildren's feeding in letters to his son-in-law and daughter, feeling no hesitation at all about voicing his opinions. Hill favored wet nursing, apparently thinking breast-feeding was too arduous for some mothers. After his daughter, Margaret Hill Morris, gave birth to twin sons in 1759, Hill expressed his approval when he learned that the boys were being wet nursed and suggested that the woman live in the Morris home. The following year, Margaret gave birth to a daughter and decided to nurse the baby herself. Hill objected strenuously, proposing that she instead put the girl "to Betty Shute's youngest daughter, some other wholesome body, or bring her up by hand."[52] Margaret Morris rejected his advice. Her husband wrote that she enjoyed nursing the child and that the baby was thriving. In this instance, Morris performed her maternal duties in a manner that would have elicited accolades from ministers, but she earned the censure of her own father.

Entangled in decisions about maternal nursing and wet nursing were issues of health, sexuality, family limitation, and race. Maternal morbidity and mortality alone did not create a demand for wet nurses, nor did maternal devotion necessarily lead women to breast-feed. To calculate the health benefits and risks of maternal nursing, families had to weigh the nutritional and physical advantages for the baby against the need for a mother to fulfill other household responsibilities and care for other children. Some observers, such as Dr. Hill, judged maternal nursing to be too exhausting and favored wet nursing. Participants may have reached different conclusions, perhaps because by choosing not to nurse, mothers put themselves in another kind of jeopardy. Lactation lengthens the interval between births, typically resulting in at least three months of amenorrhea

50 Caulfield, "Infant Feeding in Colonial America," pp. 679–81.
51 Nancy Woloch, *Women and the American Experience* (New York: Knopf, 1984), p. 23.
52 Richard Hill, *Letters of Dr. Richard Hill and His Children: or, the History of A Family as Told By Themselves,* collected and arranged by John Jay Smith (Philadelphia: T. K. and P. G. Collins Printers, 1854), pp. 173, 174, 178, 183.

and ovarian quiescence.[53] And although colonial Americans had little understanding of reproductive physiology, they were well aware that nursing
infants helped women to space their pregnancies. Families may have responded to the contraceptive effects of lactation by retaining a wet nurse in
order to increase the number of offspring. Or, they may have used lactation to limit family size or to spare a woman the physical debility that
resulted from frequent pregnancy and childbearing.

Sexual beliefs and practices also influenced decisions about infant care.
Advice books warned nursing women against sexual intercourse, hinting
that sexual excitement harmed a mother's milk and ultimately her infant.
Husbands were therefore viewed as having a critical stake in the infant-
feeding process, either because they demanded that their wives hire a wet
nurse so they could enjoy conjugal relations or because they ignored the
warnings and risked injuring their children. Doctors sometimes criticized
husbands for the presence of wet nurses or asked them to restrain their
sexual passions. William Gouge, author of a popular seventeenth-century
domestic guidebook, alleged that if husbands allowed their wives to nurse,
"where one mother now nurseth her childe, twenty would doe it."[54] In a
similar vein, the physician Hugh Smith tried to encourage men to allow
their wives to nurse, and he addressed a portion of his *Letters to Married
Women* to husbands, reminding them of the advantages of breast-feeding
for their spouses.[55]

Did women and men follow the advice about sexual self-control during
lactation, believing that restraint would assure the health of their offspring?
Or did they take advantage of the contraceptive effects of lactation to enjoy
sexual relations without fear of pregnancy? The common birth interval in
colonial America of approximately two years – several months longer than
would have been the case had breast-feeding not been the norm – supports
either explanation. However, the existing evidence points to the use of
lactation as a restraint on pregnancy, not on sexual relations. Some families, it is quite clear, deliberately used breast-feeding as a means of spacing
births.[56]

53 Lawrence, *Breastfeeding*, pp. 450–7. The contraceptive effects of lactation are influenced by
the mother's nutrition and also depend on whether the infant is completely breast-fed or
receives supplemental nutrition.
54 Cited in David Leverenz, *The Language of Puritan Feeling: An Exploration in Literature,
Psychology, and Social History* (New Brunswick: Rutgers University Press, 1980), pp. 73–4.
55 Smith, *Female Monitor*, p. 71. Historians disagree about the sexual prohibition, its parameters and its impact. See Illick, "Child-Rearing in Seventeenth-Century England and
America," pp. 310, 325–6, and n. 112; and Paula A. Treckel, "Breastfeeding and Maternal
Sexuality in Colonial America," *Journal of Interdisciplinary History* 20 (1989): 33–4. Saxton
argues that there was no prohibition on sex during lactation except for the first six weeks
after birth. Saxton, "Being Good," p. 280, n. 17.
56 Lewis and Lockridge, "'Sally has been Sick,'" pp. 7, 10. See also Ulrich, *Good Wives*, pp.
135, 138.

One of the most vivid descriptions of lactation's being used as a contraceptive comes from the diary of an eighteenth-century Virginia planter, Landon Carter, who complained bitterly about his daughter-in-law's decision to breast-feed. He objected because she was ill, and he thought she would sicken his grandchild. His daughter-in-law ignored his concerns, choosing to breast-feed, according to Carter, so that "she should not breed too fast."[57] He was well aware of his daughter-in-law's interest in controlling her fertility, having recorded in his diary her earlier efforts to induce an abortion.[58] Carter did not object to family limitation per se but to what he perceived as the detrimental effects of milk from an ailing mother who also engaged in sexual intercourse. "I have been a Parent," he wrote, "and I thought it [breast-feeding] murder and therefore hired nurses or put them [the babies] out."[59] As the days wore on, Carter recorded that his grandchild continued "to suck the poizon" from her sick mother, adding "I never knew such a vile, obstinate woman."[60] And obstinate she remained. Three years later, she fell ill again and nursed yet another infant daughter. Once more Carter complained about the "bilious mother" who refused to wean.[61]

Landon Carter was not a champion of the wet nurse so much as he was an opponent of maternal nursing. When a neighbor asked for help with her nurse, who had "something broke within her," Carter, using what appears to be a sexual slur, worried that "these creatures may be ladies of the Game, and possibly may have got foul that way." Recognizing his inability to convince his neighbor of what to do, he wrote that he wished her child had been with "some cleanly negro bubby."[62] Among upper-class Virginians, choices about wet nursing not only involved considerations of health, fertility, and sexuality, they were made with the knowledge that both slave and free wet nurses could be selected.

Wealthy Southerners' access to slave wet nurses did not necessarily translate into their frequent use. Historians remain divided on whether the African-American wet nurse was "an important adjunct in the nursery," as Wyndham Blanton argues and Julia Cherry Spruill concurs, or was no more common than white nurses in the North, as Mary Beth Norton states.[63] Clearly, though, the Southern experience was differentiated by the

57 Landon Carter, *The Diary of Colonel Landon Carter of Sabine Hall, 1752–1778,* Jack P. Greene, ed. (Charlottesville: University Press of Virginia, 1965), vol. 1, p. 511.
58 See Carter, *Diary,* vol. 2 (Charlottesville: University Press of Virginia, 1965), p. 861.
59 Ibid.
60 Carter, *Diary,* vol. 1, pp. 512, 514, 518, 520.
61 Carter, *Diary,* vol. 2, p. 765.
62 Carter, *Diary,* vol. 2, pp. 811–12.
63 Blanton argues that African-American wet nurses were commonly employed because maternal nursing was limited by frequent childbearing. Wyndham B. Blanton, *Medicine in Virginia in the Eighteenth Century* (Richmond: Garrett & Massie, 1931), p. 177. Julia Cherry Spruill also states that "employment of wet nurses was common," citing anecdotal

availability of slave "mammies" and by the ideological justifications that gradually developed to support their use. Southerners accepted cross-racial wet nursing as pragmatic, just as early settlers had turned to Native American wet nurses in times of need.[64] As the use of slave wet nurses developed into a common cultural practice, however, Southerners began to articulate arguments about its propriety. Like other aspects of racial thinking, the Southern attitude toward cross-racial nursing matured over time along with the plantation economy. Also stimulating the defense of the practice in the South were the observations and queries of visitors to the region.

Outsiders seemed to view cross-racial nursing with a mixture of fascination and disgust. In 1773, Philip Vickers Fithian, resident tutor in the family of Robert Carter III (a nephew of Landon Carter), recorded his shock upon learning that it was "common here for people of Fortune to have their young children suckled by the Negroes!" Acquaintances apparently replied to his astonishment by pointing out the frequency of the practice. As Fithian went on to note, "Dr. Jones told us his first and only child is now with such a nurse and Mrs. Carter said that wenches have suckled several of hers."[65] Other travelers also reacted with amazement, questioning whether the milk of an African-American woman influenced the character of the baby she nursed.[66] In the nineteenth century, physicians in both the South and the North would explore the issue thoroughly. In the eighteenth century, however, the Southern response remained firmly grounded on practical rather than ideological or scientific issues.

Wealthy slave owners had easy, but not necessarily certain, access to wet nurses. At times, they searched beyond their own plantations to find a wet nurse, relying, like Northerners, on newspaper advertisements. "A NURSE with a good Breast of Milk, of a healthy Constitution, and a good Character, that is willing to go into a Gentleman's Family" read a notice in

material from diaries and newspaper advertisements. Julia Cherry Spruill, *Women's Life and Work in the Southern Colonies* (Chapel Hill: University of North Carolina Press, 1938), p. 56. Mary Beth Norton rejects the argument that Southerners used wet nurses more often than did Northerners. The problem of motivation is as difficult for historians as it was for observers in the seventeenth and eighteenth centuries. Norton argues that Eliza Pickney used wet nurses regretfully. Norton, *Liberty's Daughters*, p. 91. Spruill believes that Pickney's "constitutional" explanation for not suckling her children was an "excuse."

64 Valerie A. Fildes, *Wet Nursing: A History from Antiquity to the Present* (Oxford: Basil Blackwell, 1988), pp. 128–9.

65 Philip Vickers Fithian, *Journal and Letters of Philip Vickers Fithian, 1773–1774: A Plantation Tutor in the Old Dominion*, Hunter Dickinson Farish, ed. (Charlottesville: University Press of Virginia, 1968), p. 39. Jones was Dr. Walter Jones, a Richmond practitioner, intellectual, and politician.

66 For other reactions to this custom, see Spruill, *Women's Life and Work in the Southern Colonies*, pp. 55–6; and Fildes, *Wet Nursing*, p. 141. In an interview, Mattie Logan, a former slave, recalled having been told that she had nursed on one of her mother's breasts while the mistress' child nursed on the other. George P. Rawick, ed., *The American Slave: A Composite Autobiography*, vol. 7, *Oklahoma and Mississippi Narratives* (Westport, Conn.: Greenwood, 1972), p. 187.

the *Maryland Gazette* in 1750. "Wanted by the month" began an advertisement for "A Healthy Careful Negroe Wench for a Wet Nurse" in a 1766 *Georgia Gazette.*[67] As the notices suggest, when a wet nurse could not be located among slaves, neighbors, or acquaintances, Southern (and Northern) families turned to their local newspaper.

Human milk, wrote one historian, was the most frequently advertised commodity in the eighteenth century.[68] Although the volume of notices clearly varied by locale and over time, they were indeed constant. Even in the midst of the enormous political and social upheaval caused by the British occupation of Philadelphia during the American Revolution, a notice appeared in the *Royal Pennsylvania Gazette* from "A wet nurse, who has a good breast of milk, only five weeks old, [who] would be willing to suckle a child on reasonable terms."[69] The number of notices appears to have increased at the end of the century, perhaps because the developing urban upper class could easily afford to have their children wet nursed and because, for some, employing wet nurses was a sign of status. And it is equally likely that the supply of wet nurses increased for the same reasons, as women lower down on the lengthening social ladder began to view wet nursing as a good means of earning a living.

Like others who communicated through the notice columns, wet nurses and their would-be employers evolved a kind of shorthand, which, in their case, combined the vernaculars of medicine and domestic service. Wet nurses testified to their "good health" and "full breasts of milk." Employers countered with their status as "gentlemen." The abbreviated exchanges in the press could not completely obscure the fact that wet nursing was a relationship that each participant entered into with a variety of motives.

Among free, laboring women the decision to become a wet nurse reflected an economic need that was weighed against the health of their own babies.[70] Indirect confirmation of this comes from the Quaker merchant John Reynell, who complained in a letter about a man who had thrown his wife out of the house. Reynell assumed that that would force her to wean her baby and take a job as a wet nurse.[71] Some women, of course, became wet nurses after the deaths of their infants, turning their emotional loss into an economic opportunity. Others probably delayed seeking employment until their own babies were old enough to survive without breast

67 Spruill, *Women's Life and Work in the Southern Colonies,* p. 57.
68 Calhoun attributes this statement to Schouler's *Americans of 1776.* Arthur W. Calhoun, *A Social History of the American Family From Colonial Times to the Present,* vol. 2. (New York: Barnes & Noble, 1945), p. 211.
69 Cone, *History of American Pediatrics,* p. 56.
70 Schmidt, "Health and Welfare of Colonial American Children," p. 697.
71 J. William Frost, *The Quaker Family in Colonial America: A Portrait of the Society of Friends* (New York: St. Martin's Press, 1973), p. 72.

milk. Only the most desperate mothers turned to wet nursing immediately after giving birth. If the wet nurses' infants were young, however, only the most desperate families might take them on. An employer retaining a new mother understood that the woman might favor her own offspring, if she suckled both, or suffer from excessive grief if she left her baby behind.

For both parties, a timely arrangement proved critical. Wet nurses might be needed on short notice following the death or illness of a mother or a sudden reduction in her milk supply. The women looking for work following the deaths of their babies were equally pressed; they had only a brief period in which to find a position before their milk decreased in quantity. The brevity of the newspaper notices thus disguised an intricate process in which wet nurses and families sought to make the best possible arrangement for themselves in the least possible time.

Advertisements situate wet nursing within the sphere of paid domestic employment, but they reveal little about the economics of the wet nursing business. Arrangements were private, and the marketplace was highly localized. Family records are equally difficult to decipher; some note only the amount paid to a wet nurse and fail to state whether the woman lived in the family home or in her own domicile. Other records reveal the structure of the wet nursing arrangement but omit financial details and the length of a woman's employment. For example, the 1679 business records of Robert Gibbs of Boston registers a payment of one pound eighteen shillings for suckling a child for eighteen weeks.[72] Was the child sent out or nursed at home? How did the salary compare to that paid to other domestic workers? The account books of John Pynchon, the wealthiest citizen of seventeenth-century Springfield, Massachusetts, allow for broader interpretation than the Gibbs accounts. Pynchon retained two "nurses" – probably wet nurses for his children – and over thirty domestics between 1683 and 1703. Goodwife Taylor earned twelve shillings a month for three months of nursing in 1653, and Hannah Excell earned at the same rate for four months of nursing in 1655. This was more than Pynchon paid his other female servants, but less than he paid for a lying-in nurse.[73] The wet nurses may have been married women who took babies into their own homes, whereas the domestics, typically single women, lived at service. The question remains as to whether the wages of wet nurses were high – possibly to induce women to wean their own children – or whether the value of the board and lodging given to domestics meant that the wet nurses were not well compensated. A further complication was the existence of two markets for wet nurses, one involving private families, such as the Gibbs and Pynchons, and another catering to infants under the public charge.

72 Robert Gibbs Business Records, Account book, 1669–1708. AAS.
73 Stephen Innes, *Labor in a New Land: Economy and Society in Seventeenth-Century Springfield* (Princeton: Princeton University Press, 1983), pp. 117–21, 382, 401–7.

Municipal and church authorities often hired wet nurses to suckle and care for abandoned or orphaned infants. Like the records of individual employers, accounts of these transactions are scattered and anecdotal, defining little more than the basic parameters of the arrangements. They make clear, for example, that the job of wet nursing paid satisfactorily – less than what skilled female workers could earn but enough to make a valued contribution to the family economy. In the 1730s, parishes in Virginia sent illegitimate infants to wet nurses who earned eight hundred pounds of tobacco for their work – a reflection of the local use of tobacco as currency.[74] The generosity of the payment has to be measured against the price of tobacco and the cost of renting a farm. Although no Virginia figures are available, records show that farms along the eastern shore of Maryland rented for between five hundred and six hundred pounds of tobacco during this period, and the amount of tobacco produced annually by an individual farmer typically exceeded seventeen hundred pounds.[75] A woman who earned eight hundred pounds by nursing a baby was therefore making a substantial contribution to the household.

Urban public authorities paid in cash, not kind. Between 1768 and 1787, women in Philadelphia earned five to eight shillings a week caring for infants placed out by the Overseers of the Poor. This was less than private employers reported paying wet nurses and less than the three shillings a day that male laborers could earn. Nonetheless, it was a decent wage for female domestic labor, allowing women to tend to their households and care for their children while contributing to the family welfare.[76]

The women employed by public officials may have come from a lower social class than those employed by private families, as evidenced by their willingness to accept low wages. Alternatively, they may have failed to locate a private position and settled for what the city fathers had to offer. It is almost certain that civic authorities hired women that private employers

---

74 Caulfield, "Infant Feeding in Colonial America," p. 678.
75 Paul G. E. Clemens, "Economy in Society on Maryland's Eastern Shore, 1689–1733," in Land, Carr, and Papenfuse, *Law, Society, and Politics in Early Maryland,* pp. 156–7, and Russell R. Menard, *Economy and Society in Early Colonial Maryland* (New York: Garland Press, 1985), Appendix VI, pp. 459–62.
76 Overseers of the Poor of Philadelphia, *Minutes, 1768–1774,* and Guardians of the Poor, *Minutes, September 1787 to June 1796.* PCA. A 1782 law incorporated the Overseers into a body known as the Guardians of the Poor, as part of a general overhaul of poor relief. This transition had little immediate effect on the wet nursing system. On the Philadelphia poor see John K. Alexander, *Render Them Submissive: Responses to Poverty in Philadelphia, 1760–1800* (Amherst: University of Massachusetts Press, 1980), p. 105. On wages see Gary B. Nash, *The Urban Crucible: Social Change, Political Consciousness, and the Origins of the American Revolution* (Cambridge: Harvard University Press, 1979), Table 2. Mean Wages in Philadelphia and Boston, 1725–1775, pp. 392–4. On institutional care of infants, see Samuel X. Radbill, "Reared in Adversity: Institutional Care of Children in the Eighteenth Century," *American Journal of Diseases of Children* 130 (1976): 751–61; and idem, "Centuries of Child Welfare in Philadelphia, Part I, The Seventeenth Century," *Philadelphia Medicine* 71 (1975): 279–91.

would have rejected on moral or medical grounds. Private employers shunned women with older infants because their milk was "too old," and they tried to avoid women with illegitimate children, drinking problems, or other visible vices. Public officials were not as strict, and, in addition, they offered employment to women of all races, apparently maintaining a policy of racial conformity between the wet nurses and their charges. Thus, in 1768 the Overseers of the Poor of Philadelphia sent an abandoned mulatto infant to an African-American wet nurse.[77] If white Northerners did not accept cross-race wet nursing, as the data suggest, opportunities for African-American women to find work in private homes would have been extremely limited; for this group, then, municipal employment may have been the only option.

Publicly paid wet nurses had some latitude in negotiating the terms of their work. In one instance, a woman agreed to a weekly rate of six shillings from Philadelphia's Overseers of the Poor, with the stipulation that if the infant became infected with smallpox the wage would rise to seven shillings and six pence per week.[78] The underlying assumption may have been that a sick infant required more care, that it posed a greater health risk to the wet nurse and her family, or that it was less likely to survive. The latter situation was critical. After all, when the baby died, the wet nurse became unemployed. Smart wet nurses demanded a premium for sick infants or tried to select the healthiest babies to take into their homes. In 1793 Philadelphia's Guardians of the Poor (the successors to the Overseers) found a baby left at the entry way of a private home, "in all probability deposited there by its Inhuman Mother." It was so sickly that the officials soon discovered that "no nurse would undertake to suckle it."[79]

Public authorities operated with a different set of calculations and constraints than private employers had. They had to care for the most vulnerable members of the community while carefully managing the public pocketbook. In setting rates of pay, they needed to be generous enough to attract wet nurses but not so beneficent as to entice women to abandon their own babies. For obvious reasons, Philadelphia's Overseers of the Poor tried to err on the side of caution. Their parsimony meant that they sometimes faced a shortage of wet nurses. In these instances, the infants apparently remained in the almshouse where authorities expected the residents to look after them.[80]

For women contemplating work as wet nurses, private service entailed

77 Overseers of the Poor, *Minutes, 1768–1774*, p. 26. PCA.
78 Overseers of the Poor, *Minutes, 1768–1774*, September 29, 1768, p. 33. PCA.
79 Philadelphia, Guardians of the Poor, *Daily Occurrences*, March 1792 to June 1793, June 12, 1792. PCA.
80 In 1789 the Guardians of the Poor recommended creating a foundling hospital, but it is unclear if such an institution was ever established. Alexander, *Render Them Submissive*, pp. 99, 117, and 210 n. 45.

more risks but promised greater rewards than public employment. Ann Flint, a Philadelphia woman, accepted an offer of nine shillings a week to wet nurse the child of Alice Harper in 1768. The rate exceeded that paid from civic coffers, but the payments never arrived. Flint, having no other recourse, left the infant with the Overseers of the Poor.[81] As Flint learned and other women may have surmised, although public authorities paid at low wages, workers were at least assured of receiving them. Arrangements with a stranger probably posed the greatest risk, whereas the surest position was employment by a wealthy and well-known family. One fortunate wet nurse worked for Stephen Girard, a leading Philadelphia merchant whose wife gave birth in 1791 while a "lunatic patient" at the Pennsylvania Hospital. Girard sent the infant to the country and paid the wet nurse ten shillings a week, twice what public authorities offered.[82] The Flint and Girard cases illustrate the complexity of the private wet nurse marketplace, which employed both urban and rural women and served a broad spectrum of employers. The rich, it appears, favored (and could afford) rural placement, whereas poorer urban families or single mothers looked to local wet nurses.

Girard's selection of a rural wet nurse and the wages he paid her suggest that women living in the country earned a premium. Like the Bostonians who sent their children to wet nurses living in rural Massachusetts communities, residents of Philadelphia apparently believed in the beneficial effects of country living and had parallel apprehensions about the detrimental influences of urban life. Nothing validated their fears more than the 1793 outbreak of yellow fever, which claimed the lives of over four thousand Philadelphians and sickened many thousands of others.

Many residents fled the city, and those who remained behind struggled to care for the dead and dying. Margaret Hill Morris, whose father had been so eager for her to avoid breast-feeding, assumed responsibility for five orphaned grandchildren after her son and daughter-in-law perished in the epidemic. The youngest child, her namesake, went out to a wet nurse. As the epidemic raged on, Morris described the situation in a letter to her father, depicting the "fifty-two orphan children whose parents have died in the present calamity, now under the care of the committee," among them "sixteen infants put to wet nurses."[83]

Morris referred to a citizens' committee organized to respond to the medical and social dislocations of the epidemic. Among its leaders was Stephen Girard, who helped the committee establish both a hospital for the

81 Overseers of the Poor, *Minutes, 1768–1774,* June 23, 1768. PCA.
82 Francis R. Packard, *Some Account of the Pennsylvania Hospital from Its First Rise to the Beginning of the Year 1938* (Philadelphia: Engle Press, 1938), p. 49. For examples of wages paid by Philadelphia's Guardians of the Poor, see Guardians of the Poor, *Minutes, September 1787 to June 1796.* PCA.
83 Hill, *Letters,* pp. 374, 377, 379, and 388.

sick and a home for orphaned infants and children. The older children lived with a matron and several assistants in the home; wet nurses cared for the youngest infants. Altogether the committee aided 192 "helpless innocents," approximately 25 percent of whom were nursing babies.[84] The epidemic experience proved that whatever the strain on public resources, however bleak the prospects for survival in the midst of a devastating outbreak of disease, city officials and benevolent institutions accepted standard medical knowledge that a wet nurse was the best substitute for the maternal breast.

The medical, civic, and public use of wet nurses by the citizens' committee during the yellow fever epidemic contrasts with the many instances in which wet nursing was a private, temporary act of personal generosity. Wet nursing was situated structurally along a variety of axes. As a social custom, it ranged from an act of friendship to one of paid labor to one inextricably linked to a system of plantation slavery. As a form of labor, it was an arrangement that could last as briefly as a day or as long as over a year, with varying rates of pay. The continuum of demand ranged from need – arising from the death or illness of a mother – to choice. Similarly, the continuum of employers stretched from private families to public agencies. A geographic continuum existed as well; some wet nurses lived with their employers, whereas others took babies into their own homes. In each instance of wet nursing, the axes crossed at different points, like lines from a crudely drawn star. Social critics and physicians saw these individual arrangements as a constellation and characterized its boundaries and its luminosity at various historical moments. However, to understand wet nursing at its most fundamental, experiential level, it is necessary to explore individual instances of wet nursing and judge the meaning of the wet nursing relationship to all involved: the suckling, the employer, the wet nurse, and the wet nurse's family.

The diary kept by Elizabeth Sandwith Drinker, the wife of a prosperous Philadelphia merchant and manufacturer, offers an opportunity to view and dissect three instances of wet nursing. Drinker, the mother of eight, nursed five of her children and retained wet nurses for three others. She recorded in detail her decisions and experiences, offering a window into nursery relations in eighteenth-century Philadelphia. Her private writings, covering almost fifty years, reveal complex beliefs about infant nurture and maternal responsibility, as well as about the consequences of employing wet nurses.

84 *Minutes of the Proceedings of the Committee Appointed on the 14th of September 1793 by the Citizens of Philadelphia, the Northern Liberties and the District of Southwark to Attend and Alienate the Sufferings of the Afflicted with the Malignant Fever Prevalent in the City and Vicinity* (Philadelphia: Printed by the Order of the City Council, 1848). The periodic reports of the committee mention between thirty-eight and forty-four infants "at nurse."

Drinker did not hire wet nurses in order to escape her duties, as wealthy women were often accused of doing. Wet nurses suckled her children only when she herself could not perform the task. In fact, she seems to have embraced the maternal ideology espoused in the religious, medical, and domestic literature. Yet, the overlap between Drinker's private writings on domesticity and public sentiment is deceptive. Drinker's interest in maternal nursing went beyond simply fulfilling her moral obligation; like other women, she used lactation as a means of controlling the size of her family.[85] For her, maternal nursing and employment of wet nurses were conscious acts shaped sometimes by immediate needs and other times by long-term goals. Furthermore, the situation with each infant was unique.

Drinker nursed her second child, Ann (called Nancy), for six months, until the summer of 1764, and then, for reasons left unexplained, she sent her to live in the Frankford home of wet nurse Nanny Harper. The Drinkers maintained a country home in Frankford (just outside of Philadelphia), and throughout the summer Elizabeth Drinker called on Harper, the wife of a blacksmith, regularly. She also sent her carriage to bring Nanny Harper and baby Nancy to her summer home for visits. After the Drinkers returned to Philadelphia in the fall, visits became less frequent. However, in October, after only ten months of nursing, Drinker ordered Harper and baby Nancy to Philadelphia so that weaning could begin. Ten months of nursing was short by medical standards and the briefest period of nursing given any of the Drinker children.[86] Perhaps Drinker missed her daughter.

The severing of the physical ties between Nanny Harper and baby Nancy did not signal an end to cordial relations between the adult women. In November, Drinker, her husband, and her two children rode their sleigh out to the country to call on the Harpers. The following summer, with the Drinkers again in residence in Frankford, the families paid regular visits, including one at the end of the season that allowed Nanny Harper to say goodbye to her former nursling.

Despite the ties of friendship, Nanny Harper worked for the Drinker family: they paid her, they determined for a time where she lived, and they oversaw her labors. Harper was the mother of two children, George, born in 1762, and Benjamin, born in 1764, the same year as the Drinker daughter.[87] Whether Harper weaned her son in order to suckle Drinker's daughter, whether she became a wet nurse after Benjamin finished nursing, or whether she nursed both babies at once is unclear, although the fact that

---

85 Drinker's interest in lactation as a form of contraception appears at various places in her diary, and she makes a point of recommending it to her daughter. Elaine F. Crane, "The World of Elizabeth Drinker," *Pennsylvania Magazine of History and Biography* 107 (1983): 11–12.

86 Elizabeth Sandwith Drinker, Diary, 1734–1807. HSP. On the age at which the Drinker children were weaned, see Crane, "The World of Elizabeth Drinker," p. 27.

87 Unpublished file on Philadelphia Harpers. Genealogical Society of Pennsylvania. HSP.

Harper was hired in the summer suggests the latter. Physicians recommended that women avoid weaning in the hottest months of the year, when infants were most likely to fall ill with cholera infantum – the name given to the gastrointestinal ailment that dehydrated and often killed young babies. If Harper ceased nursing her own baby in order to suckle Drinker's, she put her own baby at risk, and the likely reason was money.

Relationships in the nursery spanned a vast social continuum. At one extreme lay the plantation mistress and the slave who suckled her baby. At the opposing end was the nursing mother who suckled the hungry child of a friend, neighbor, or relative. Between the slave and the friend was the paid wet nurse, characterized in the medical and religious literature as a poor woman with few virtues other than her milk. The stereotype was grounded in the realities of female domestic employment and by the existence of poor women who squeezed out a living taking in foundlings. As a result, society's expectations of these women were low. Abigail Adams seemed startled to find that a woman suckling an orphaned boy was "very decent, respectable," and "healthy looking," adding she was "above the common level of such persons here."[88] As Adams discovered and as the case of Nanny Harper illustrates, there were significant variations among the women employed as wet nurses. Still, Elizabeth Drinker never attained the same level of intimacy with or developed the same respect for her other wet nurses. Her relationship with Harper stands in sharp relief to her later experiences, which more closely resembled traditional service arrangements. Perhaps the ties between the Drinkers and Harpers were forged by their shared Quaker religion and by their common residence in Frankford.[89]

After the birth of her sixth child, Henry Sandwith, Drinker again employed a wet nurse. As in the case of baby Nancy, Drinker nursed her child for several months before hiring help. In this instance, she fell ill while in residence in Frankford during the summer of 1771, and, obeying a doctor's orders, she hired a wet nurse for her nine-month-old son. Drinker "called on" Sally Oats, visited again the next day, and, apparently satisfied, took her "little lamb" to Oats four days later. After watching him nurse, she departed. Returning in the afternoon she found the boy in "high good humour." Thereafter she visited almost daily, stopping at the Oats home with friends or family members during the remainder of her stay in Frankford. When she returned to the city in the fall, she frequently arranged for Oats and the baby to make overnight visits. Finally, in February

88 Cited in Claire Elizabeth Fox, "Pregnancy, Childbearing and Early Infancy in Anglo-American Culture, 1675–1830" (Ph.D. diss., University of Pennsylvania, 1966), pp. 223–4.
89 On the use of wet nurses in Quaker families, see Frost, *The Quaker Family*.

1772, Drinker ordered Oats to begin weaning, and in March young Henry returned home to Philadelphia.[90]

Although Drinker followed the doctor's orders in regard to her own health, she did not consult with physicians about finding or supervising wet nurses. She made arrangements on her own and managed the care of her babies either by regular visits or direct supervision. When her eighth child, Charles, required a wet nurse, Drinker, then ensconced in her city house, searched for a wet nurse willing to live with the family.

Drinker initially nursed Charles herself, as was her custom, and probably because, at age forty-six, she was hoping to prevent any more pregnancies. Five days after his birth, however, Charles developed a sore mouth, which prevented him from nursing for nine days. In the interim, Drinker's milk diminished. She then retained Rachael Bickerton, a neighbor and the wife of a shoemaker, to come to her home four or five times a day to suckle the baby, while she continued to breast-feed as best she could.[91] At the same time, she searched for full-time help. After four weeks of work, Bickerton became ill with ague (fever), and Drinker arranged to hire a replacement, Nancy Pool, a young widow. Fate intervened again when Pool became too ill to take up her position. Drinker then hired Elizabeth Scott, but within two days she too succumbed to sickness. Rather than helping Drinker, Scott required four days of nursing care, suffering two "smartt fits" as Drinker looked after her. Scott's replacement, Betty Larkey, managed to stay on the job for a week before being dismissed as unsuitable. With understandable exasperation, Drinker wrote of breast-feeding that "it is a favour to be able to do that office oneself – as there is much trouble with nurses." Ultimately, she did resume the office herself, nursing Charles until he was twenty-six months old, the longest period she nursed any of her children.[92]

In many respects Drinker's relations with her wet nurses resembled her relations with other household employees. Accustomed to managing a live-in household staff of indentured and salaried servants as well as temporary employees, Drinker treated them all as members of an extended family, caring for them in times of illness and assisting them in times of need. She was equally capable of firing them, and she became accustomed to having them depart on short notice. Tending to Elizabeth Scott during

90 Drinker, Diary, July 17, 1771–March 8, 1772. HSP.
91 The Bickertons lived at 290 South Front Street and the Drinkers at 110 North Front Street, an easy "commute" for Rachel Bickerton. James Hardie, *The Philadelphia Directory and Register* (Philadelphia: Printed by the Author, 1794).
92 Drinker, Diary, October 28, 1781. HSP. The periods of nursing for each Drinker child were calculated by Crane. Crane, "The World of Elizabeth Drinker," Table I, p. 27. Crane's listings for Elizabeth Drinker's age at the birth of each of her children are off by one year. Elaine Crane, personal communication.

her illness or dismissing Betty Larkey as unsuitable seemed of no great consequence. However, when Drinker employed married women with homes and families of their own the relationship was necessarily different from that between a mistress and her live-in help. That Harper and Oats did not board in the Drinker home strongly suggests they were on sounder financial footing than servants earning wages.

For Drinker, sending her babies to wet nurses was, very simply, a means of providing nourishment; she did not view it as a way to relinquish her maternal duties. She visited her children regularly, monitored their health, and determined when they would be weaned. Other mothers reported the same kind of vigilance. In 1785, Mary Badger, the wife of a minister in Newport, Rhode Island, described a visit to her eight-month-old son who was being cared for by a wet nurse and noted her plans to take the boy home when he reached the age of one year. While he was absent from the household she carefully monitored his development, recording at one point that he had "already a number of teeth."[93]

Wet nursing, as experienced by Elizabeth Drinker and others, was a private relationship that challenged the description in the public discourse and was equally at odds with the private, informal wet nursing relationships that occurred beyond the gaze of social critics.[94] Drinker hired wet nurses out of need, not choice, defying the received wisdom that wealthy women used wet nurses to escape maternal duties and preserve their ties to fashionable society. Her wet nurses were not the mercenary social outcasts described in the imported literature. Two of them, Nanny Harper and Nanny Oats, appear to have been the "ruddy cottagers" Benjamin Rush recommended. The others were urban women, one of whom had a home of her own and three of whom lived temporarily in the Drinker household, much like any other domestic servant.

Drinker governed the nursery, just as she governed the household. She fired one wet nurse; four others came and went from her life according to their usefulness. One woman, uniquely, remained a peripheral part of her life after the wet nursing relationship ended. In no case did Drinker stop to ponder the meaning of wet nursing or the moral character of the wet nurse; she judged her employees by their work.

Just as Drinker's visible experience with wet nursing differed from rhetorical wet nursing, so too did it stand apart from informal wet nursing. Unlike women who relied on neighbors to suckle their infants at times of

93 Mary Badger to Mary Harrod, December 29, 1785. Robert E. Moody, ed., *The Saltonstall Papers, 1607–1815* (Boston: Massachusetts Historical Society, 1972), vol. 1, p. 534.
94 For a late eighteenth-century example of informal wet nursing see Mary Beth Norton's discussion of a woman who offered to breast-feed another woman's child along with her own so that the woman would be free to canvass for contributions to support the revolutionary troops. Norton, *Liberty's Daughters*, p. 180.

acute need – an arrangement that implied possible reciprocity – Drinker participated in wet nursing only as a consumer of services. She had no need to feel gratitude toward her wet nurses or to note the details of their lives, their families, or their characters; the women were fleeting figures who played only a cameo role in the nursery.

Colonial Americans participated in a discourse on wet nursing as well as observing the private relations between wet nurses and their employers. The discourse was about motherhood, womanhood, God, and home; the relationships were based on equally fundamental concerns: mortality, morbidity, infant health, sexuality, and family economics. In the nineteenth century, reality and rhetoric became more closely intertwined insofar as both responded to the rise of bourgeois domesticity and to the creation of an urban working class. Moreover, a native medical and domestic literature appeared that presented a new kind of motherhood, a new kind of wet nurse, and a new form of nursery relations. Elizabeth Drinker viewed her wet nurses as sometimes troublesome; later generations would see wet nurses as dangerous. Drinker wrote unsentimentally of maternal nursing that "it is a favour to be able to do that office oneself." By contrast, nineteenth-century mothers would describe suckling as an ennobling activity.

2

The new motherhood and the new view of wet nurses, 1780–1865

Thirty years after Elizabeth Drinker gave birth to her last child, another mother of eight published anonymously the first American book to deal exclusively with the raising of children: *The Maternal Physician* (1811). The author, Mary Palmer Tyler, sounding like a latter-day Cotton Mather, approached the question of maternal nursing in light of its moral value. Joining the chorus of those singing its praises, she urged mothers to "undergo every thing short of death or lasting disease" to nurse their babies. Still, like the medical authorities she cited, Tyler advised employing a wet nurse temporarily if the mother was unable to satisfy the hunger of her newborn or permanently if the mother could not nurse at all.[1] Little had changed in the rhetoric of infant feeding or the rationale for employing wet nurses. The reality, however, was different.

Motherhood, as the discussions of Tyler and her contemporaries suggest, was being recontoured in the postrevolutionary era. The moral weight placed on maternal nursing grew heavier as women assumed even greater responsibility for child rearing and as child rearing was given greater emphasis in republican America. Overwhelming women's search for child-rearing advice was a flood of domestic treatises and popular medical guidebooks, all dealing with infant nurture. In this literature, the wet nurse appears in a new guise. As she crossed the threshold of her employer's home, bringing with her the taint of her environment and her flawed character, the wet nurse became a potential threat as well as a possible savior.

One physician who expressed the new view of wet nurses was William Potts Dewees. "Perhaps nothing displays the selfishness of the nurse in such strong relief," he wrote, "as the tyranny with which she attempts to

---

1 [Mary Palmer Tyler,] *The Maternal Physician; A Treatise on the Nurture and Management of Infants, From the Birth Until Age Two Years Old* (New York: Isaac Riley, 1811), pp. 12–14. A second edition – a sign of the book's popularity – was published in 1818. On the maternal physician, see Charles E. Rosenberg, "Introduction," *The Maternal Physician* (reprint; New York: Arno Press, 1972), unpaged.

govern the whole house – every body, and every thing."[2] Dewees, a professor of midwifery at the University of Pennsylvania, described the social relations between wet nurses and their employers in the language of the early republic. In Dewees's view, the wet nurse threatened to subvert the household commonwealth by substituting domestic tyranny for the natural hierarchy of the family. Furthermore, the wet nurse epitomized the threat to gender conventions posed by working-class women, for, according to Dewees, she sought not only to earn a living but also to gratify her "wayward pleasures." Fusing the language of politics with the politics of gender and class, Dewees articulated a new interpretation of nursery relations.

In the nineteenth century, descriptions of wet nurses became a means for elucidating the maternal deficiencies of poor women, in contrast to the virtues of middle-class mothers. A developing doctrine of motherhood stressed that the fate of children rested not just in God's hands, but in those of women. And the home, increasingly viewed as a private sphere separated from commercial enterprises, became a mother's workshop. Opening the nursery door to a stranger, an unknown wet nurse – possibly a woman of deficient character – was, therefore, a risk.

The growing suspicion of the poor and their increasing cultural and geographic separation from the middle class had many consequences for the practice of wet nursing. Elizabeth Drinker hired neighbors to wet nurse her children and maintained cordial relations with at least one of them; later generations hired strangers. One result was that direct supervision of wet nurses came to be seen as vital by both physicians and lay advisors, as well as by private families. Experts no longer advocated sending babies to the country, and middle- and upper-class families no longer did so. Good mothering, they believed, required that the nursery be closely watched. Yet, by making wet nursing a form of live-in domestic service, employers brought a new population of women into the wet nursing business. No longer was wet nursing a job performed by rural married women with homes of their own; instead, it was a temporary occupation for poor urban mothers. The perceived risk of wet nursing was thus increased, as the poor were seen as medically threatening and morally lax. And this perception, in turn, heightened maternal vigilance.

Between the American Revolution and the Civil War, the idea and reality of motherhood was reconfigured by a demographic transition, by changes in the economy, and by the creation of a new domestic ideology. White families living on farms as well as those in cities began limiting their

---

2 William Potts Dewees, *A Treatise on the Physical and Medical Treatment of Children*, 2d ed. (Philadelphia: Carey & Lea, 1826), pp. 59–60.

fertility over the course of the nineteenth century.[3] In 1800 white American women bore an average of 7.04 children; by 1860 the number fell to 5.21, and it would continue to fall thereafter.[4] Among the reasons for this decline offered by demographers were the decreasing availability of farmland, the impact of urbanization along with an increase in the number of individuals engaged in industrial and commercial enterprises, the growing access to education, and the more difficult to define transformation known as modernization.[5] Modernization was not an engine of change per se, but a reflection of how new economic, political, and social realities structured personal and family life.[6] Women spent less time being pregnant, nursing, or rearing the young, and their experience of mothering encouraged a new cultural interpretation of motherhood. It became less extensive but more intensive.

On-going economic transformations resulted in new conceptualizations of home and work.[7] Ideally, wives and mothers remained outside the paid labor force. Moreover, the home, although materially, emotionally, and functionally intertwined with the marketplace, came to be viewed as a separate domain.[8] Within it, women engaged in social reproduction –

3 For an analysis of the literature on the demographic transition and the methods used to limit fertility, see Carl N. Degler, *At Odds: Women and the Family in America from the Revolution to the Present* (New York: Oxford University Press, 1980), pp. 178–249. One study that links decreasing family size to the shifting economy is Mary P. Ryan, *Cradle of the Middle Class: The Family in Oneida County, New York, 1790–1865* (Cambridge: Cambridge University Press, 1981), pp. 55–7, 184; 249, Table A.6; 267, Table E.1. On the Southern exception to the decreasing size of families, see Sally G. McMillen, *Motherhood in the Old South: Pregnancy, Childbirth, and Infant Rearing* (Baton Rouge: Louisiana State University Press, 1990), pp. 32–3. On the ideological framework of sexual control, see Nancy F. Cott, "Passionlessness: An Interpretation of Victorian Sexual Ideology, 1790–1850," *Signs: A Journal of Women in Culture and Society* 4 (1978): 210–36; and Daniel Scott Smith, "Family Limitation, Sexual Control, and Domestic Feminism in Victorian America," *Feminist Studies* 1 (1973): 40–57.

4 Mary P. Ryan, *Womanhood in America*, 2d ed. (New York: New Viewpoints, 1979), p. 96. The most thorough analysis of this demographic transition remains Yasukichi Yasuba, *Birth Rates of the White Population in the United States, 1800–1860: An Economic Study* (Baltimore: Johns Hopkins University Press, 1962). Yasuba demonstrates the rural decline in fertility, a point reiterated by Tamara K. Hareven and Maris A. Vinovskis, eds., *Family and Population in Nineteenth-Century America* (Princeton: Princeton University Press, 1978), pp. 5–7.

5 Maris A. Vinovskis, *Fertility in Massachusetts from the Revolution to the Civil War* (New York: Academic Press, 1981).

6 Richard D. Brown, *Modernization: The Transformation of American Life, 1600–1865* (New York: Hill & Wang, 1976).

7 On the links between the changing conceptions of home and work, see Jeanne Boydston, *Home and Work: Housework, Wages, and the Ideology of Labor in the Early Republic* (New York: Oxford University Press, 1990). On domesticity see Glenna Matthews, *"Just a Housewife": The Rise and Fall of Domesticity in America* (New York: Oxford University Press, 1987), pp. 50–65.

8 Discussion of the separation of spheres is extensive. See, for example, Nancy F. Cott, *The Bonds of Womanhood: "Woman's Sphere" in New England, 1780–1835* (New Haven: Yale University Press, 1977); Degler, *At Odds*, pp. 26–51; and Barbara Welter, "The Cult of True Womanhood: 1820–1860," *American Quarterly* 18 (1966): 151–74. An analysis and critique of this concept can be found in Linda K. Kerber, "Separate Spheres, Female

endowing their offspring with physical well-being and the character traits needed for economic success.

The work of mothering began when children were at a tender age. In 1838 the writer Lydia Sigourney reminded mothers of their "dominion over the unformed character of the infant" and invited them to "write what you will upon the printless tablet with your wand of love."[9] Sigourney's emphasis on the malleable character of infants epitomized the emerging theory of child rearing, in which nurture supplanted fear as the critical operating principle. Calvinist belief in the innate evil of children slowly eroded.[10] Rather than break the will of their offspring, mothers, many social observers commented, should seek to lead their children to righteousness. Nancy Cott's study of the private writings of New England women found surprising congruence between advice and practice.[11] Writing in 1813, one woman expressed little doubt that "if mothers would begin with their children when they are young, they might mould them into any frame they chose."[12] The effect of such efforts is uncertain, but the women who tried to follow the new model clearly developed what Southern historian Suzanne Lebsock calls "a passionate attachment to their children."[13]

Historians have bestowed a variety of labels on the emerging ideals of the nineteenth century: republican motherhood, the cult of domesticity, moral motherhood, imperial motherhood, to mention a few.[14] The most critical historical insight lies not in naming the cultural transformation,

Worlds, Woman's Place: The Rhetoric of Women's History," *Journal of American History* 75 (1988): 9–39.

9 Lydia H. Sigourney, *Letters to Mothers* (Hartford: Hudson & Skinner, 1838), p. 10.

10 Bernard Wishy, *The Child and the Republic: The Dawn of Modern American Child Nurture* (Philadelphia: University of Pennsylvania Press, 1968), pp. 11–49. Barbara Leslie Epstein, *The Politics of Domesticity: Women, Evangelism, and Temperance in Nineteenth Century America* (Middletown: Wesleyan University Press, 1981), pp. 81–4.

11 Cott, *Bonds of Womanhood*.

12 Peggy Dow, "Vicissitudes, or the Journey of Life; and Supplementary Reflections to the Journey of Life," in Lorenzo Dow, *History of Cosmopolite . . .* (Cincinnati: Anderson Gates & Wright, 1859), p. 669 cited in Cott, *Bonds of Womanhood*, pp. 88–9. Cott cites a number of other New England women discussing what she terms "the vocation of motherhood." See pp. 84–98.

13 Suzanne Lebsock, *The Free Women of Petersburg: Status and Culture in a Southern Town, 1784–1860* (New York: Norton, 1985), p. 159.

14 Ruth H. Bloch, "American Feminine Ideals in Transition: The Rise of the Moral Mother, 1785–1815," *Feminist Studies* 4 (1978): 101–26; Linda K. Kerber, *Women of the Republic: Intellect and Ideology in Revolutionary America* (Chapel Hill: Published for the Institute of Early American History and Culture by the University of North Carolina Press, 1980); Jan Lewis, "Mother's Love: The Construction of an Emotion in Nineteenth-Century America," in Andrew E. Barnes and Peter N. Stearns, eds. *Social History and Issues in Human Consciousness; Some Interdisciplinary Connections* (New York: New York University Press, 1989) pp. 209–29; Mary P. Ryan, *The Empire of the Mother: American Writing about Domesticity, 1830–1860* (New York: Copublished by the Institute for Research in History and Haworth Press, 1982); and Welter, "Cult of True Womanhood." For a discussion of Southern women and child-centered homes, see Lebsock, *The Free Women of Petersburg,* pp. 159–61.

however, but in explicating its development in the context of the emergence of an urban bourgeoisie distinct from both the wealthy, merchant-dominated elite and the masses of families dependent upon low-wage labor.[15] The cultural hegemony of the new urban middle class would express itself in many forms. Among the most influential was the remaking of motherhood as a vocation imbued with social meaning, yet seemingly removed from the social nexus of the marketplace.

For wet nursing, the creation of this new, largely urban middle class had critical consequences. First, families began to expect that wet nursing would take place in the homes of employers, who could carefully oversee the daily development of their offspring. Second, as the employment of servants became a critical index of middle-class status, wet nursing was framed by the conventions of domestic service. Third, the growing cultural isolation of the working class led to the characterization of wet nurses as dangerous. More than other servants, wet nurses could threaten the sanctity of the home because they strongly influenced the life of the family's most vulnerable member. They also entwined the sacred space of the nursery with the cash economy and with the world of the working class. Finally, the middle class's perception that the city was unhealthy and that they and their children were particularly vulnerable to its perils accentuated the fear that wet nurses conveyed disease. It also forced mothers and, later, doctors to make every effort to insure that the wet nurses were healthy. This meant that, over time, wet nursing arrangements came to be mediated bv physicians. The wet nurse's path from servant to medical resource was long and twisted, however, fenced in by the expectations of employers and, eventually, by those of doctors.

Domestic service work remained the most common occupation for women in the nineteenth century, although both the composition of the household labor force and the nature of the work itself changed because of the emerging industrial economy and the increasing pace of urbanization. In 1820, 8 percent of the U.S. population lived in urban areas; by 1870 the

15 On the rate of urban growth, see U.S. Bureau of the Census, *Historical Statistics of the United States: Colonial Times to 1970, Bicentennial Edition, Part 2* (Washington, D.C.: U.S. Government Printing Office, 1975). On the development of a middle-class culture and the widening gulf between classes, see Stuart M. Blumin, *The Emergence of the Middle Class: Social Experience in the American City, 1760–1900* (Cambridge: Cambridge University Press, 1989); and Karen Halttunen, *Confidence Men and Painted Women: A Study of Middle-Class Culture in America, 1830–1870* (New Haven: Yale University Press, 1982). Neither book emphasizes the role of servants who helped to define a household as middle class even as they also brought aspects of lower-class life into this newly created domestic sphere. This concept is elaborated in Faye E. Dudden, *Serving Women: Household Service in Nineteenth-Century America* (Middletown, Conn.: Wesleyan University Press, 1983). For analysis of women in urban America, see Barbara J. Berg, *The Remembered Gate: Origins of American Feminism: The Woman and the City, 1800–1860* (New York: Oxford University Press, 1978); and Christine Stansell, *City of Women; Sex and Class in New York, 1789–1860* (New York: Knopf, 1986).

figure was 25 percent.[16] Early in the nineteenth century the predominant model of service was one of "hired help," in which women and girls assisted rural families in producing for the marketplace; later, domestic work in private urban households became the standard form of service.[17] The corollary to this in terms of wet nursing was a shift from informal, temporary arrangements to the practice of hiring wet nurses to live with a family for extended periods of time.

Accompanying changes in the structure of service was a shift in the population of servants. Native-born servants began to be replaced, first by Irish and later by Scandinavian and German immigrants.[18] The consequences for employers of wet nurses can be seen in an 1861 letter written by Elizabeth Cabot, a wealthy Boston matron. After her sister-in-law's wet nurse had "given out," Cabot canvassed immigrant enclaves to find a replacement:

> I roused up and trotted over, and thought I would raise a wet nurse in the village and dressed forthwith and started in the carryall with Powell, invaded *four* Irish mansions, succeeded in raising a nurse and a woman to take her baby and sent her off with Powell into town to be examined by Sam and go to Lillie.[19]

A comparison of Cabot's expedition with Elizabeth Drinker's eighty years earlier reveals several differences. Drinker relied on her own judgment in assessing potential wet nurses; Cabot seemingly sought the advice of a physician – the unidentified Sam. More significantly, Drinker hired neighbors or acquaintances, whereas Cabot crossed an abyss of social class by "invading" an Irish neighborhood to find a wet nurse.

As Cabot's recollection suggests, the geographic and social distance between the working poor and the middle and upper classes was expanding. The well-to-do gradually retreated from the urban core and clustered together in neighborhoods of increasing homogeneity. The poor had their own districts, which by the 1840s were labeled slums and seen as wells of poverty, social pathology, and disease.[20] That the offspring of the well-to-do sometimes drank, literally, from such wells could be deeply troubling.

16 Bayrd Still, *Urban America: A History with Documents* (Boston: Little, Brown, 1974), p. 76.
17 Dudden, *Serving Women*, pp. 1–103.
18 David M. Katzman, *Seven Days a Week: Women and Domestic Service in Industrializing America* (Urbana: University of Illinois Press, 1981).
19 Elizabeth (Dwight) Cabot to Ellen Twistleton, April 8, 1861. In Elizabeth (Dwight) Cabot, *Letters* (Boston: Privately printed, 1905; New Haven: Research Publications, microform), pp 220–1.
20 Blumin, *Emergence of the Middle Class*; David Ward, *Poverty, Ethnicity, and the American City, 1840–1925: Changing Conceptions of the Slum and the Ghetto* (Cambridge: Cambridge University Press, 1989), pp. 13–45. Epidemic diseases highlighted the problem of the slum. See Charles E. Rosenberg, *The Cholera Years: The United States in 1832, 1849, and 1866* (Chicago: University of Chicago Press, 1962); and John Duffy, *The Sanitarians: A History of American Public Health* (Urbana: University of Illinois Press, 1990). Residential segregation of the poor was, of course, the obverse of the on-going residential segregation

The fear was not entirely unjustified; cities were unhealthy, and the young were at greatest risk. Overall, life expectancy at birth declined in the half century before the Civil War, and one reason was the excess mortality in urban areas. The concentration of population, the contamination of food and water, and the poverty of the urban lower classes combined to shorten the length of life, in large measure by producing an excess of infant mortality.[21] Nineteenth-century statisticians demonstrated convincingly that it was the poor and particularly their children who suffered disproportionately from urban ills. Indeed, one consequence of the increased mortality was an expanding supply of wet nurses, as poor women whose infants had died offered their milk in the marketplace. Yet, for many decades the popular belief persisted that the rich were most vulnerable because of their high living. Wealth, the argument went, led to ill health, whereas the poor enjoyed the advantages of a vigorous life.[22] Even when this notion had largely faded, vestigial elements of it remained, most notably in the belief that some wealthy women found it difficult to suckle their children, although poor mothers could do so easily.

As was the case in the eighteenth century, the number of families relying on wet nurses is beyond calculation. Two studies of childbearing and infant care suggest that maternal nursing predominated among the well-to-do, with wet nursing a second choice and artificial feeding a distant third. Antebellum mothers in the urban North, Sylvia Hoffert suggests, found in breast-feeding a source of power, self-esteem, and autonomy. An analysis by Sally McMillen of seventy-three families in the antebellum South yielded similar conclusions. Only fourteen of the families relied either partially or exclusively on wet nurses.[23] The small samples of families in both studies makes it difficult, however, to generalize from the results.

Assessing the demand for wet nurses in nineteenth-century cities, towns, and rural areas therefore remains a matter of inference. Maternal deaths in childbirth remained a critical factor, as they had been in the eighteenth

of the rich. See Edward Pessen, *Riches, Class, and Power before the Civil War* (Lexington: D. C. Heath, 1973), pp. 169–204; and William H. Pease and Jane H. Pease, *The Web of Progress: Private Values and Public Styles in Boston and Charleston, 1828–1843* (New York: Oxford University Press, 1985), pp. 1–11.
21 R. W. Fogel, "Nutrition and the Decline in Mortality since 1700: Some Additional Preliminary Findings," National Bureau of Economic Research, Working Paper no. 1802, cited in Samuel H. Preston and Michael R. Haines, *Fatal Years: Child Mortality in Late Nineteenth-Century America* (Princeton: Princeton University Press, 1991), p. 51.
22 Richard A. Meckel, *"Save the Babies": American Public Health Reform and the Prevention of Infant Mortality, 1850–1929* (Baltimore: Johns Hopkins University Press, 1990), pp. 20–1.
23 On infant feeding in the urban North, see Sylvia D. Hoffert, *Private Matters: American Attitudes toward Childbearing and Infant Nurture in the Urban North, 1800–1860* (Urbana: University of Illinois Press, 1989), p. 148 n. 34, and pp. 163–4. For the South see McMillen, *Motherhood in the Old South*, pp. 111–34; and Sally McMillen, "Mothers' Sacred Duty: Breast-feeding Patterns among Middle- and Upper-Class Women in the Antebellum South," *Journal of Southern History* 51 (1985): 333–56.

century. The 1850 census reported that 2 percent of the deaths of white women occurred in childbirth, although the rate varied considerably from a low of 1.2 percent in New Hampshire to a high of 5.4 percent in Florida.[24] In some instances, the babies probably perished along with their mothers; in others, the surviving infants needed to be fed, either by a wet nurse or, if necessary, by artificial means. Of course, social and economic resources played a critical role in determining the method.

Another driving force in the demand for wet nurses was, as it had been in earlier periods, maternal morbidity. For the nineteenth century as for the eighteenth, the definition and magnitude of maternal morbidity remain imprecise. In addition to the women who were physically, mentally, or physiologically incapable of feeding their infants, there were others who suffered from a sense that nursing was simply too enervating. Popular literature increasingly defined middle- and upper-class urban women as frail. Some women no doubt applied the diagnosis to themselves and found a ready-made excuse to avoid nursing. As in the eighteenth century, the line between needing a wet nurse and wanting one easily blurred.

Another issue, sexuality, disappeared from popular discussion. The medical literature no longer addressed men and asked them to practice self-restraint during the period that their wives were nursing, and it no longer mentioned the subject to women. A veil of modesty descended. Yet, some remained concerned that lower-class wet nurses would continue to be sexually active and thus harm their milk. This was another reason for changing the venue of the work from the wet nurses' homes to the homes of their employers.

Some women frankly rejected breast-feeding. A study of the small town of Rockdale, Pennsylvania, in the antebellum years uncovered a network of upper-class women who customarily employed wet nurses to lighten their nursery responsibilities. Though the prescriptive literature would define these mothers as selfish and the wet nurses they retained as dangerous, from the women's own perspective it was simply a matter of custom.[25] On the spectrum of wet nurse employers, the Rockdale elite stood at an extreme. They were wealthy, not middle class; lived in a small town, not a city; and were accustomed to managing large staffs of servants, including wet nurses. Yet, even in the small village of Rockdale, the signs of social distance between wet nurses and their employers and the problems of wet nurse management were becoming apparent.

---

24 McMillen, *Motherhood in the Old South,* Appendix 1, Table III.
25 On the Rockdale sisterhood, see Anthony F. C. Wallace, *Rockdale: The Growth of an American Village in the Early Industrial Revolution* (New York: Knopf, 1978), pp. 22–32. Wallace describes the wet nursing of Harriet's infant, as well as the situation of Anna Lammont, whose wet-nursed infant forgot her while she was on a long trip.

In 1857, Clementina Smith of Rockdale described the "baby show" she had recently witnessed at the home of her sister, Harriet, the mother of a newborn.[26] In rapid succession the household hired two wet nurses who, due to unforeseen events, briefly brought their own infants to reside in the home. Although Smith ultimately regarded the situation with amusement, for a time it proved to be a taxing reminder that dependence on a wet nurse brought with it a unique set of problems.

The mutual obligations between upper-class mistresses and their servants still compelled the kind of attention given by Elizabeth Drinker to her servants seventy years earlier. When the first wet nurse, Mary, developed infections in her breasts she was quickly relieved of her duties, but she remained in the household to be looked after as she convalesced. Smith spent "anxious days and nights" engaged in "the hardest nursing I ever did" helping the woman to recover.[27] Over several weeks Smith reported on Mary's treatment, on the success of her replacement, and on the progress of her sister's baby. Treatment of Mary's breasts included repeated lancings and the application of several breast pumps – common therapies that may have discouraged some women from even attempting to suckle their own infants lest they be subjected to similar treatments if they experienced any difficulties.

As Mary recovered from her illness (and perhaps her treatment), her successor, a Welsh wet nurse, joined the household, bringing her baby with her for reasons of expediency. Employers, as a rule, did not allow wet nurses to keep their own babies with them. They did not want another child in the household, fearing that the wet nurse would favor her own baby over her assigned charge. Clearly, an exception had been made, and Mary knew it. She became jealous and demanded that she too be allowed to have her child with her, ostensibly to help draw her milk. At this juncture the "baby show," as Smith described it, began. The house was crowded with infants. Nevertheless, the arrangement had no ill effects on Harriet's baby, who was reportedly "thriving." However, the family quickly took command of the situation, returning Mary's baby to her own nurse and sending the child of the Welsh wet nurse out to board. The peace proved to be short-lived. Mary's infant fell ill, was brought back to her, and died shortly after its arrival.[28]

Smith's patient care of Mary and consideration for her baby did not blind her to what she saw as the woman's defects of class, character, and religion. Mary, Smith believed, lacked the necessary stoicism when faced

26 Clementina Smith to Sophie du Pont, January 22, 1857. W9–26035. HML.
27 Ibid.
28 Clementina Smith to Sophie du Pont, January 17, 1857, W9–26033, Clementina Smith to Sophie du Pont, January 22, 1857, W9–26035; Clementina Smith to Sophie du Pont, February 7, 1857, W9–26037. HML.

with pain, and the appropriate response when faced with tragedy. When Mary first became sick, Smith admitted that she supposed "no suffering is more intense."[29] Nonetheless, she expressed exasperation in terms that belied her sympathy and betrayed her true sentiments: "That class of people have little self control or patience in sickness." Mary's torment following the death of her infant also puzzled Smith, who wrote that "she rather disappoints not to have relief mixed up with a sort of maternal instinct of pain in not having been with the child."[30] Had a middle-class woman failed to grieve for her infant, she would have stood in violation of every stricture of moral motherhood. When a poor woman was seen anguishing over the loss of her baby she evoked a far different response. Smith maintained an emotional distance from Mary's tragedy, concerned only with helping to keep order in her sister's house.

Although the paternalism of an older system of servant–mistress relations still existed, clearly the fault lines of religion and class had ruptured in the nursery. Smith never identified Mary as the mother of a baby; she saw her only as a slightly hysterical and often disruptive member of the lower class. Following the burial of Mary's child, Smith complained of the "difficulties getting the truth about her" and remarked that the other servants, including her replacement, harbored "a protestant bitterness against her."[31] Religion not only isolated Mary from her fellow servants, it also marked her as untrustworthy and in need of careful management.

For Smith and her sister, a lifetime of experience provided all the training necessary for coping with this brief episode. For mothers of smaller means and less practice, with no family members to guide them or with a diminished confidence in their own abilities to manage a nursery, help was available. Domestic manuals, home medical books, medical textbooks, and, eventually, family physicians, stood ready to advise in the selection and day-to-day management of wet nurses.

The wave of bourgeois domesticity that crested in Europe in the eighteenth century broke over the American shore in the decades preceding the Civil War, creating not only a new view of middle-class motherhood but also a new view of wet nurses. These beliefs appeared in their fullest expression in the domestic and medical literature. The books offered interpretations of the roles of mothers as well as sometimes fanciful descriptions of nursery relations and are, therefore, a lens through which one can view the transformation of the early nineteenth-century household. The literature refracted the theme of increasing class estrangement by consistently juxtaposing the nurturing middle-class mother against the threaten-

29 Clementina Smith to Sophie du Pont, January 17, 1857, W9–26033. HML.
30 Clementina Smith to Sophie du Pont, February 7, 1857, W9–26037. HML.
31 Ibid.

ing lower-class wet nurse. At the same time, the literature magnified what was seen as the emerging distinction between scientific knowledge and practical experience, suggesting a division that would not be fully manifested until the late nineteenth century. But as a lens the literature was sometimes clouded. It obscured the most fundamental and obvious fact about nursery relations – that each encounter was unique. Finally, the popular and medical literature, written for a middle-class readership, was blind to the existence of both municipal wet nursing and the informal arrangements working-class women made among themselves.

Popular literature exalted the home as the seedbed of spiritual wealth, needing only proper cultivation by wives, mothers, and daughters.[32] Literate women could not escape the deluge of advice on home management and child rearing, some of it barely concealed in novels, much of it freely offered in household manuals. In urging women to follow the precepts of modern motherhood, writers assumed from religious authorities the task of defining the importance of women's roles in the nursery. On the surface, the advice echoed earlier recommendations. The writers lauded women who breast-fed, reprimanded those who chose not to, and detailed the exceptional circumstances that required a wet nurse. In these texts, the vilification of the "fashionable lady" – the straw woman of domestic literature – continued unabated. Yet, if the tune was familiar, the words resonated with new force in an era of ennobled motherhood. Mrs. J. Bakewell, author of *The Mother's Practical Guide* (1843), offered both inspiration and jeremiad: "Happy the mother who can suckle her infant; she who has not the power to do so is deprived of one of the greatest maternal pleasures, while her toils and anxieties are more than doubled."[33] Similar appeals to maternal duty appeared in fiction. In *Two Lives; or, To Seem and To Be* (1846) the popular novelist Maria McIntosh described a dissolute American woman living in Paris who found it "quite impossible" to "fulfill the two characters of a lady of fashion and a nursing mother." Her choice of a dissolute lifestyle led, predictably, to an early and tragic death.[34]

As did the novelists, the authors of advice books sometimes referenced their own experiences and invoked themes of personal sacrifice. "Heaven has crowned my endeavors with success," wrote Mary Palmer Tyler, "why then may I not show my gratitude, by presenting to the matrons of

---

32 For a discussion of the literature – its main concepts and its change over time – see Bloch, "American Feminine Ideals in Transition"; Cott, *Bonds of Womanhood*, pp. 63–4; and Ryan, *The Empire of the Mother*, pp. 97–8 and passim.

33 Mrs. J. Bakewell, *The Mother's Practical Guide*, from 2d ed. London (New York: G. Lane & P. P. Sanford, 1843), p. 31.

34 Maria J. McIntosh, *Two Lives; or, To Seem and To Be* (New York: D. Appleton, 1846, American Fiction Series, microfilm), p. 293. See also Nina Baym, *Woman's Fiction: A Guide to Novels by and about Women in America, 1820–1870* (Ithaca: Cornell University Press, 1978).

my country the fruits of my experience."[35] Tyler's book explained how she successfully nursed and reared eight children, including one child whose suckling caused her such excruciating pain that her friends advised her to wean the baby.[36] Her message was quite clear: she had suffered for her children; others should do the same.

Even as domestic writers brought the language of the pulpit into the parlor, they subtly moved maternal responsibility out of the realm of the sacred. In sandwiching advice about babies between hints for wash day and cooking instructions they suggested that not the Almighty, but mothers were the chief architects of their infants' welfare.

Catherine Beecher's enormously popular *Treatise on the Domestic Economy* (1841) exemplified the secularization of infant care. She placed her faith in a rational approach to the problems of household management in general and was strikingly unsentimental on the subject of nursery organization. Her book, which addressed subjects ranging from charity to the care of parlors, included a chapter on the care of infants that quoted liberally from the medical literature. Uniquely, Beecher refrained from reprimanding those mothers who did not suckle their infants and chose instead to hire a wet nurse.[37] Here close observation may have substituted for personal experience, as Beecher had no children. However, her younger sister and fellow author Harriet Beecher Stowe bore five children in the first seven years of her marriage and seven altogether.[38] For Stowe, in at least one instance, using a wet nurse proved to be a necessity.

Stowe retained the wet nurse to suckle her son Charles Edward, born in 1850.[39] In a letter to another sister, Sarah, Stowe complained about problems with her breasts that had caused her incessant pain and described the "healthy young Irish woman" who was nursing her child.[40] The woman had her flaws; according to Stowe, she "didn't know how to do anything" and was "very slack and slovenly" – charges not infrequently lodged against the Irish servants who streamed into the United States in the middle

---

35 Tyler, *The Maternal Physician*, p. 6.
36 Tyler, *The Maternal Physician*, pp. 10–12; for descriptions of other women who nursed despite their pain and illness, see Degler, *At Odds*, pp. 79–80.
37 Catherine Beecher, *A Treatise on Domestic Economy* (reprint of 1841 ed.; New York: Schocken Books, 1977), pp. 207–24. See also Katherine Kish Sklar, *Catherine Beecher: A Study in American Domesticity* (New York: Norton, 1976), pp. 151–67.
38 Stowe, known around the world as the author of *Uncle Tom's Cabin*, wrote other novels and religious books and coauthored with her sister Catherine Beecher, *The American Woman's Home, or Principles of Domestic Science . . .* (New York: J. B. Ford, 1869).
39 It is possible that some of her other children were wet nursed. A letter from Catherine Beecher mentions that one of Harriet's twin daughters had been "put out for the winter." Catherine Beecher to Mary Beecher Perkins, 1838. Cited in Kathryn Kish Sklar, "Introduction," Beecher, *Treatise on Domestic Economy*, pp. viii and xvii n. 5.
40 Harriet Beecher Stowe to Sarah Beecher, December 17, 1850. Harriet Beecher Stowe papers, Folder 9A, SLRC. Stowe nursed her son herself before turning to a wet nurse.

of the nineteenth century.[41] Nevertheless, the baby apparently thrived on her milk, and Stowe kept the woman in her home for three months. As in earlier decades, the gap between private experiences and public expectations remained a broad one. Stowe settled for a less than ideal wet nurse, satisfied that her baby remained in good health.

Medical writers viewed the nursery in a different light than did domestic authorities, emphasizing health above order. Their guidebooks addressed a wide range of topics but generally advised the family to adhere to the rules of proper hygiene and right living, to carefully diagnose and treat the ailments that plagued them, and when necessary, to concoct and use tonics and other remedies. European books, especially William Buchan's *Domestic Medicine,* remained extraordinarily popular in the United States.[42] Another favorite medical advisor was the Scottish physiologist and phrenologist Andrew Combe, whose book, *The Management of Infancy,* was cited by Catherine Beecher and by the feminist Elizabeth Cady Stanton.[43] Combe's book was imported and later reprinted in the United States.

Although foreign writers seem to have had a certain cachet in addition to their long track record in the marketplace, homegrown authors also found an expanding place on the family bookshelf. In the nineteenth century, American physicians began producing books that reflected their own practices and their knowledge of local needs. Among the home medical guidebook writers were practitioners from various sectarian schools of medicine, such as those who preached reliance solely on botanical cures. Orthodox medical practitioners (sometimes known as regulars, or allopaths) also produced a multitude of books. The lucky writers, who found a niche for their works, had their volumes regularly reprinted. Comparing the successive editions on the topic of wet nursing reveals both the increased attention to the subject and the enhanced focus on the needs of urban readers.

In contrast to their European counterparts, the early editions of American popular health guides were largely silent on the subject of wet nursing. James Ewell, a Savannah physician whose early work, *The Planter's and Mariner's Medical Companion* (1807), was intended for residents of "warm climates," stated simply that if an infant could not receive milk from its mother, or from "a healthy woman who laid in about the same time," the

41 Hasia R. Diner, *Erin's Daughters in America: Irish Immigrant Women in the Nineteenth Century* (Baltimore: Johns Hopkins University Press, 1983).
42 Charles E. Rosenberg, "Medical Text and Social Context: Explaining William Buchan's *Domestic Medicine," Bulletin of the History of Medicine* 57 (1983): 22–42.
43 Elizabeth Cady Stanton, *Eighty Years and More: Reminiscences, 1815–1897* (reprint; New York: Schocken Books, 1971), p. 115. Combe's work was reprinted in several American editions after his death; Stanton must have read an imported volume. See Andrew Combe, *The Management of Infancy, Physiological and Moral,* 1st Am. ed. from 10th London ed. (New York: D. Appleton, 1871).

best choice would be the milk of a goat.[44] Horatio Gates Jameson, author of the popular *The American Domestick Medicine; or, Medical Admonisher* (1817), remained mute on the subject of wet nurses, as did John Gunn, whose treatise on domestic medicine appeared in 1830. Gunn, a Knoxville, Tennessee, physician, wrote for frontier residents who had little financial or geographic access to full-time hired wet nurses.[45]

In later decades, revised versions of the popular medical manuals appeared, aimed at an expanded and increasingly urban audience that was more familiar with wet nurses and more willing to embrace the emerging ideas of female debility. An enlarged and revised edition of Ewell, published in 1856, informed readers that "It has been improperly imagined that all mothers ought to be nurses." Such a false belief, the book continued, could result in harm to both mother and child.[46] Gunn's extraordinarily successful book was similarly transmogrified. Eastern publishers significantly revised his book to appeal to an urban constituency, adding new material on infant feeding and a somber discussion of wet nursing, which, like other popular works of the day, castigated upper-class women who let others care for their children.[47] The editors understood that wet nursing was a subject of greater interest to the urban well-to-do than it had been for the farmers and shopkeepers on the trans-Appalachian frontier.

In books written in the 1840s and 1850s, a new theme emerged in the discussion of wet nursing: the threat of the dangerous stranger.[48] The subject inspired both the popular and the medical imagination, combining the growing alienation of the middle and upper classes from the urban poor with more specific fears about disease. The 1848 edition of the home medical guide written by the botanic practitioner Wooster Beach used the term "stranger" in reference to wet nurses who communicated "loathsome and fatal diseases" and gave milk "rendered unwholesome by age or other causes."[49] With increasing specificity, physicians such as Beach outlined the problems of infant feeding, linking them to an expanding perception

44 James Ewell, *The Planter's and Mariner's Medical Companion* . . . (Philadelphia: Bioran, 1807), p. 266.
45 Horatio Gates Jameson, *The American Domestick Medicine; or, Medical Admonisher* . . . (Baltimore: F. Lucas & J. Robinson, 1817); and John Gunn, *Gunn's Domestic Medicine, or Poor Man's Friend, In the Hours of Affliction, Pain and Sickness* (Knoxville: The Author, 1830). On Gunn's work and influence, see Charles E. Rosenberg, "John Gunn: Everyman's Physician," in Charles E. Rosenberg, ed., *Explaining Epidemics and Other Studies in the History of Medicine* (Cambridge: Cambridge University Press, 1992), pp. 57–73.
46 James Ewell, *The Medical Companion, or, Family Physician* . . . 11th ed. enlgd. (Philadelphia: Keen & Lee, 1856), p. 488.
47 Criticisms of rich mothers and poor mothers alike can be found in John C. Gunn, *New Family Physician: or Home Book of Health* . . . , 200th ed. rev. and enlgd. (Cincinnati: Wilstach, Baldwin, 1880), p. 590.
48 The problem of strangers is discussed in Halttunen, *Confidence Men and Painted Women*.
49 Wooster Beach, *The American Practice Condensed or, the Family Physician* . . . , 14th ed. (New York: James McAlister, 1848), p. 631.

that the well-to-do were vulnerable to the afflictions of the lower classes and suggesting that solutions lay in the careful application of medical as well as practical knowledge.

The fullest expression of the idea of medical management of infant feeding appeared in seven pediatrics books published between 1825 and 1850. As a collective achievement, they signaled a decreasing reliance on foreign authorities, the gradual maturing of the American medical community, and the growing intellectual ambitions of certain members of the medical profession.[50] Unlike the authors of popular medical books, the physicians who wrote pediatrics manuals addressed clinical subjects and employed technical language in a discourse aimed at fellow practitioners. However, the books also found a popular readership, as self-doctoring remained the rule in many homes and as popular writers began to refer their readers to the new medical literature. For example, both the physician William Alcott and the writer and reformer Lydia Maria Child suggested that mothers consult Dewees's *Treatise on the Physical and Mental Treatment of Children* (1825), although Alcott complained that the book was too expensive.[51] Alcott found a competing volume, James Stewart's *A Practical Treatise on the Diseases of Children* (1841), more erudite but believed it was of use only to practitioners. Stephen Tracey, author of *The Mother and Her Offspring* (1853), also cited Stewart, and physician Caleb Ticknor, author of a popular medical book, referred readers to Dewees and to John Eberle's *A Treatise on the Diseases and Physical Education of Children* (1833).[52]

It is tempting to portray the textbook authors as exemplars of modern science in contrast to the more populist physicians who wrote home health guides, but this accords too much to the former and suggests too wide a knowledge gap among the various practitioners. As historian Charles Rosenberg has noted, all Americans, physicians and laypersons alike,

50 The textbooks are cited in Thomas E. Cone, Jr., *History of American Pediatrics* (Boston: Little, Brown, 1979), pp. 78–83. They are George Logan, *Practical Observations on Diseases of Children* . . . (Charleston: A. E. Miller, 1825); William Potts Dewees, *A Treatise on the Physical and Medical Treatment of Children* (Philadelphia: H. C. Carey & I. Lea, 1825); John Eberle, *A Treatise on the Diseases and Physical Education of Children* . . . , (Cincinnati: Corey & Fairbank, 1833); James Stewart, *A Practical Treatise on the Diseases of Children* (New York: Wiley & Putnam, 1841); D. Francis Condie, *A Practical Treatise on the Diseases of Children* (Philadelphia: Lea & Blanchard, 1844); John Forsyth Meigs, *A Practical Treatise on the Diseases of Children* (Philadelphia: Lindsay & Blakiston, 1848); and Charles Delucena Meigs, *Observations on Certain of the Diseases of Young Children* (Philadelphia: Lea & Blanchard, 1850).
51 Lydia Maria Child, *The Family Nurse; or Companion of the Frugal Housewife* (Boston: Charles J. Hendee, 1837), p. 3. Child also quoted from the *Maternal Physician*, p. 36. William A. Alcott, *The Young Mother's Medical Guide in Children's Diseases*, 2d ed. enlgd., (Boston: P. R. Marvin, 1848), p. 21. On Alcott see Charles E. Rosenberg, "Introduction" to William A. Alcott, *The Physiology of Marriage* (reprint; New York: Arno, 1972).
52 Stephen Tracey, *The Mother and Her Offspring* (New York: Harper, 1853), p. 203; and Caleb B. Ticknor, *A Guide for Mothers and Nurses in the Management of Young Children* . . . (New York: Taylor & Dodd, 1839), p. iv.

shared a vernacular healing tradition, an understanding of the body in health and disease, and a knowledge of various remedies.[53] What distinguished analyses of infant feeding in medical textbooks from those found in popular guides was not their science, but rather their belief in medical authority. The pediatrics books were beginning to assert that the nursery was a medical domain as much as it was a domestic space.

The new textbooks offered a more expansive and less moralistic assessment of employer's needs. Whereas popular writers championed mothers who overcame all varieties of pain and suffering to breast-feed their babies and popular medical guides similarly exalted maternal sacrifice, the textbook authors paid homage to ideal mothers, but also enumerated the conditions that prevented women from nursing. Cincinnati practitioner John Eberle explained that a mother with either insufficient or bad milk, a disease, or a painful condition could not nurse, and therefore a wet nurse had to be obtained.[54] Without explicitly sympathizing with women who considered breast-feeding immodest, wearisome, or déclassé, the long lists of exemptions implicitly sanctioned the women who chose to defy convention, enabling them to frame their decision as a medical necessity rather than a personal choice. The inventory of medical excuses had the effect of endorsing the use of wet nurses without contradicting the physicians' basic objections to hired substitutes.

A belief that middle- and upper-class women were weak vessels who could not fulfill their biological duties was a distinguishing characteristic of both the popular and the professional medical literature. Doctors had begun to suspect that some middle- and upper-class women lacked the physical stamina necessary to withstand the pain of childbirth and therefore required anesthesia. Similarly, they surmised that well-to-do women found breast-feeding more difficult than did lower-class women.[55] Ticknor argued that "women of the higher classes frequently possess such extremely sensitive and excitable temperaments as will render it imprudent for them to suckle their own children."[56] Under the circumstances, it was best to ask the doctor to find a wet nurse.

The pediatrics textbooks endorsed wholeheartedly the notion that families needed direct medical guidance in matters of child rearing, including the hiring of wet nurses. Ideally, the physician would hire the wet nurse. Failing that, the family would refer to a medical textbook to help them select a proper candidate. Wet nurses were to be treated not simply as

53 Rosenberg, "John Gunn: Everyman's Physician," pp. 62–70.
54 Eberle, *Treatise on the Diseases and Physical Education of Children*, p. 33.
55 On upper-class women lacking stamina for birth, see Hoffert, *Private Matters*, pp. 67–8; and Judith Walzer Leavitt, *Brought to Bed: Childbearing in America, 1750 to 1950* (New York: Oxford University Press, 1986), p. 126.
56 Ticknor, *Guide for Mothers and Nurses*, p. 92.

servants, but as individuals capable of transmitting either health or disease; they had to be judged by medical standards.

With the heightened concern for infant nurture among middle-class women, the argument for medical control would become increasingly compelling. Simultaneously, the notion that a wet nurse was simply a household servant came to be viewed as fundamentally and dangerously flawed. The full expression of this belief would not occur until the late nineteenth century, in the context of a changing population of wet nurses and their increasing institutionalization and medical scrutiny. But the first steps were taken in the antebellum years as doctors outlined a new protocol for hiring wet nurses.

In selecting wet nurses physicians scrutinized their health, their milk, and their children. The ideal candidate, of course, was free of evidence of disease. Women with eruptions suggestive of venereal infection, with swollen' necks that hinted at scrofula (tuberculosis of the lymph glands, usually those of the neck), or with a history of convulsions were to be weeded out. Failure to do so could have tragic consequences. Dewees, in obvious reference to venereal infections, recounted two cases of babies acquiring "the most loathsome and horrible of all diseases" from their respective wet nurses. He also discussed an episode in Scandinavia involving a wet nurse who infected an entire family, including the father, mother, three children, a maid servant, and two clerks – a pattern of transmission that leaves much to the reader's imagination. Dewees's intention in recounting this near-epidemic episode was not to frighten employers away from wet nurses, although it may well have had that effect. Instead, he wanted to upbraid families who hired wet nurses without "previous inquiry into [their] character."[57]

The possibility of contracting a venereal disease from a wet nurse was real, and frightening. In an 1845 letter to her mother, Laura Lenoir Norwood of Hillsboro, North Carolina, expressed her dread of employing a wet nurse. "I can't feel reconciled to the idea," she wrote, believing she would have "never had one if my children had not done so badly on feeding, and now I feel ten times more averse to it than ever." Norwood's reluctance stemmed from a previous "narrow escape" from a wet nurse infected with a venereal disease.[58] Infant feeding, her case illustrates, raised fundamental medical questions about the transmission of disease and the protection of health. With venereal disease perceived to spread upward

57 Dewees, *Treatise on the Physical and Medical Treatment of Children*, p. 60.
58 Letter from Laura Lenoir Norwood to her mother cited in Erna Olafson Hellerstein, Leslie Parker Hume, and Karen M. Offen, eds., *Victorian Women: A Documentary Account of Women's Lives in Nineteenth-Century England, France, and the United States* (Stanford: Stanford University Press, 1981), p. 218.

from the lower classes, the hiring of wet nurses took on a heightened danger as the social class of workers fell.

Fulfilling the demand for thorough examinations of potential wet nurses proved difficult because investigations violated codes of morality and modesty. It was easy for the authors of textbooks to explain the need to scrutinize a woman's breasts and nipples. But how could an inspection take place in an era in which medical professionals approached the female body with reluctance and when most physicians did not yet view women giving birth as part of their clinical training?[59] The recommendation that the doctor examine a woman's milk and pay attention to the quantity, appearance, and color seems equally unlikely to be followed, as did the suggestion that the doctor taste the milk to determine if it was sufficiently "sweet."[60] Such actions moved the doctor far beyond the bounds of proper professional decorum and gentlemanly behavior.

It was far simpler to rely on the traditional means of discovering a wet nurse's health: viewing her baby. Careful inspection of the infant helped to rule out the presence of a communicable disease, provided evidence that the woman gave milk capable of nourishing a child, and allowed prospective employers to see if the wet nurse's infant was close in age to the suckling. Many doctors believed that young infants could not consume "old milk," commonly defined as having come from women who had nursed for six months or more. Constitutionally, physicians asserted, old milk did not suit the needs of a young baby, and physiologically, it became more likely that the wet nurse had resumed menstruating or possibly become pregnant.[61] Both conditions, physicians believed, were detrimental to the milk's quantity and quality.

The age limit, however, proved difficult to enforce in light of the uncertain supply of wet nurses and the family's interest in finding a wet nurse who suited not only the baby but the needs of the entire household. In an 1858 article in the *American Medical Monthly,* William H. Cummings complained of a shortage of wet nurses, lamenting that in cities there were "not enough to supply the demand," and in the country they could

59 On the viewing of women giving birth, see Virginia G. Drachman, "The Loomis Trial: Social Mores and Obstetrics in the Mid-Nineteenth Century," in Susan Reverby and David Rosner, eds., *Health Care in America: Essays in Social History* (Philadelphia: Temple University Press, 1979), pp. 67–83; and Leavitt, *Brought to Bed,* pp. 40–50.

60 Ticknor, *Guide for Mothers and Nurses,* p. 102; Stewart, *Practical Treatise on the Diseases of Children,* pp. 189–90.

61 The English physician Burns, whose work was reprinted in several American editions, suggested that families refrain from hiring wet nurses who have nursed for some months "as the milk is apt to go away in some time, or become bad." John Burns, *The Principles of Midwifery; Including the Diseases of Women and Children,* rev. and enlgd. (Philadelphia: Hopkins & Earle, Fry & Kammer, 1810), p. 381. See also M. K. Hard, *Women's Medical Guide; Being a Complete Review of the Peculiarities of the Female Constitution . . .* (Mt. Vernon, Ohio: Cochran, 1848), p. 217; and J. Meigs, *Practical Treatise on the Diseases of Children,* p. 219.

"scarcely ever be obtained."[62] Perhaps the scarcity accounted for the singular case of a woman who employed the same wet nurse for three of her infants. At the mother's direction the wet nurse weaned one baby just in time to begin nursing the new arrival.[63] The arrangement, though highly unusual and counter to medical advice, allowed the family to solve several problems at once: it kept a trusted woman ready for service at a time when wet nurses were perceived as both scarce and dangerous.[64]

The new maternal ideology that anointed mothers as the molders of the health and character of their children ironically served to vest greater power in wet nurses.. Writing in *Godey's Lady's Book,* the educator Almira Phelps conceded that even if the mind could not be transfused from one soul to another, the "moral character of the future man may be influenced by the treatment he receives at the breast and in the cradle."[65] Such potential power could not be granted lightly. A mother needed to be absolved of responsibility for feeding her baby, not simply permitted to abdicate her role. And the need for this absolution ultimately required the doctors to determine first, whether a woman could breast-feed and, second, if she could not, who would be hired to take her place. As the ideology of middle-class maternity grew more fixed, the rules governing the nursery became more rigid.

A key change involved the placement of the infant. Under the new regimen babies no longer went to wet nurses in the country but lived at home under the watchful gaze of their mothers. Even though urban living was recognized as less healthy than country life, only one of the textbook authors explicitly endorsed outplacement. Philadelphia physician D. Francis Condie believed, "A country residence for a nurse has one important advantage," explaining "it indemnifies, in some degree, the infant for its removal from the maternal breast, particularly when the mother inhabits the confined and illy ventilated streets of a crowded city."[66] His colleagues and many families strongly disagreed.[67] The need to oversee the work of the wet nurse far outweighed the benefits of country air. Physicians placed

---

62 William H. Cummings, "On a Substitute for Human Milk," *American Medical Monthly* 9 (1858): 196.

63 Tracey, *The Mother and Her Offspring,* p. 204. The author admitted that this situation was "rare."

64 This discussion draws from Mary Douglas, *Purity and Danger: An Analysis of Concepts of Pollution and Taboo* (London: Routledge & Kegan Paul, 1980).

65 Almira H. Phelps, "Remarks on the Education of Girls," *Godey's Lady's Book* 18 (1839): 253. Quoted.in Anne L. Kuhn, *The Mother's Role in Childhood Education: New England Concepts, 1830–1860* (New Haven: Yale University Press, 1947), p. 57.

66 Condie, *Practical Treatise on the Diseases of Children,* p. 37.

67 Discussions of outplacement can be found in Edward H. Parker, *The Handbook for Mothers; A Guide in the Care of Young Children,* 2d ed. rev. (New York: Hurd & Houghton, 1867), p. 59; and Tracey, *The Mother and Her Offspring,* p. 208. For an example of a child sent out to a wet nurse for weaning from the mother, see Boydston, *Home and Work,* pp. 114–15.

aside their scientific understanding of the deleterious effects of urban living, echoing the opinions of domestic advisors that no woman who expected to exert a strong moral influence over her children could send an infant away to be reared in the home of a stranger.

The effects of the new geographic imperatives proved significant. First, urban wet nurses came from a different social class than their rural counterparts. As a result, the wet nursing vignettes in the medical and popular literature became stylized presentations of urban class antagonisms. Second, and more critically, the new arrangement typically meant separating the wet nurse from her own child. The literature thus began to depict wet nurses who missed their babies and took desperate measures to visit them. A frequent scenario involved a woman who clandestinely visited her child after putting her suckling into a deep sleep. Dewees reported a case in which a wet nurse applied laudanum – tincture of opium – to her breasts to quiet the baby and make time for an afternoon visit.[68] Lydia Maria Child, a domestic expert, offered a fuller explanation of the laudanum problem:

If the nurse have her own child with her, she is naturally tempted to give it a greater proportion of nourishment; if the child be removed, there is the painful consideration of deriving benefit from the privations and sacrifices of another; however conscientious she may be, it is more difficult to perform her duties patiently and well for mere money, than it is from instinct, or feeling; hence the great dangers of injuring a babe by putting it to sleep with laudanum.[69]

The motherly desires of wet nurses demanded fear, not reverence. If they tried to insure the future for their own babies, by suckling them first or making a brief visit, they posed a threat to their employers' infants.

In Child's account there were two possibilities: allowing a wet nurse to keep her child – something most employers frowned upon – or making her cast the infant aside. A third possibility was, of course, hiring a woman whose infant had died. Physician John Eberle favored this plan, thinking that a mother who had "no child of her own to take care of" was safer than one who would somehow find a way to express her feelings for her own baby.[70] The scheme had a serious drawback, however; without an infant to inspect, many doctors and employers had no way of determining whether a potential wet nurse was healthy and whether she produced good milk.

Even as they stood accused of maternal feelings, wet nurses also faced charges that they acted from greed alone. Eberle warned that women who lacked sufficient milk might resort to clandestine feedings in order to retain their situations and more importantly, their income. The life of a nursling,

68 Dewees, *Treatise on the Physical and Medical Treatment of Children*, pp. 57–9.
69 Child, *The Family Nurse*, p. 39.
70 Eberle, *Treatise on the Diseases and Physical Education of Children*, p. 33.

he alleged, was "often sacrificed to the secret practices of a mercenary and unprincipled nurse."[71] Mrs. C. A. Hopkinson, author of *Hints for the Nursery* (1863), provided a graphic account of a wet nurse whose milk failed after eight or nine months, causing the infant to starve. A physician misdiagnosed the problem and recommended sending the complaining baby to the seashore with his wet nurse. Only a chance encounter with a nursing mother, during which the baby "screamed and stretched out his arms to the woman," allowed the family to discern the truth.[72] The saga presented the evil counterpart to the wet nurse who missed her own baby – the wet nurse who sacrificed her suckling in order to fatten her purse. Wet nursing, all parties knew, was a lucrative job, and a woman was well advised to keep it as long as she could.

Wet nurses, the literature suggested, acted as both instinctive mothers and instinctive entrepreneurs. Indeed, it was instinct that was thought to separate middle-class from lower-class mothers. The former reared their children by following moral precepts, by rationally determining how to nurture them, and by consciously instilling in them proper bourgeois values. Lower-class women in general and wet nurses in particular also had strong feelings for their children, but their feelings were steeped in instinct, not enlightened motherhood. And, Condie alleged, emotions such as "grief, envy, hatred, fear, and jealousy" could alter a wet nurse's milk and ultimately destroy the child and the family.[73]

The characterization of wet nurses in the prescriptive literature as instinctive mothers and instinctive entrepreneurs was more accurate than the authors might have realized. Records from the Orphan Society of Philadelphia reveal both the pragmatism and sentimentality of women who wet nursed the offspring of other working women. The cases also reveal that municipal employment of wet nurses continued in the nineteenth century much as it had existed in the eighteenth century, with local authorities turning over abandoned babies to women willing to accept a small stipend to care for them. More critically, the records show that although the vicissitudes of working-class life forced women to earn what they could, the emotional dimensions of the job sometimes overcame material considerations.

The shift from placing infants in rural homes to live-in wet nursing spawned a two-tiered system of infant care. The offspring of the well-to-do were suckled in their homes; the offspring of wet nurses were placed

71 Ibid.
72 Hopkinson was equally critical of a mother whose milk failed but was reluctant to hire a wet nurse. Mrs. C. A. Hopkinson, *Hints for the Nursery or, The Young Mother's Guide* (Boston: Little, Brown, 1843), pp. 29–30, 33–4.
73 Condie, *Practical Treatise on the Diseases of Children*, p. 35.

with other women. Harriet Smith, for example, reported that the wet nurses working for her sister had their babies sent out to other wet nurses. Working in an informal system of care, home-based wet nurses were of little interest to doctors or domestic writers. They did, however, concern municipal authorities, for when they failed to be paid for their work, they handed their charges over to the town. In 1830, for instance, wet nurse Grace McDernish sent the infant in her care to the Philadelphia Orphan Asylum after the child's father died and the payments stopped.[74] Jane Courtney, another Philadelphia wet nurse, also attempted to turn her suckling over to the authorities when its father died, but she was persuaded to keep the girl after the Guardians of the Poor of Philadelphia promised her fifty cents a week.[75]

When sentiment collided with self-interest, the latter typically won, but there were exceptions. Some wet nurses kept babies long after the payments for their maintenance ceased to arrive. Philadelphian Matilda Thorne, hired to wet nurse a girl whose mother went to New York to work as a wet nurse, received only two payments despite repeated efforts to collect what she was owed. Rather than send the infant to the city's care and earn a stipend suckling another baby (or perhaps being paid to continue her work), she simply continued to rear the girl on her own for several years before depositing her at the Orphan Society.[76] Thorne was not alone in her generosity. After Hugh Devine's mother died, he was kept "on charity" by his nurse Lydia Vannater until he turned five.[77] Had Thorne or Vannater turned the babies over to authorities and perhaps taken in another child from the Guardians of the Poor, they could have earned fifty cents a week. It was not a large sum – the amount equaled the stipend given to the indigent and was less than the seventy-five cents to one dollar per week usually paid to servants – but it was, at least, something.[78] Keeping the infants abandoned to their care meant a loss of income for the women and the additional costs of rearing the child.

Despite the cases just noted, wet nursing arrangements among the working class were largely invisible. Few physicians or domestic experts knew or cared that poor women sometimes voluntarily mothered abandoned babies. Although the relationships between Vannater and Thorne and the

---

74 Orphan Society of Philadelphia, Admittance Book, 1815–1833, p. 626. HSP.
75 Orphan Society of Philadelphia, Admittance Book, 1815–1833, p. 261. HSP.
76 Orphan Society of Philadelphia, Folder "Admitting and Binding Indentures, 1815–," document signed by Matilda Thorne, March 1825. HSP.
77 Orphan Society of Philadelphia, Admittance Book, 1815–1833, p. 597. HSP.
78 Philadelphia's poor laws were revised in 1828 to limit outdoor relief. It is unclear whether this influenced the practice of taking in babies. Priscilla Ferguson Clement, *Welfare and the Poor in the Nineteenth-Century City: Philadelphia, 1800–1854* (Rutherford, N.J.: Fairleigh Dickinson University Press, 1985), pp. 70, 79. On wages see Matthew Carey, "Essays on the Public Charities of Philadelphia . . . ," *Miscellaneous Essays* (Philadelphia: Carey & Hart, 1830), pp. 193–4.

infants they suckled began in the marketplace, they concluded in the private household. In a sense, both women were acting like middle-class mothers – making the tender rearing of a child a vocation. Yet, their actions were grounded in emotion; after all, they overlooked their own rational, economic interests. Although Vannater and Thorne were not instinctive entrepreneurs – a charge often lodged against wet nurses – they were instinctive mothers – a fact that set them apart from the middle-class ideal.

The social dichotomies of motherhood presented in the medical and popular literature reflected a larger reality of deepening social class divisions and functioned as propaganda for the emerging ideal of middle-class motherhood. Still, the descriptions hardly qualify as an accurate analysis of the relationships that arose between wet nurses and employers. The aim of the literature was not to chronicle the possibilities or exceptions, but to share and shape the modern understanding of home, family, and health. Thus, the literature presented an abstract, schematic view of wet nurses and wet nursing.

Personal accounts bring additional factors into view, including the way in which the perception of wet nurses intersected with the popular understanding of unmarried motherhood and household service. As wet nursing became, increasingly, a job for poor single mothers, the contemporary understanding of morality entered into the equation. Some considered wet nurses to be inherently depraved and would hire one only if a child's life was at stake. Others, in the context of a growing moral reform movement, saw single wet nurses as victims rather than as sinners. Attorney Richard Henry Dana, Jr., described the efforts of the Boston physician Charles H. Stedman on behalf of a domestic, Elisa Butler, who had become pregnant after being raped by the son of her employer. Stedman found the woman a place to live during her confinement, and, after she delivered, he found her a wet nursing job where she was permitted to keep her baby. Thereupon Dana became involved, suing the father of Butler's child and winning a settlement for her.[79]

Whereas in Butler's case employment as a servant led to a brief career as a wet nurse, in most other instances the pattern was reversed. A wet nurse who did a satisfactory job, learning the household routine and caring capably for the baby, might be kept on after the baby was weaned, sparing the family the need to find new help. Despite the logic and practicality of this progression, medical and popular guidebooks never portrayed wet nursing as a back door to a domestic position. Still, such shifts in status did take place. One example occurred in the home of Emma Elizabeth Sullivan Stuart.

79 Robert F. Lucid, ed., *The Journal of Richard Henry Dana, Jr.*, vol. I (Cambridge: Harvard University Press, 1968), pp. 137–8.

Stuart was not a typical middle-class mother or the kind of woman addressed by medical writers; she was the wife of a retired partner in John Jacob Astor's Pacific Fur Company and thus a woman accustomed to managing a large household staff. Nor was she the mother of an infant; she was a grandmother.[80] For Stuart, employment of a wet nurse was a necessity born of tragedy. After her daughter died of puerperal fever in 1853, she brought her infant granddaughter Kate and the baby's wet nurse Maria from her daughter's home in New Jersey to her home in Detroit. On whether Maria had been found with the assistance of a physician or whether she had been examined in terms of her health and her morals, Stuart remained silent. Similarly, Maria's personal situation evoked no comment, although it seems doubtful that Maria would have moved from New Jersey to Michigan if she had a financially stable home and family. Most likely she was, like a growing number of wet nurses, a single mother, but this fact drew no notice or reproach from her employer. The only fact about Maria that Stuart recorded was her religion: Catholic. As nativism flared up in street fights and political skirmishes, Maria's religion could hardly have escaped notice. At the same time, the burgeoning supply of Irish workers meant that Stuart's experience was far from unique.

In the early months of her employment, Stuart found Maria to be an estimable helper, and she believed Maria to be equally fond of her. Therefore, when Maria became worried about her family, Stuart instructed her son in a letter to inquire about their welfare. She reminded him that Maria was "a most valuable, excellent woman, at least towards us." Her judgment later soured when she came to suspect that Maria had lied about her past.[81]

Maria had told the Stuarts that her own baby had died, but when she asked to have her wages forwarded, Stuart conjectured that she had in fact entrusted the baby to her sister's care. The moral implications of this exchange did not escape Stuart; she recognized that it was the infant left behind by Maria "whose milk has made a fine healthy child of ours." It troubled Stuart enough to raise the question as to whether Maria had abandoned her baby, but she made no further inquiries. Rather, she focused on Maria's presumed dishonesty. It left her "a little humbugged" and caused her to weigh the economics of her displeasure: "Were her wages $10.00 – very well – but $15.00 we should want a new wet nurse."[82]

The devotion of Maria to baby Kate exerted a strong influence on Stuart's judgment. She admitted that "Were she Maria's own, she could not love her any better." The baby reciprocated these feelings. Despite the

80 Robert Stuart, *Stuart Letters of Robert and Elizabeth Sullivan Stuart and Their Children, 1819–1864*, vol. 2 (Privately printed, 1961), pp. ix–x, n. 587.
81 *Stuart Letters*, pp. 603, 613.
82 Ibid., p. 613.

misgivings about the emotional capacity of wet nurses expressed in so many printed sources, firm bonds between the women and their sucklings did develop. In Maria's case, these sentiments and her familiarity with the household proved strong enough to keep her employed in the Stuart home after she had weaned the baby.[83]

Maria did not retain her new position for long, however. When she refused to wash the parlor dishes, thereby setting a dangerous example for the other servants, Stuart discharged her. She wrote to her son that Maria had been an excellent wet nurse and that she would "unhesitatingly have given her a high recommendation."[84] Undoubtedly, the shift from wet nurse to servant had made Maria's position more tenuous. Behavior that could be overlooked in a wet nurse could not be ignored in a servant. A woman with nutritious milk whose care of an infant seemed satisfactory (and who was difficult to replace on short notice) had to be allowed a certain latitude for misconduct, so long as it did no harm to the child. A common household servant lacked this bargaining chip.

The servant model fit the job of wet nursing imperfectly; or, more precisely, wet nursing was a clumsy adaptation. One reason was that wet nurses had more power than did other household workers. When a child was dependent upon a wet nurse's milk, her threat to quit, demand for more comfortable quarters, or request for a better diet might have to be met. This was the "tyranny of the household" that Dewees described. Still, the strategic position of wet nurses should not be overestimated. Employers could threaten to fire the women – leaving them without a means to support their own babies – or they could promise a successful wet nurse that she would be kept on in some other capacity when her nursing days ended. In the bourgeois household, mistresses, not servants, were ultimately in control.[85] Wet nurses did not dictate to their employers, they simply made the best bargains they could, under the circumstances.

In the wake of the redefinition of motherhood, the meaning of wet nursing and the perception of wet nurses changed. Wet nurses came to be viewed under the same harsh light once cast only on the women who hired them. The authors of popular tracts portrayed them as morally deficient women who traded their duties to their children for money and who stealthily infiltrated the nurseries of the middle class. If individual employers did not always share their trepidation, if the employers' daily experi-

83 Ibid.
84 *Stuart Letters*, p. 692.
85 For a discussion of the nineteenth-century transformation in domestic labor relations from "benevolent maternalism" to "bourgeois freedom," see Carol Lasser, "The Domestic Balance of Power: Relations Between Mistress and Maid in Nineteenth-Century New England," *Labor History* 28 (1987): 5–22.

ences were mediated by expectations about servants and by hopes for the health of their own babies, they were not unaware of the gulf between themselves and their temporary employees. In the middle decades of the nineteenth century this division would grow wider, as increasing numbers of privately employed wet nurses came from the ranks of institutionalized single mothers.

3

Finding "just the right kind of woman": The urban wet nurse marketplace, 1830–1900

In 1881, physician Jerome Walker published a novel entitled *The First Baby: His Trials and the Trials of His Parents,* an account of one family's experiences in rearing a young infant.[1] The book, an extended didactic discussion of a popular subject, was thinly disguised as fiction so that it could compete in a market crammed with advice literature. In one segment, the hero, Robert Matthews, accompanied by the faithful family physician, Dr. Lyons, undertakes an extensive journey in search of a wet nurse. The trip is only moderately successful, leading Lyons to lament the absence of a "systematic effort to furnish the persons most needing wet nurses with just the right kind of woman."[2]

Walker's novel accurately delineates the complexity of the urban wet nurse marketplace, in which public facilities, private entrepreneurs, and benevolent organizations vied to supply families with wet nurses. At the core of the expanding layers of wet nurse suppliers was a wet nurse labor force increasingly composed of poor, single mothers. These were not the "right kind of women" referred to by Dr. Lyons. However, as the novel's characters and real-life families recognized, the wet nurse population was shaped not by the demands of employers and the preferences of physicians, but by the conditions of life and labor for urban, working-class women.

The evolution of the marketplace between 1830 and 1900 reflected three separate, simultaneous trends, beginning with the commercialization of domestic service. This brought intelligence offices (employment agencies for servants) into the wet nurse business. A second trend was the institutionalization of unwed mothers, which brought civic shelters and benevo-

---

1 Jerome Walker, *The First Baby: His Trials and the Trials of His Parents* (New York: Brown & Derby, 1881), p. 85.
2 Ibid. Walker made this same point in a medical journal, noting both the difficulty of procuring healthy, even-tempered wet nurses with good milk and the lack of a "well-regulated system" for finding suitable candidates. Jerome Walker, "Practical Points in the Medical Care and Nursing of Children," *Sanitarian* 2 (1874): 17.

lent organizations into the business of placing wet nurses. Finally, the medicalization of childbirth and of infant-welfare programs also created new venues for hiring wet nurses.

The development of new sources for wet nurses did not displace the old ones; rather, they reflected a change in the structure of demand. Working-class families still sought wet nurses for their babies through word-of-mouth and via newspaper advertisements. It was the well-to-do who began to eschew informal arrangements negotiated individually in favor of formal arrangements made through intermediaries. In essence, the market began to be both rationalized and segmented.

To find a wet nurse, employers, or physicians working on their behalf, visited a few local purveyors, investigated the available candidates, selected one, and negotiated a price either with the intermediary, the wet nurse, or both. Rationalization meant that the process of hiring a wet nurse became easier, governed, so to speak, by tacit rules and marketplace protocols. It was not, however, without difficulties. An examination of the old and the new sources for wet nurses makes clear that each had its limitations. It also reveals that among the most critical considerations for families seeking wet nurses were those of convenience, reliability, and degree of medical supervision.

The First Baby, which Walker claimed was "a novel on which to hang facts," provides the best introduction to the wet nurse marketplace. The wet nursing section of the book begins with the infant's mother suffering a bout of pneumonia, leading the father, Robert Matthews, and Dr. Lyons to begin their odyssey. They cull names from the local newspaper, the *New York Herald,* and set out on a round of visiting, interviewing several candidates in rapid succession. The first, an obviously Irish "Mrs. Malone," displays a healthy, but dirty, baby. The second, "Mrs. Hughes," meets all the necessary conditions but one: the baby she shows off was borrowed from a sickly neighbor, leaving readers to conclude that her own infant either had died or was too ill to be shown. Finally, on their third visit, an acceptable wet nurse is found, the ominously named "Mrs. Badall," whose own baby had died of convulsions at the age of one week. In accepting her, Dr. Lyons breaks ranks with the medical orthodoxy that demanded that a successful candidate have a healthy baby to examine. Nonetheless, Matthews offers her twenty-five dollars a month and installs her in his home.

Mrs. Badall's tenure proves brief. She is fired after a visit from her drunken husband upsets both her and her milk. The author, like many physicians and members of the public, assumed that human milk was a volatile substance that could become toxic as a result of the lactating woman's strong emotions and, by implication, sexual activity.[3] The death by convulsions of Mrs. Badall's baby now seems, in retrospect, suspicious, an allusion to what might have happened to the Matthews child had it continued to suckle her milk. Walker's tale stands as a clear warning to the reader: even when they are selected with the aid of a doctor, wet nurses pose serious risks.

The novel illustrates in sequence the succession of wet nurse sources that emerged in the nineteenth century, as well as the limitations of each. After Mrs. Badall's departure, Matthews runs his own advertisement in the newspaper and arranges for Dr. Lyons to do the same. They are unsuccessful, forcing them into the streets in search of a candidate. They go first to a fancy intelligence office catering to the "Fifth Avenue crowd" and charging a steep five dollars for a wet nurse referral. Lyons inspects and rejects each woman offered for his examination, noting in passing that after wet nurses find work, their own infants are dispatched to institutions. Whether the fictional hero means to criticize private entrepreneurs who trafficked in wet nurses, the wet nurses who callously allowed the disposal of their babies, the employers who were parties to this practice, or all three of them remains unclear. The narrator makes only this brief aside, unwilling perhaps to implicate the physicians tacitly involved in the arrangement.

The continuing quest for a suitable wet nurse provides Walker with additional opportunities to instruct and warn his readers. A second intelligence office receives low marks because the proprietress keeps no records, and a third fails to pass inspection, foiling the good intentions of its three "ladylike" owners. Lyons advises these women to hire a physician to screen the candidates on their list. To underscore his point, he recites the familiar cautionary tale of the wet nurse discovered to have a venereal disease. The message to readers could not have been clearer: intelligence offices can recruit wet nurses, but only a physician can determine their fitness to serve.

Lyons and Matthews subsequently shift their search from employment agencies to institutions. They visit homes and asylums, including the municipal hospital, St. Anthony's Retreat, and several private maternity homes. At last they locate an acceptable employee with a comforting biblical name, Sarah. Unfortunately, what the Matthews family hopes will be the resolution to their crisis and the end of their pursuit proves to be neither. Sarah remains on the job only briefly. During her term of service the family tolerates reluctantly her excessive demands for food and drink.

3 See, for example, John Eberle, *A Treatise on the Diseases and Physical Education of Children*, 2d ed. (Cincinnati: Corey & Fairbank, 1834), p. 35; D. Francis Condie, *A Practical Treatise on the Diseases of Children*, 6th ed. rev. (Philadelphia: H. C. Lea, 1868), p. 35; J. Forsyth Meigs, *A Practical Treatise on the Diseases of Children* (Philadelphia: Lindsay & Blakiston, 1848), p. 219; and J. Lewis Smith, "Recent Improvements in Infant Feeding," *Transactions of the American Pediatric Society* 1 (1889): 89.

Ultimately, her overindulgence decreases her milk supply, necessitating her removal from the home.

The First Baby illustrated several of the problems intrinsic to wet nursing: the troublesome types of women seeking work, the poorly managed intelligence offices, and the uncertainty of judging the character of potential candidates. A woman might be free of disease, but she might also lack sound judgment and self-control. The evocatively named Mrs. Badall had married a drunk; "tall, healthy, clean and lady-like," Sarah could not curb her appetite. Equally distressing, there were no simple means for finding a suitable wet nurse; individuals were left to scour the city, hiring the best women they could get and hoping the arrangement would last.

For the Matthews family, the answer to their predicament and, by implication, the answer for others as well, is a respectable "American" woman – Mrs. Leonard – who nurses their baby during the day. At night, the infant, by now five months old, drinks from a bottle. As a literary device, Mrs. Leonard allows Walker to proceed to his next chapter and to his next child-rearing dilemma. The practical ramifications were another matter. Few families wanted a woman who nursed only during the day. More critically, a part-time wet nurse defied the lessons learned from Mrs. Badall's brief stay. The novel's criticism of Mrs. Badall suggested a deep distrust of married wet nurses, whose milk could be easily excited by sexual intercourse. Mrs. Leonard, whose name and designation as "respectable" strongly insinuate she was married, was presumably not immune to such excitement. Having reviewed the options for families in search of wet nurses and the problems with the practice itself, Walker simply wrote his way out of a corner, without providing any practical guidance for his readers. Or perhaps that was his message: that wet nursing arrangements were difficult to make, difficult to keep, and often haphazard.

As *The First Baby* suggests, newspapers continued to be a vital resource for both wet nurses and their prospective employers. A cheap means for communicating women's needs and hopes, newspaper advertisements functioned, in the words of historian David Katzman, as "the literature of the servant class."[4] Wet nurses, like servants of all types, placed the majority of notices.[5] Their two- and three-line advertisements were, in fact, the only words they wrote into the historical record, and these tell, in an abbreviated form, some of the reasons why they entered the wet nursing trade.

Despite their offering the direct statements of wet nurses, the notices'

---

4 David M. Katzman, *Seven Days a Week: Women and Domestic Service in Industrializing America* (New York: Oxford University Press, 1978), p. 99.
5 Daniel E. Sutherland, *Americans and Their Servants: Domestic Service in the United States from 1800 to 1920* (Baton Rouge: Louisiana State University Press, 1981), p. 18.

Table 3.1. *Advertisements in the* Philadelphia Public Ledger,
1837–1897

Year	By wet nurse	By family	By agency	Total
1837	11	3	3	17
1847	118	49	12	179
1857	226	125	7	358
1867	241	111	1	353
1877	126	62	4	192
1887	18	11	4	33
1897	8	6	—	14

Note: Advertisements were counted only the first time they appeared.
Source: Philadelphia Public Ledger.

limitations as historical sources are manifold. Their brevity disguises the
enormously varied personal situations that led wet nurses and families to
communicate their wants and needs in this way, their truthfulness is uncertain at best, and their results are unknowable. The wet nurses and employers who formed relationships as a result of the short phrases published in a
local paper are absent from the historical record; there is no way to know
either which advertisers found jobs or how they fared in those positions.

Nevertheless, newspaper advertisements for wet nurses do yield insights.
They show the growing influence of the intelligence offices, which placed
increasing numbers of notices; the popular resistance to certain medical
ideas involving the examination of wet nurses' babies, and the ways in
which race and ethnicity structured demand. They also reveal the language
through which wet nurses and families communicated their interests, including the idioms in which health, morality, and ethnicity were asserted
or obfuscated. Additionally, the notices make clear that whereas wet nursing itself was a national phenomenon, the wet nurse marketplace was
highly localized and often idiosyncratic.

The advertisements testify to the existence of an informal marketplace
that expanded in the midnineteenth century and shrank rapidly in the
century's closing decades. This is apparent in two noncomparable samples
of advertisements, one from the *Boston Evening Transcript* and one from the
Philadelphia Public Ledger.[6] Both papers were regularly consulted by fami-

6 Advertisements from the *Boston Evening Transcript* were counted the first time they appeared on the first Tuesday, Thursday, and Saturday of each month for every fifth year
  from 1861 to 1896 inclusive. Advertisements in the *Philadelphia Public Ledger* were counted
  daily, the first time they appeared, every tenth year from 1837 to 1897 inclusive.

Table 3.2. *Sample of advertisements in the* Boston Evening Transcript, *1861–1896*

Year	By wet nurse	By family	By agency	Total
1861	15	1	12	28
1866	5	1	12	18
1871	12	2	10	24
1876	19	3	23	45
1881	8	7	31	46
1886	4	3	1	8
1891	4	1	2	7
1896	3	—	—	3

Note: Advertisements were counted on the first Tuesday, Thursday, and Saturday of each month, the first time they appeared.
Source: Boston Evening Transcript.

lies looking for servants and by servants looking for work.[7] In 1837 only 17 notices for and by wet nurses appeared in the *Philadelphia Public Ledger.* Two decades later, in 1857, advertisements peaked at 358, and in 1867 there were 353. Subsequently, the numbers plummeted; in 1897 there were only 14.

In the *Boston Evening Transcript* the number of notices crested in 1876 and 1881 and, as in Philadelphia, showed a precipitous drop in the last years of the century. The ebb in advertising probably reflected the fact that poor single women were being siphoned off into institutional settings.

The notices document a shift from placing out infants to having wet nurses live in their employers' homes. Of the eleven advertisements from wet nurses in the *Philadelphia Public Ledger* in 1837, eight came from women seeking to take in a baby to nurse. "Wanted, a child to wet nurse" read a notice from July 1837, which went on to offer more particulars:

A healthy young English woman having abundance of milk, wishes to take a child to wet nurse at her own house – every attention will be paid to the comfort of the child, as she is living in a quiet and healthy house, and has nothing to engage her time except her own child which is three months old.[8]

7 For characterizations of nineteenth-century newspapers and their readers, see Frank Luther Mott, *American Journalism: A History, 1690–1960,* 3d ed. (New York: MacMillan, 1962); and Oswald Garrison Villard, *The Disappearing Daily: Chapters in American Newspaper Evolution* (New York: Knopf, 1944).
8 *Philadelphia Public Ledger,* 18 July 1837.

By 1897 none of the women advertising in the same newspaper suggested taking a baby into her home; all the women sought live-in positions. "Wet Nurse – Healthy young mother wants place," reads a typical example.[9]

The 1837 advertisement and the one published sixty years later both refer to the medical fitness of the wet nurse – the primary concern of employers. The 1837 advertisement offered repeated assurances about the woman's health, baby, and home. The 1897 advertisement, by contrast, was extraordinarily pithy; it contained no hints as to the woman's background or personal circumstances. Perhaps all parties assumed that claims of health would be verified by a physician. After all, a woman who boasted of a fresh breast of milk might have recently weaned her one-year-old child, and the woman who asserted she was in good health might harbor syphilis. As physicians played a more active role in the selection of wet nurses, and as the subject of infant feeding moved from the domestic to the medical domain, employers were becoming increasingly suspicious of women who promoted themselves as "healthy" but could not verify their claims.

During the heyday of wet nurse advertising in the 1850s, 1860s, and 1870s, women typically emphasized four qualities: good health, upstanding character, plentiful milk, and milk that was fresh. The appearance of these latter characteristics suggests that medical demands had begun to penetrate popular thinking. Indeed, with a growing emphasis on the medical inspection of wet nurses prior to their employment, doctors became critical players in an increasing number of transactions. They advertised on behalf of patients seeking work and also represented the interests of employers. "Wanted, a child to wet nurse by a lady who has lost her own baby," began an advertisement from a Philadelphia physician in 1857.[10] A notice placed by Dr. E. Wilson, also of Philadelphia, asked for "a wet nurse with a recent breast of milk and good city references."[11]

Despite the claims about medical fitness, the advertisements showed a degree of popular resistance to one of the emerging themes in the medical literature – the need to hire a woman with a living child. Physicians almost uniformly regarded it as crucial to examine the wet nurses' babies for signs of health. Ignoring this demand, being unaware of it, or perhaps believing that employers had a different standard, a number of the advertisers forthrightly announced that their infants had died. Similarly, many of the employers, particularly in the antebellum years, made choices that ran counter to medical advice, requesting a wet nurse without "encumbrance" or, more openly, a woman "who had lost her baby." Clearly, the widespread perception that a woman without a child would pay more attention to her

9 *Philadelphia Public Ledger*, 24 April 1897.
10 *Philadelphia Public Ledger*, 17 August 1857.
11 *Philadelphia Public Ledger*, 9 September 1857. In this case it is unclear whether Dr. Wilson sought a woman to suckle his own child or that of a patient.

Table 3.3. *Advertisements in the* Baltimore Sun, *1875*

By wet nurse	Number	By family	Number
Work out	43	Live in	57
Work in home	6	Baby placed out	2
Either situation	3		
Total	52		59

Note: Advertisements were counted only the first time they appeared.

Source: Baltimore Sun.

suckling continued to shape private practices. In revealing this conflict between medical theory and popular practice, the newspaper notices offer a window into an otherwise obscure world and serve as a counterweight to the prescriptive literature.

Another unique characteristic of the advertisements is their ability to illuminate local conditions and customs as well as more general marketplace trends. Boston had the highest ratio of servants to employers of any city in the country – 1 servant for every 3.5 families in 1870 in contrast to a national ratio of 1 to 7.[12] Under such conditions, intelligence offices proliferated, and many made active use of newspaper advertisements, eliminating the need for families or, more importantly, for wet nurses to place their own notices. In the 1876 *Boston Evening Transcript* sample, employers placed only 3 advertisements, wet nurses placed 19, and intelligence offices, 23. By contrast, in the 1877 *Philadelphia Public Ledger,* only 4 of the 192 advertisements involving wet nurses came from intelligence offices, with the vast majority, 126, from individual women.

In the South, where intelligence offices were less common, employers took a more active role in announcing their needs. A one-year sample from the *Baltimore Sun* in 1875 indicates a rough parity between the advertisements placed by employers in search of wet nurses – fifty-nine – and those from wet nurses who were seeking work – fifty-two. An additional notice came from the Maryland Lying-In Asylum, indicating that it had wet nurses available for hire. Another distinctive and possibly regional difference was that some families continued to send babies to live with wet nurses. Two Baltimore employers expressed an interest in having the wet nurse take the baby into her home, six wet nurses looked for babies to take in, and three wet nurses indicated a willingness to work either at home or in service.

12 Sutherland, *Americans and Their Servants*, p. 89.

Essentially, the two-, three-, or four-line newspaper advertisements display a marketplace for wet nurses configured by patterns of immigration, ethnic stereotypes, and racial prejudice, as well as by medical thinking and local domestic practices. The most prominent regional and local patterns appeared, not surprisingly, in references to race and ethnicity. Between 1830 and 1870 immigrants streamed into American cities, where many of the women took positions in service. Well aware of popular prejudice against the Irish women who rapidly came to dominate the marketplace, wet nurses who advertised in the *Boston Evening Transcript* sometimes pointedly described themselves as American, English, or Scottish. Notices in the *Philadelphia Public Ledger* specified the German backgrounds of the potential wet nurses – evidently an indication of what was perceived to be the most-favored immigrant group. Families made their preferences known as well. "Wanted, a wet nurse, German preferred," began a notice in the *Philadelphia Public Ledger* in 1867.[13] The owners of intelligence offices also understood the demand for women of specific backgrounds, choosing appropriate names for their businesses. The "Protestant Agency" and the "Swedish Employment Office," both of Boston, and the "American Agency" of Philadelphia explicitly assured prospective employers that no taint of rum or Romanism would defile their homes. Given the size of the immigrant population and the extensive evidence of Irish wet nurses in institutional records, it seems that the names of the agencies disguised rather than dictated the ethnic makeup of the wet nurse labor force.

Whereas the subject of a wet nurse's nativity permeated the medical discourse and infused the advertising, the topic of race was conspicuously absent. In the North, where the population of white servants far surpassed that of African-Americans, families may have assumed that white women were writing and answering the notices unless otherwise stated. One rare example of racial identification appeared in the *Philadelphia Public Ledger* from a Dr. Rosell, a self-identified mulatto physician, who noted the availability of a "responsible colored woman."[14]

In the South, other factors appear to have accounted for the patterns of advertisements. Notices in the *Baltimore Sun* in 1875 for domestic servants of all types nearly always specified the preferred race. Yet, only 5 of the 111 notices referring to wet nurses mentioned a racial preference (white), and only 2 women provided their racial identification. In New Orleans, the Southern city with the largest proportion of white domestic workers, racial preferences for wet nurses were almost always omitted.[15] Possibly the

13 *Philadelphia Public Ledger*, 7 January 1867. For other examples see *Philadelphia Public Ledger*, 4 January 1867; and idem, 22 May 1867.
14 *Philadelphia Public Ledger*, 1 February 1867. The advertisement misspells Rosell's name as Rosel. Rosell is identified in the 1870 manuscript census as mulatto.
15 This conclusion is drawn from an examination of all advertisements for wet nurses published in the *New Orleans Daily Picayune* in 1856 and from a survey of advertisements

Southern tradition of cross-race wet nursing in the antebellum years made race an unimportant qualification, or individual time constraints outweighed concerns about race. A notice in the 1859 *Charleston Courier,* for example, forthrightly announced: "Wanted immediately, a wet nurse, white or colored, without a child. Good recommendations would be satisfactory."[16] Furthermore, it is possible that references to race were covert rather than overt and that the addresses listed by wet nurses obliquely informed employers of their demographic characteristics. An advertisement by a wet nurse in the *New Orleans Daily Picayune* in 1856 sent interested parties to "Reverend N. C. Pridham, Rector of St. Peter's Church on Esplanade Street."[17] Local readers undoubtedly knew who belonged to the congregation.

Historian Deborah Gray White asserts that some antebellum families developed a custom of hiring white wet nurses and that this practice may have continued into the late nineteenth century.[18] Yet, the ability of families to select their wet nurses according to race depended in part on the structure of the local labor market. With nine out of ten African-Americans living in the South, and with African-American women in towns and cities actively seeking domestic employment in the postwar years, the South's wet nurse labor force undoubtedly included many nonwhite women.[19] This led, in turn, to the development of a Southern perspective on wet nursing.

The Southern view of wet nursing differed from the Northerner's perspective in several critical ways. First, the use of wet nurses among wealthy antebellum women appears to have been a more common pattern in the South than in the North, even though, like their Northern counterparts, Southern mothers were told that suckling their offspring was a duty. Second, Southern wet nursing included not only the use of African-American nurses for white infants but also occasional instances in which plantation mistresses nursed the infants of slaves. With the wealth of a plantation measured in slaves and with infant mortality rates high, the loss

in the following years. On the ratio of African-American and white servants in New Orleans and elsewhere, see Sutherland, *Americans and Their Servants,* p. 51.

16 Cited in Sally G. McMillen, *Motherhood in the Old South: Pregnancy, Childbirth, and Infant Rearing* (Baton Rouge: Louisiana State University Press, 1990), p. 125. McMillen believes that haste was a key reason that the wealthy Southern families she studied welcomed any healthy candidate, white or black, slave or free. Wet nursing by slave women and the attitudes of plantation mistresses toward their own nursing duties is also discussed in Elizabeth Fox-Genovese, *Within the Plantation Household: Black and White Women of the Old South* (Chapel Hill: University of North Carolina Press, 1988), pp. 279–80, 431 n. 35.

17 *New Orleans Daily Picayune,* 1 January 1856.

18 Deborah Gray White, *Ar'n't I a Woman?: Female Slaves in the Plantation South* (New York: W. W. Norton, 1985), p. 54.

19 On the postwar labor market position of African-American women, see Jacqueline Jones, *Labor of Love, Labor of Sorrow: Black Women, Work, and the Family from Slavery to the Present* (New York: Vintage, 1986), pp. 110–15.

of a slave infant was calculated in dollars as well as sentiment.[20] Third, cross-race wet nursing led Southerners to evolve a fixed and ultimately modern notion of heredity – that parents endowed their offspring with certain physical traits at the time of conception. Northerners had a different perspective.[21] Some went so far as to argue that the wet nurse could endow her suckling with her character. For obvious reasons, Southerners rejected this view altogether. In 1825 South Carolina physician George Logan published one of the first American medical treatises on the diseases of infants. In it he firmly refuted the belief that milk shaped character. Choosing classical examples to make his point, he explained that "among the ancients Diodorus relates, the intemperance of Nero and the sanguinary character of Caligula were imbibed from their nurses" but that he rejected this as "heathenish superstition" that "has now but few advocates."[22] Finally, the character of "mammy" served in important symbolic ways to underscore the idea that Southern children were valued regardless of race. In the antebellum years she emerged as a symbol of harmony – the woman who, by nursing infants black and white, created an organic plantation family.[23] In the postwar decades, the sentimentalization of "mammy" continued, helping to enshrine the idea of a contented past and to add further pathos to the idea of the "lost cause."[24] But the degree to which the "mammy" ideal, or even the preference for wet nurses of a particular race, shaped the marketplace is not revealed in the advertisements in Southern newspapers.

An analysis of newspaper advertisements leaves many other questions unanswered as well. What were the cultural expectations regarding wet nurses? Who responded to the notices – the family hiring the wet nurse or a physician working on their behalf? If the family undertook the task, what questions did they ask the wet nurse? Did they try to determine her health or the condition of her child? If they did, on what did they base their examinations – common knowledge about wet nurses, advice in popular medical books, or the suggestions of a physician? Were there differences in social class between the families who placed the advertisements and those who answered them? And what distinguished those employers who used the newspapers to find a wet nurse from those who visited institutions or intelligence offices?

Ultimately, newspaper notices proved inefficient and of dubious reliabil-

20 Fox-Genovese, *Within the Plantation Household*, pp. 234–5, 279–80.
21 Mark H. Haller, *Eugenics: Hereditarian Attitudes in American Thought* (New Brunswick: Rutgers University Press, 1963), p. 53.
22 George Logan, *Practical Observations on Diseases of Children, Comprehending a Description of Complaints & Disorders Incident to the Early Stages of Life, and a Method of Treatment* (Charleston: A. E. Miller, 1825), p. 22.
23 Fox-Genovese, *Within the Plantation Household*, pp. 191–2 and passim.
24 White, *Ar'n't I a Woman?*, pp. 46–61.

ity. Waiting for an employer to call, a would-be wet nurse who had lost her baby might see her milk supply diminish. Waiting for an acceptable wet nurse to answer their notice, a family might be tormented by the screams of a hungry baby or suffer the consequences of ineffective artificial feeding. More critically, the service offered in print – fresh milk supplied by a healthy wet nurse – often turned out to be less than advertised. Under the circumstances, intelligence offices and private maternity homes seemed to be a practical alternative. They had more candidates available and in the case of the maternity home, sometimes provided a medical reference or the chance to make an examination.

The owners of intelligence offices and maternity homes understood the profit-making potential in linking wet nurses and employers, although each business operated primarily for other purposes. Intelligence offices commercialized the placement of domestic servants, and wet nurses represented an extremely small portion of the business. The limited but critical role of maternity homes in the wet nurse marketplace displayed the entrepreneurial spirit of midwives who recognized that women could pay the expenses of their confinement by going out to service. Given the essentially private nature of both businesses, their small size, and the lack of formal oversight, it is difficult to measure their collective contribution to the marketplace. Nevertheless, anecdotal reports make clear that both had a part to play.

In her 1873 novel, *Work,* Louisa May Alcott acidly characterized intelligence offices as "the purgatory of the poor."[25] Most were simple neighborhood shops run by saloon keepers, shopkeepers, and other small-scale entrepreneurs.[26] Many operated outside the law, charging fees in excess of those allowed or failing to obtain a license. Despite the costs, frustrations, and illegalities, they proved popular over the long term. An inquiry in the early twentieth century revealed that 50 percent of the domestics and 34 percent of the employers made use of them.[27] Although traditional household servants were their stock-in-trade, employment agencies also supplied wet nurses. An advertisement in the *Boston Evening Transcript* informed readers that Miss M. T. Finn's Select Registry for Wet Nurses and Female Help had "twelve very healthy wet nurses" on hand. Their milk, according to the notice, ranged in age from one week to seven months, and all the

25 Louisa May Alcott, *Work: A Story of Experience* (reprint; New York: Schocken Books, 1971), p. 16.
26 On intelligence offices see Faye E. Dudden, *Serving Women: Household Service in Nineteenth-Century America* (Middletown, Conn.: Wesleyan University Press, 1983), pp. 79–87; Katzman, *Seven Days a Week,* pp. 101–7; and Sutherland, *Americans and Their Servants,* pp. 19–21, 71–4.
27 Gail Laughlin, *Domestic Service* (Washington, D.C.: U.S. Government Printing Office, 1901), p. 755.

women came with good references.[28] In Philadelphia, Odell's Intelligence Office offered a wet nurse to those who called between 9 a.m. and 2 p.m.[29]

Intelligence offices helped maintain the fiction that wet nursing was a form of household service, subject to the same rules and drawing from the same pool of workers. Like newspaper advertisements, they situated wet nursing in the domestic domain rather than in the world of medicine. Sitting among cooks, maids, and parlor girls, the wet nurses presented themselves as simply another category of household help. Yet, all participants knew otherwise. Whereas few families would openly employ as a domestic servant a woman known to have given birth out of wedlock, single motherhood failed to disqualify a wet nurse. Still, families had to be wary. Although Mrs. Finn promised "very healthy wet nurses," few savvy employers would put much credence in her words.

Maternity homes were similarly suspect institutions. According to contemporaries, maternity homes operated in a shadowy realm. "George Ellington," the pseudonymous author of the 1869 exposé *The Women of New York or the Under-World of the Great City,* claimed that maternity homes served wealthy women seeking to disguise their fall from the path of virtue.[30] Some may have done so. Most, however, seem to have been run by midwives catering to women too poor to give birth at home, disqualified from admission to lying-in hospitals by a previous out-of-wedlock pregnancy, or unwilling to accept the disgrace of giving birth in an almshouse infirmary. Whatever the economic rank of their patients, that maternity homes housed unwed mothers and that they were often places in which women obtained abortions contributed to the public's perception of them as, in the words of historian Morris Vogel, "accessories to vice and degradation" and "adjuncts to brothels."[31] Nevertheless, despite their shady reputations, they were a convenient source for wet nurses.

To make money, maternity home operators either charged a fee for their services upon a woman's admission or received their due after the woman left to find a place at service – with wet nursing being the logical occupation for the mother of a newborn child. In an annual report, the directors of the Boston Lying-In Hospital made harsh reference to one of their competitors, a disreputable "resort" that kept a woman's baby as collateral for the one hundred dollars she owed for her care.[32] A physician lodged a similar complaint, claiming that "many wet-nurses who apply at agencies

28 *Boston Evening Transcript,* 2 June 1881.
29 *Philadelphia Public Ledger,* 18 June 1877.
30 George Ellington [pseud.], *The Women of New York or the Under-World of the Great City* (New York: New York Book Co., 1869), pp. 397–8. Like other antebellum social critics, Ellington aimed many of his barbs at "fashionable women."
31 Morris J. Vogel, *The Invention of the Modern Hospital, Boston, 1870–1930* (Chicago: University of Chicago Press, 1980), p. 13.
32 Boston Lying-In Hospital, *Forty-third Annual Report* (Boston, 1876), p. 9.

have been confined by midwives who keep lying-in establishments and are sent out as wet-nurses by those women to earn money to pay the expenses of confinement."[33] In spite of this, at least one leading pediatrician, Isaac Abt, formed a lasting partnership with the owner of a maternity home.

In his autobiography, *Baby Doctor* (1944), Abt recalled a midnight search for a wet nurse many decades earlier that concluded when he drove his horse and buggy to the door of a local maternity home. Standing outside, he dickered with its feisty proprietress:

"I've got to have a wet nurse," I told her. "Right away." "Is that so," she drawled. Coming out on the stoop she turned and looked critically at her front windows. "Well, I've got to have some new lace curtains." "You'll get them," I promised. "Where's the wet nurse?"

From then on, Abt sent the woman a set of new lace curtains annually. A good source of wet nurses, his story implied, required constant cultivation.[34] Moreover, a discrete maternity home may have furnished a seemingly more genteel candidate than the local almshouse could have.

Unlike intelligence offices, maternity homes linked wet nursing to childbirth rather than to domestic service. Customers could be certain that the women they hired had recently given birth and accordingly had milk that was "fresh." Nevertheless, the implied motto of the maternity home, like that of the intelligence office and the newspaper advertisement, was *caveat emptor*. For this reason, perhaps, maternity homes faced growing competition from other institutions supplying wet nurses, including lying-in hospitals, homes for fallen women, and public shelters. The distinguishing feature of all of these facilities was the presence of a matron or doctor who kept the candidates under surveillance and could ostensibly vouch for their morals and their health.

In the nineteenth century, wet nursing became a multilayered enterprise, with several tiers of wages. On the bottom rung of the ladder were poor, institutionalized women living in almshouses and other public shelters who were coerced into suckling abandoned babies – an enterprise that met with little success. A step above them were poor women with homes of their own who, in order to earn a small stipend, took in babies placed out by civic authorities. The next level consisted of women with homes of their own who made private arrangements to suckle babies. Among the infants left in their care were those belonging to wet nurses employed by private families. Ironically, the highest ranking group – in terms of pay – were the women who gave birth out of wedlock and

33 Joseph Edcil Winters, "The Relative Influences of Maternal and Wet Nursing on Mother and Child," *Medical Record* 30 (1886): 511.
34 Isaac Abt, *Baby Doctor* (New York: McGraw-Hill, 1944), p. 85.

78   *A social history of wet nursing*

through good luck escaped the public asylum for work in a private family. Had they not been hired, they might have remained in the almshouses nursing abandoned babies. Instead, they were brought up from the depths of poverty into the nurseries of the well-to-do. It was this group of workers, of course, who were so often vilified in the medical and domestic literature.

The efforts of a municipal shelter in Boston, the City Temporary Home, demonstrate how public officials played a role in aiding both women seeking babies to nurse at home and those in search of live-in positions. Operating as a kind of halfway house, the Temporary Home cared for women in transit from the Tewksbury Almshouse and other welfare institutions to jobs at service.[35] In addition, the Home maintained a list of women seeking work as wet nurses or in other positions.

Like private reformers, Boston public officials attempted to classify and distinguish between the worthy and the unworthy poor. The Home claimed to serve only "deserving persons." A woman giving birth out of wedlock for the first time was given refuge; a woman who had transgressed a second time was to be turned away.[36] The dividing line had the effect of bringing the policies of the Home in line with those of private benevolent establishments and of marking the women placed out as "redeemable" rather than condemned.

Of course, the majority of women had, in contemporary terms, "fallen." Betsy McFarlaine, a typical resident and former almshouse denizen, worked a farm in the community of Fall River, Massachusetts, until she became pregnant by a fellow employee. She gave birth at the Bridgewater Almshouse, moved three days later to the Tewksbury Almshouse – which had facilities for children – and from there went to the City Temporary Home.[37] Between 1862 and 1864, McFarlaine and one hundred other Temporary Home residents left the facility to become private-duty wet nurses.

Most of the women found work quickly. Twenty-eight of the fifty-two for whom data are available found work within a week of their arrival, and by the end of a month another fifteen had found jobs. After their employment ended, eighteen of the women returned to the Temporary Home for a brief period and found new wet nursing positions; four came back to

35 Eighteen of the women arrived at the Temporary Home after a stay in a public shelter, four came from a private facility, and eight came from some other kind of institution. Eighteen appear to have had no previous affiliation. Calculated from the records of the Boston Overseers of the Poor, City Temporary Home Records, Box 16, Folder 1. MHS.
36 On the Temporary Home see "Ordinances, Rules, and Regulations as to the Overseers of the Poor, Charity Building and Temporary Home" (Boston, 1869), p. 18; and *Directory of Charitable and Beneficent Organizations* (Boston, 1880), pp. 6, 21.
37 Boston, Overseers of the Poor, City Temporary Home Records, May–December 1862, p. 79. Box 16, Folder 1. MHS.

Table 3.4. *Placement of wet nurses discharged from the Boston City Temporary Home, 1862–1864*

	Number	Percentage
Wait for first placement		
Less than one week	28	57.1
1–2 weeks	6	12.2
3–4 weeks	9	18.4
5–6 weeks	2	4.1
7 weeks and over	4	8.2
Total	49	100
(Missing cases	52)	
Wait for second placement		
Less than one week	8	44
1–2 weeks	7	39
3–4 weeks	0	0
5–6 weeks	2	11
7 weeks and over	1	6
Total	18	100

Source: Records of the Boston Overseers of the Poor, City Temporary Home, Box 16, Folder 1, MHS.

look for work a third time. The patterns of arrivals and departures illustrate the ways in which women used the civic facility to negotiate the labor market and find shelter between jobs.

The ability to suckle an infant lifted women out of severely regimented institutional life into a relatively high-paying position. At the Temporary Home it was forbidden to talk or to sing loudly, to smoke, or to drink. The residents retired each night by nine o'clock after dreary meals of tea and bread in the morning and rotating dinners that included beef stew, bread, and potato every Monday, Thursday, and Saturday.[38] No wonder the women in the Temporary Home and those in similar facilities chose to live in private homes when the opportunity arose. And no wonder that many wet nurses were accused of looking upon these positions as opportunities for culinary indulgence. As one pediatrician was quoted as saying, wet nurses viewed their jobs "as one would regard 'a land which flows with milk and honey' and where 'roasted pigeons fly into the mouth,'

38 The daily diet of the residents and rules of the house are spelled out in "Ordinances, Rules, and Regulations," p. 21.

Canaan and America at once, – and where there is no end of things to eat."[39]

In making the leap from institution to private household each wet nurse negotiated her own price. The records reveal a wage scale that ranged from less than one dollar a week to over three dollars. The variation may have reflected the fact that women at the lower end of the scale had employers who paid the costs of boarding out their babies, whereas the best-paid women were responsible for covering this expense themselves. However, with an average weekly pay of over two dollars, the women discharged from the Temporary Home earned better wages than the typical domestic – who received an average of $1.85 per week in 1860. Indeed, their earnings compared favorably with those of the foreign-born factory hands in the nearby Lowell textile mills, whose net income, after paying board, was about two dollars.[40] Women who made wet nursing a career or, as one physician termed it, "a business," earned a fair amount of criticism, but a decent amount of money.[41]

Whether the moral gatekeeping or the presence of a matron to screen and observe inmates helped attract employers is uncertain, but the records show that families of all social classes looked to the Temporary Home for wet nurses. Despite tarnished reputations as former almshouse residents and single mothers, the women found employment with some of the wealthiest families in the city. Fifteen of the thirty-eight employers for whom occupations were recorded were professionals, and a substantial portion came from the city's elite. Among them were Mrs. William C. Codman, wife of the president of the Lawrence Fire Insurance Company; John Tisdale Bradlee, a merchant; and Francis D. Denny, a lawyer.[42] Employers several rungs lower on the social ladder also appeared on the register, including sixteen lower-level white-collar workers and seven

39 Abraham Jacobi quoted in Edward P. Davis and John M. Keating, *Mother and Child* (Philadelphia: J. B. Lippincott, 1893), p. 91. For a midnineteenth-century perspective, see Joseph Laurie, *The Parent's Guide: Containing the Diseases of Infancy and Childhood and Their Homeopathic Treatment,* ed. and with additions by Walter Williamson (New York: W. Radde, 1853), p. 31.
40 Stanley Lebergott, *Manpower in Economic Growth; The American Record since 1800* (New York: McGraw-Hill, 1964), Table A-26, p. 542; Thomas Dublin, *Women at Work: The Transformation of Work and Community in Lowell, Massachusetts, 1826–1860* (New York: Columbia University Press, 1979), Table 11.12, p. 197. Dublin's table gives the mean daily pay. The figure of $3.40 presumes a six-day week. Dublin cites board fees averaging $1.375 per week in 1850. (p. 188).
41 Joseph Edcil Winters, "The Relative Influences of Maternal and Wet Nursing on Mother and Child," *Medical Record* 30 (1886): 512.
42 Boston, Overseers of the Poor, City Temporary Home Records, May–December 1862; January–July 1863; and August 1863–March 1864. Box 16, Folder 1. MHS. Occupational rankings come from Stephen Thernstrom, *The Other Bostonians: Poverty and Progress in the American Metropolis, 1880–1970* (Cambridge: Harvard University Press, 1973), Appendix B, "On the Socioeconomic Rankings of Occupation," pp. 289–302. The occupations of employers were traced through city directories for Boston and its surroundings.

Table 3.5. *Wages earned by wet nurses discharged from the Boston City Temporary Home, 1862–1864*

Wages[a]	Number	Percentage
Less than $1.00	2	10
$1.00–$2.00	7	37
$2.01–$3.00	6	32
Over $3.00	4	21
Total	19	100
(Missing cases	82)	

[a]Wages given for first placement only.
Source: Records of the Boston Overseers of the Poor, City Temporary Home, Box 16, Folder 1, MHS.

workers in skilled, semiskilled, or blue-collar occupations. Among the latter were Police Captain Hough and foundry worker Darius Crosby.[43] The occupational range suggests that the availability of wet nurses rather than their cost made the Temporary Home an attractive emporium. It also provides evidence that wet nursing met a need that spanned a broad social spectrum. Families of all income levels experienced a mother's death or disability and subsequently chose the best substitute they could, a wet nurse. Even the wet nurses hired out of the Temporary Home sought to place their own babies with wet nurses. In at least eight instances, their babies went to women who registered at the Temporary Home in the hopes of finding a baby.

The history of Boston's City Temporary Home illustrates several aspects of social welfare in the nineteenth century: the erection of new institutions for housing the destitute, the segregation and classification of the dependent poor, and the enduring interest in restricting welfare eligibility in order to force individuals to work.[44] From the standpoint of civic officials, a woman who had milk to sell had no reason either to mix with the idle and dissolute in the almshouse or to receive a stipend (then termed "outdoor relief") for herself and her child. She belonged at service. Admittedly,

43 Boston, Overseers of the Poor, City Temporary Home Records, May–December 1862, p. 82; August 1863–May 1864, p. 49. Box 16, Folder 1. MHS.
44 On asylum building in the nineteenth century, see David J. Rothman, *The Discovery of the Asylum: Social Order and Disorder in the New Republic* (Boston: Little Brown, 1971); for a general analysis of welfare and the state, see Michael B. Katz, *In the Shadow of the Poorhouse: A Social History of Welfare in America* (New York: Basic Books, 1986).

civic officials coerced destitute women into separating from their own infants at a tragically early age. In this regard, they were no worse than profiteering maternity home operators and far less greedy than the owners of intelligence offices who made the wet nurses pay for the privilege of finding work. For public officials and private entrepreneurs alike, wet nursing was at bottom a financial enterprise in which consideration of the wet nurse's infant played no role.

For doctors, who were increasingly involved in wet nursing at the institutional and private levels, and for reformers, the separation of a mother and her baby proved problematic. Physicians knew that the results were often fatal. Reformers reached the same conclusion about the inadvisability of separating mothers and infants, but they did so on different grounds, constructing the issue as one of morality, rather than mortality.

Homes for fallen women comprised another sector of the wet nurse marketplace. Their collective mission was neither profit nor protection of the public purse. Instead, they sought to inculcate good work habits and maternal virtues in women thought likely to develop neither. Benevolent shelters established in the nineteenth century thus entered the wet nursing business through a back door, as their founders and matrons sought placements for their residents and patients in order to make them self-supporting.

Historians have ascribed a great many motives for the flowering of benevolence in the nineteenth century, from the bolstering of upper-class hegemony to a covert attack on the sexual double standard, from the exercise of social control to an expression of capitalism.[45] Given the diver-

45 Some of these arguments are elucidated in Thomas L. Haskell, "Capitalism and the Origins of Humanitarian Sensibility, Part I," *American Historical Review* 90 (1985): 339–61; and "Capitalism and Humanitarian Sensibility, Part 2," *American Historical Review* 90 (1985): 547–66; T. J. Jackson Lears, "The Concept of Cultural Hegemony: Problems and Possibilities," *American Historical Review* 90 (1985): 567–93; Carroll Smith-Rosenberg, "Beauty, the Beast, and the Militant Woman: A Case Study in Sex Roles and Social Stress in Jacksonian America," *American Quarterly* 23 (1971): 562–84; and Anthony F. C. Wallace, *Rockdale: The Growth of an American Village in the Early Industrial Revolution* (New York: Knopf, 1978).

The issue of gender and benevolence has been studied through general analysis and in terms of individuals, peer groups, and institutions. See Virginia Drachman, *Hospital with a Heart: Women Doctors and the Paradox of Separatism at the New England Hospital, 1862–1969* (Ithaca: Cornell University Press, 1984); Peggy Pascoe, *Relations of Rescue: The Search for Female Moral Authority in the American West, 1874–1939* (New York: Oxford University Press, 1990); and Virginia Anne Metaxas Quiroga, *Poor Mothers and Babies: A Social History of Childbirth and Child Care Hospitals in Nineteenth Century New York City* (New York: Garland, 1989). For a general analysis of women's benevolent activities see Anne M. Boylan, "Women in Groups: An Analysis of Women's Benevolent Organizations in New York and Boston, 1797–1840," *Journal of American History* 71 (1984): 497–523; Lori D. Ginzberg, *Women and the Work of Benevolence: Morality, Politics, and Class in the Nineteenth-Century United States* (New Haven: Yale University Press, 1990); Nancy A. Hewitt,

sity of the programs that developed, the clients who they served, and the women who were involved, however, no single explanation is adequate, nor are the arguments mutually exclusive. Case histories reveal how benevolent institutions embodied many conflicting ideologies and how they changed over time. Rescue homes, for example, often portrayed their clients as the innocent victims of men's sexual urges. But, simultaneously, they also labeled the rescued women as agents in their own downfall, as immoral women who needed to be resocialized to accept middle-class norms of sexual restraint.[46] From this perspective, the women entering service from the shelters for fallen women were not independent entrepreneurs like the wet nurses who advertised in the newspapers; instead, like residents of city facilities, they were part of the "dangerous poor." Their entrance into an institution stripped away any pretense the women might have made to accidental misfortune; it replaced the autobiographical accounts in the wanted column that began "lost my baby" with implied tales of seduction and abandonment. Mitigating this effect were the assurances of the institutions' matrons that the women under their care had fallen only once, that they had been morally rehabilitated, and that they had behaved properly while in residence.

The records of the Protestant Home of Philadelphia and of its sister charity, the Christian Home, reveal how small private benevolent organizations operated within the wet nurse marketplace. The Protestant Home, which opened in 1881, cared for white, unmarried mothers in the hopes of preventing them from abandoning their babies. At the same time, the shelter welcomed foundlings into its fold. Women remained in the Protestant Home until places at service could be found for them and arrangements made for their children. When possible, the foundlings went to adoptive homes. The Christian Home, located in the heart of Philadelphia's red-light district, "rescued" pregnant unmarried women, trained them, and found them respectable jobs. Residents typically remained until their confinements; after the births of their children, they went to the Protestant Home to await placement as domestics.[47]

The Protestant Home combined aspects of an intelligence office, a city temporary home, and an infant asylum. Like an intelligence office, it sent

Women's Activism and Social Change: Rochester, New York, 1822–1872 (Ithaca: Cornell University Press, 1984); and Kathleen D. McCarthy, *Noblesse Oblige: Charity and Cultural Philanthropy in Chicago, 1849–1929* (Chicago: University of Chicago Press, 1982).
46 Regina G. Kunzel, *Fallen Women, Problem Girls: Unmarried Mothers and the Professionalization of Social Work, 1890–1945* (New Haven: Yale University Press, 1993).
47 The Protestant Home and the Christian Home were agencies, now defunct, affiliated with the Protestant church in Philadelphia. The names of the agencies have been disguised to protect the identities of the clients. The records of the agencies are the property of a private Philadelphia social work agency affiliated with the Protestant church and are housed at the Temple University Urban Archives.

women out to work in domestic positions, including that of wet nurse. Like an infant asylum, it cared for abandoned babies. And, like a temporary home, it provided a place to live. Hard work earned the women a recommendation and the right to leave their infants in the facility when they took a private position. Philosophically as well as programmatically, the Protestant Home united several popular beliefs, situating its efforts at the nexus of moral reform and public welfare. It attempted to redeem its female inmates through prayer and a regimented life, and it also adopted a welfare model based on a belief in the regenerative value of work. Within this framework, wet nursing was a small but nonetheless vital aspect of daily life in the institution.

The Protestant Home both consumed and supplied wet nurses. Between 1882 and 1887, the matron of the Home recorded in her diary twenty-five visits from private employers seeking wet nurses; she accommodated only eight of them. Other disappointed visitors to the Protestant Home included six families who asked to have their wet nurses' babies admitted and three women who requested that the shelter admit their babies so they could accept jobs as wet nurses. Even the babies cared for at the Protestant Home had inquiries made on their behalf. Three women asked to wet nurse them in their homes, and four men asked to borrow babies to "help draw" milk from their wives' breasts. The matron granted the various requests when possible, giving priority to the needs of the residents.[48] The Home, after all, existed to care for unwed mothers and unwanted babies.

The majority of women residents had only enough strength, milk, or interest to nurse their own offspring. The matron therefore had to find women willing to enter the shelter and suckle babies, putting herself in direct competition with the private employers who lured away her resident wet nurses. Occasionally, to her relief, nursing women applied for admission. Of the nineteen noted in the records, only one was turned away. However, high turnover kept her busy, as women left without notice, quit after receiving permission to look for work, or were dismissed for insubordination. In six instances, the matron visited the city almshouse to recruit new wet nurses. She also sought candidates at the Philadelphia Infant's Home and at the Philadelphia Temporary Home.[49] Her expeditions reveal the permeability of the public and private welfare systems, and, in later records, the avenues of exchange ran in two directions. By the early twentieth century, Protestant Home residents often left with their

---

48 Calculated from the "Protestant Home" Diary, February 1882–August 1883; Diary, August 21, 1883–January 1, 1887; House Records, June 1881–April, 1884; House Records, November 1884–December 1890, and the *Annual Reports*. TUA.
49 These figures are calculated from the "Protestant Home" Diary, February 28, 1882–August 20, 1883; and Diary, August 21, 1883–January 1887. TUA.

Table 3.6. *Requests regarding wet nurses at the Protestant Home, 1882–1887*

	Number
Request	
Family seeking to hire wet nurse	25
Women seeking admission as wet nurses	19
Family wanting wet nurse's baby admitted	6
Wet nurse wanting baby admitted	3
Woman wanting to borrow baby to "draw" breast	4
Woman wanting to take in baby to wet nurse	3
Total	60

Source: "Protestant Home" Diaries, February 1882–August 1883, August 21, 1883–January 1, 1887; House Records, June 1881–April 1884, and November 1884–December 1890, TUA.

babies to go to work in the Infant's Home or to go to placements arranged through the local Children's Aid Society.[50]

Other wet nurses came to the Protestant Home from the Christian Home, and on a few occasions, the Christian Home's inmates also went to work as wet nurses in private homes. Between 1897 and 1903, long past the heyday of the wet nursing business, the records list several such arrangements. A leading industrialist, for example, hired a wet nurse from the Christian Home, even though residence in the facility signified destitution and, more certainly, was evidence of past immorality.[51] Perhaps employers believed that the moral environment within a church-run shelter imbued wet nurses with proper humility and work habits and that the taint of the almshouse or the brothel could be worn off by prayer sessions and discipline. They had no guarantee, however. Hiring a wet nurse placed a family in a difficult position in terms of assessing the woman's health and morals.

Ironically, it was not the moral complications haunting employers that removed rescue homes from the wet nursing business, it was the objections raised by the leaders of the homes. They wanted to cease participating in the wet nurse supply business in order to ignite the flames of maternal duty in the unwed mothers they served. According to the philosophy articulated

50 "Protestant Home" Register, January 1900–September 1907. TUA.
51 "Christian Home" Register of Inmates, 1893–1920, and House Records, January 1898–December 1899. TUA.

in the closing decades of the nineteenth century, the moral regeneration of fallen women depended upon encouraging their love for their own children. Mothers and babies were not to be separated, and petitions for wet nurses were to be refused. As Kate Waller Barrett, the well-known general superintendent of the National Florence Crittendon Mission, argued, "Mothering [banished] selfishness and shallowness and self will," allowing a woman to transfer her affections from the man who deceived her to her child.[52] Numerous institutions and even individuals followed this policy. The Boston civic activist and writer Margaret Deland, for example, took in sixty girls from the New England Hospital over a four-year period and kept all but six or seven from "slipping back into the gutter." Deland believed she was helping bring women closer to their babies.[53] In the context of a broad-based commitment to keeping mothers and babies united, many national organizations as well as state laws began to forbid their separation.[54]

The policy may well have developed in response to the rising rate of illegitimacy and in the hope that by encouraging mothers to stay with their babies, the crisis would subside.[55] It also reflected the growth of national organizations serving what contemporaries referred to as "fallen women" or "ruined girls." The Salvation Army, the Women's Christian Temperance Union, and, most notably, the Florence Crittendon Missions joined the nineteenth-century crusade to aid single mothers by erecting small, locally run shelters.[56] The directors of these facilities typically refused

52 Kate Waller Barrett, "Maternity Work – Motherhood as a Means of Regeneration," in National Florence Crittendon Missions, *Fourteen Years Work Among 'Erring' Girls* (Washington, D.C.: National Florence Crittendon Missions, 1897), pp. 52–4.
53 Margaret Deland, *Golden Yesterdays* (New York: Harper & Bros., 1941), pp. 153–9.
54 Rickie Solinger, *Wake Up Little Susie: Single Pregnancy and Race before Roe v. Wade* (New York: Routledge, 1992), pp. 150–1.
55 Limited demographic data suggest that after a decline in the first half of the nineteenth century, rates of both out-of-wedlock and premarital pregnancies began to climb in the second half of the century. Daniel Scott Smith, "The Long Cycle in American Illegitimacy and Prenuptial Pregnancy," in Peter Laslett, Karla Oosterveen, and Richard M. Smith, eds., *Bastardy and Its Comparative History: Studies in the History of Illegitimacy and Marital Nonconformism in Britain, France, Germany, Sweden, North America, Jamaica, and Japan* (London: Edward Arnold, 1980), pp. 370–2. The link between rates of premarital pregnancy and rates of illegitimacy is described in Daniel Scott Smith and Michael S. Hindus, "Premarital Pregnancy in America, 1640–1971: An Overview and Interpretation," *Journal of Interdisciplinary History* 4 (1975): Figure 1, pp. 538–9, and 561.
56 For a discussion of the responses to illegitimacy and the terms applied to the mothers, see Joan Jacobs Brumberg, " 'Ruined' Girls: Changing Community Responses to Illegitimacy in Upstate New York, 1890–1920," *Journal of Social History* 18 (1984): 247–72; Kunzel, *Fallen Women, Problem Girls*; Marian J. Morton, "Seduced and Abandoned in an American City, Cleveland and Its Fallen Women, 1869–1936," *Journal of Urban History* 11 (1985): 443–69; idem, "Fallen Women, Federated Charities, and Maternity Homes, 1913–1973," *Social Service Review* 62 (1988): 448–64; idem, *And Sin No More: Social Policy and Unwed Mothers in Cleveland, 1855–1990* (Columbus: Ohio State University Press, 1993); and Michael W. Sedlak, "Youth Policy and Young Women, 1870–1972," *Social Service Review*

requests for wet nurses, expecting that the women would keep and rear their babies. In Chicago, for example, the Erring Woman's Refuge shifted from a policy of separating mothers and babies to one of encouraging women to keep their children.[57] Three rescue homes in Cleveland – one run by the Salvation Army, another sponsored by the Catholic Diocese, and the third established by the Women's Christian Association – also embraced a policy of keeping women and babies united.[58] Nevertheless, some facilities, such as the Christian Home and Protestant Home in Philadelphia and the Anchorage, a Women's Christian Temperance Union home in Elmira, New York, resisted the new imperatives and continued to follow an older tradition.[59]

The effects of these new policies on the mothers and babies are difficult to measure. It seems certain that some new mothers lost the opportunity to engage in high-wage work as wet nurses and thus to escape institutional life. At the same time, the mothers' loss was their infants' gain: the babies were neither left behind in asylums nor shipped off to relatives, friends, or other caretakers, and thus their chances of survival increased. Indeed, the low survival rate of the infants and the lack of adoptive families for babies judged "illegitimate" was one reason public authorities tried to halt the separation of mothers and babies.[60]

Equally difficult to gauge is how changes in the placement practices of benevolent institutions influenced the wet nurse marketplace. The growing interest in the reclamation of fallen women probably diminished the number of wet nurses available from private shelters in the late nineteenth century, but the loss may have been made up by the growing number of women who went out to wet nursing service from lying-in hospitals and infant asylums. The expansion of institutions housing mothers and babies meant that families turned away from one door could knock on another.

The development of lying-in charities in the nineteenth century reflected many of the same forces that impelled the construction of other facilities for mothers and infants: an expansion in female benevolence and a desire to aid poor but worthy women. With a steady stream of women passing through their wards, lying-in hospitals were in a good position to offer employers a sizable selection of wet nurses, all of whom had been scrutinized by physicians. Another advantage of a wet nurse hired from a lying-in hospital was the age of her milk: she had, by definition, a baby

---

56 (1982): 448–64. On Salvation Army rescue homes, see Edward H. McKinley, *Marching to Glory: The History of the Salvation Army in the United States of America, 1880–1980* (New York: Harper & Row, 1980), pp. 54–5.
57 Sedlack, "Youth Policy," p. 452.
58 Morton, "Fallen Women," pp. 62–4; and *And Sin No More*.
59 Brumberg, " 'Ruined' Girls," pp. 260–1.
60 Solinger, *Wake Up Little Susie*, p. 150.

that was less than three weeks old. True to their mission to provide medical care rather than moral reform, the hospitals discharged women after a brief recovery period.

The vast majority of lying-in patients were unwed mothers. Initially, to distinguish themselves from disreputable maternity homes, lying-in facilities drew the line at admitting unwed mothers, but a dearth of patients soon forced them to enlarge the scope of their mission to include assistance to women who had made "a single mistake." The directors of the New York Female Asylum for Lying-In Women, for example, which opened a facility in 1823, complained that the almshouse indiscriminately mixed the "virtuous and the vicious." Unlike many benevolent institutions that aimed to redeem the fallen, the directors of the Asylum for Lying-In Women hoped to aid "reputable married females" who presented a certificate of marriage and a character reference.[61] They found few candidates and by 1831 capitulated, changing their policies to include unmarried mothers and to provide home deliveries – which rapidly outnumbered hospital births by a wide margin. Between 1823 and 1899 the outdoor department handled 20,764 deliveries, whereas only 7,052 women bore children in the Asylum.[62] Many of those who gave birth in the facility were unmarried women who later sought work as wet nurses.

Other lying-in facilities faced similar problems in trying to limit their admissions to married women. The Boston Lying-In Hospital opened in 1832 with a promise to assist only married and recently widowed women. A circular assured prospective donors that the Hospital "gives no encouragement to vice, furnishes no excuse for improvidence, offers no asylum for the dissolute."[63] The restrictions and a recurring epidemic of puerperal fever – a deadly postpartum infection – resulted in a shortage of patients and fees, forcing the hospital to close its doors in 1856.[64] Six years later,

61 Mrs. Rev. Thomas. Mason, "Account of the Organization of the New York Asylum for Lying-In Women in 1823." Manuscript. NYHS. See also Thomas F. Cock, "History of the New York Asylum for Lying-In Women," 1894, manuscript. NYHCMC; and Virginia A. Metaxas Quiroga, "Culture and Class Conflict at the New York Asylum for Lying-In Women, 1823–1850," *Transactions and Studies of the College of Physicians of Philadelphia*, Ser. V 11 (1989): 105–21. Admissions posed several issues for the hospital beyond the question of morality. The board was informed by the Commissioners of the Almshouse that if they admitted women who were not citizens, they would be liable for the support of the children of those women. Board of Managers Minutes, New York Asylum for Lying-In Women, vol. 1, p. 25. NYHCMC.
62 Board of Managers of the Old Marion Street Maternity Hospital, *Seventy-sixth Annual Report* (New York, 1899), p. 9. In 1894 the New York Female Asylum for Lying-In Women officially became the Old Marion Street Maternity Hospital.
63 Board of Trustees, Boston Lying-In Hospital, "Public Statement," April 5, 1832. FACLM. On the stigma attached to maternity hospitals, see Vogel, *The Invention of the Modern Hospital*, p. 20.
64 "Boston Lying-In: Its Past, Present, and Future" (Boston, 1890). On the effects of puerperal fever on childbirth practices, see Judith Walzer Leavitt, *Brought to Bed: Childbearing in America, 1750 to 1950* (New York: Oxford University Press, 1986), pp. 155–65.

another Boston facility, the New England Hospital for Women and Children, began providing medical, surgical, and obstetrical services and serving as a site in which female physicians could train and work. The founders, haunted perhaps by the failure of the Boston Lying-In or simply more pragmatic, welcomed "fallen women" into the maternity wards, openly serving "those who came to Boston to hide their condition and spare their friends the mortification of seeing an illegitimate [birth] among them." Their indulgence did not extend to women giving birth out of wedlock for a second time.[65] When the Boston Lying-In Hospital reopened in 1873, it embraced a similar policy, mixing "respectable women" with "that class whom maternity makes outcasts."[66] The moral rhetoric remained potent, but the goal shifted from excluding immoral women to uplifting them.

The consequences of the admissions policies for families hiring wet nurses were clear: when they or their physicians called at the hospital gate, they knew they would probably come away with a woman widely considered to have transgressed. The woman sitting on the bench in the basement of an intelligence office or living behind the lace curtains of the maternity home could at least keep up the pretense of respectability, offering a claim of marriage or widowhood. The woman hired from a lying-in hospital or public shelter could not maintain even this charade.

The stain of illegitimacy did not, however, deter employers. From the beginning, the leaders of the New York Female Asylum for Lying-In Women resolved to benefit the community by supplying wet nurses.[67] Careful screening at the time of admission, observation by the matron of their "tempers and dispositions," and examination by the physician at the time of delivery assured families of the health and character of the wet nurses they retained. In 1828, the managers proudly announced, "Of fifty who have been discharged from the house . . . , 23 have obtained places as wet nurses in respectable families."[68] The Boston hospitals also attracted families and doctors seeking wet nurses. The New England Hospital for Women and Children boasted of the frequency with which physicians visited the hospital to find wet nurses, and the annual reports of Boston

65 New England Hospital for Women and Children, *Fifth Annual Report* (Boston, 1868), p. 10. See also Ednah D. Cheney, "Private Charities in Boston," *Proceedings of the National Conference of Charities and Corrections* 8 (1881): 89; and Drachman, *Hospital with a Heart*.
66 Boston Lying-In Hospital, *Forty-second Annual Report* (Boston, 1875), pp. 6–7. A comparison of the two hospitals found that worthiness of patients was a more significant factor at the New England Hospital for Women and Children than at the Boston Lying-In and that patients at the Lying-In were poorer. See Regina Markell Morantz and Sue Zschoche, "Professionalism, Feminism, and Gender Roles: A Comparative Study of Nineteenth Century Therapeutics," *Journal of American History* 67 (1980): 577.
67 Cock, "History of the New York Asylum for Lying-In Women," pp. 57, 67.
68 Managers of the New York Asylum for Lying-In Women, *Fifth Annual Report* (New York, 1928), p. 3.

Lying-In Hospital listed 284 wet nurses discharged between 1873 and 1908.[69]

Although lying-in hospitals shared a heritage of benevolence with shelters for women, they represented a different branch of social welfare. The medical mission of the hospital meant that women were to be delivered and allowed to convalesce, but once recovered, they and their infants were discharged, regardless of whether they had a place to go. On Christmas Eve 1827, the New York Female Asylum for Lying-In Women sent Mrs. Fagan and Mrs. Kelly to positions as wet nurses; a more unfortunate woman left for the almshouse.[70] In later years, the Asylum, still unwilling to become a refuge, looked to the Society for the Improvement of Domestic Servants to aid women about to be discharged.[71] Boston institutions followed a similar policy; women went into service within a few weeks of their admission. Anna Kinney left the New England Hospital for Women and Children only twelve days after the birth of her son. The boy went to a boarding place and was later adopted; she went out to work as a wet nurse.[72] Other women, unable to find a position and having no place to go, departed for the Massachusetts Infant Asylum, which employed wet nurses to suckle foundlings. Some, after a brief sojourn working in the Asylum, traveled on to work in private homes.

Infant asylums, like lying-in hospitals, had a complex relationship to the private wet nurse marketplace. They aimed to aid motherless babies and prevent abandonment by allowing single mothers to suckle foundlings in exchange for the opportunity to live in the facility and nurse their own infants. Physicians often criticized such efforts, claiming they led to unnecessarily high infant-mortality rates. When medical professionals succeeded in gaining control over the institutions, they often rejected congregate care, substituting a system of outplacement of healthy babies. When reformers held the upper hand, however, the goal of rescuing women remained paramount, and group care of infants continued.

An example of an infant shelter and wet nurse service run by reformers was the Nursery for the Children of Poor Woman, which opened in New

---

69 New England Hospital for Women and Children, *Fifth Annual Report* (Boston, 1868), p. 16; and Boston Lying-In Hospital, *Annual Reports*
70 New York Female Asylum for Lying-In Women, Visiting Committee, Board of Managers, vol. 1, December 25, 1827. NYHCMC.
71 New York Female Asylum for Lying-In Women, Visiting Committee, Board of Managers, vol. 1, May 8, 1827. NYHCMC. The minutes were probably referring to the New York Society for the Encouragement of Faithful Domestic Servants, founded in 1825 and having an overlapping membership.
72 Records of the New England Hospital, 1866–1902, Maternity Cases, April 15, 1869. FACLM.

York City in 1854 expressly to serve the offspring of wet nurses.[73] The Nursery's founder, Mary Delafield Du Bois, understood the difficult choices faced by wet nurses, having been awakened to the issue, she claimed, by the near tragedy of Mary Ennis.

As Du Bois recounted, Ennis's employer paid her extra wages in return for a promise never to visit her own infant. Ennis kept the bargain, but with evident difficulty. Her longing for her child became noticeable to a nurse visiting the household, who volunteered to check on the baby. The nurse found Ennis's infant lying in rags in the squalid basement room of its caretaker – a woman dying of smallpox. Rescued and vaccinated, Ennis's infant survived. Alerted to the cruelties of wet nursing by this tale, Du Bois established her Nursery, with priority for admission going to the offspring of wet nurses and other daytime places reserved for the children of working women.[74]

The Nursery was an instant success. Demand for admission rapidly outstripped the number of places available as wet nurses removed their babies from other accommodations and brought them to the Nursery. One mother admitted a child suffering a severe injury due to neglect in its expensive boarding home; another woman sent her blind infant who had been mistreated by other caretakers.[75] Wet nurses' employers paid a twenty-five-dollar fee to have the infants enter the Nursery. To keep the infants well fed, Du Bois offered other women the chance to exchange nursing for shelter. Women earned a place for their babies by spending three months in residence suckling a Nursery baby as well as their own. After completing their terms they were free to leave their infants and go out to service. Candidates admitted under this plan underwent a medical examination and submitted both a certificate of good character and a marriage license – documentation not required by facilities for foundlings.[76]

Not only did the Nursery have higher standards of admission, it offered something that most infant shelters could not: wages. For their labors in the institution, the wet nurses received three forms of payment: six dollars

---

73 For a later account of women's clash with physicians, see Marion Hunt, "Women and Childsaving: The St. Louis Children's Hospital, 1879–1979," *Missouri Historical Society Bulletin* 36 (1980): 65–79.
74 Quiroga, *Poor Mothers and Babies*, pp. 60–1. Knowing of the demand for quality care and fearing that women might take advantage of them, the Nursery managers pointedly informed mothers using the day nursery that children not picked up at the end of the day would be sent to the almshouse. A later account from 1872 suggests this policy was modified when the facility began operating as a hospital rather than a day nursery. J. F. Richmond, *New York and Its Institutions, 1609–1872* (New York: E. B. Treat, 1872), p. 393.
75 Nursery for the Children of Poor Women, *Second Annual Report* (New York, 1856), pp. 4–5.
76 *New York Tribune*, 20 July 1878; and *Constitution, By-Laws, and Regulations of the Nursery for the Children of Poor Women* (New York, 1854).

per month, a good conduct letter from the matron that helped them later find private employment, and the prerogative of leaving their infants in the Nursery when they found work.[77] In attempting to convince women to nurse babies, the Nursery resembled an infant asylum. In its moral gatekeeping, it echoed the policies of other benevolent institutions. In its demand for medically certified candidates, the Nursery showed itself to be at the forefront of the medicalization of wet nursing. Nevertheless, the Nursery of the Children of Poor Women conceived of itself as a benevolent organization serving needy women and children, not as a medical facility.

To help sustain itself financially, the Nursery opened a wet nurse placement bureau that operated in the same fashion as a commercial intelligence office. Each day resident wet nurses looking for private positions as well as other interested wet nurses gathered for an open-house viewing. Employers called between 11 a.m. and 1 p.m., inspected potential candidates, and after selecting one, paid the Nursery five dollars. Dissatisfied customers could return within ten days to choose another wet nurse without charge.[78] In 1857, eighty-nine wet nurses found work through the Nursery; in 1858, the number peaked at ninety-four. Placements fell off in the ensuing years and waxed and waned thereafter as the institution's mission changed.

Although the Nursery welcomed the premiums provided by the placement service and undoubtedly benefited from the good will of wealthy employers who found healthy wet nurses with relative ease, the upper-class managers who directed the facility were quick to castigate the women who chose private duty wet nursing over institutional service. Like many of the domestic and medical writers, the managers saw the women's decision as stemming from a lack of maternal instinct, a selfish desire for wealth (or what the managers termed high wages), and an interest in a "luxurious life" in service. Their criticisms encapsulated perfectly the bourgeois construction of motherhood and showed remarkably little understanding of the realities of working-class life. As private employees, wet nurses who went out to work from the Nursery earned twelve dollars a month, paid five dollars for the care of their children, and netted an impressive seven dollars. This was top dollar in the New York City servant market, according to the editors of *Harper's Weekly* in 1857, and much more than most working women earned.[79] Institutional service, although

77 Nursery and Child's Hospital, *Fifth Annual Report* (New York, 1859), p. 3; and Quiroga, *Poor Mothers and Babies,* p. 69.
78 When the Nursery ran short of candidates, it advertised for more. See Nursery for the Children of Poor Women, *Third Annual Report* (New York, 1857), pp. 25–6.
79 *Harper's* reported in an 1857 article that newly arrived immigrant women demanded top wages of seven dollars a month. "The New York Labor Market: Female House Servants," *Harper's Weekly* 1 (1857): 418–19. Stansell's assessment of wages in New York City suggests that rates were far lower, an estimated one dollar per week between 1845 and 1860. Even for skilled workers in the shirtmaking trade, top dollar was only twelve dollars

Table 3.7. *Wet nurses placed
by the Nursery and Child's
Hospital, 1857–1871*

Year	Number
1857	89
1858	94
1859	NA
1860	43
1861	17
1862	21
1863	NA
1864	NA
1865	48
1866	22
1867	34
1868	NA
1869	47
1870	43
1871	60

Source: Annual Reports, Nursery and Child's Hospital.

still lucrative, netted women only six dollars a month and required them to live under the watchful eyes of the matron. From the perspective of the institution's leaders, the wages earned in private service seemed insufficient compensation for leaving an infant behind. The wet nurses, however, made a different calculation of the costs and benefits.

The Nursery for the Children of Poor Women might have survived for years outside the world of medicine, offering a combination day nursery and program for the offspring of wet nurses, had Du Bois not developed a grander vision. After three years of operation as a Nursery she rechristened it the "Nursery and Child's Hospital." Two years later, a neighborhood dispensary for children was added, and the institution subsequently expanded to include both a lying-in asylum and a home for the reception of illegitimate children. In less than two decades, Du Bois's residence for the children of wet nurses evolved into a medical facility with a broader constituency and grander aims. Although doctors had been on the staff

per month. Christine Stansell, *City of Women: Sex and Class in New York, 1789–1860* (New York: Knopf, 1986), p. 272 n. 9 and Table 2, p. 226.

from the beginning, as the role of the institution changed, they demanded a greater voice in creating its policies.

The employment of wet nurses became a touchstone in a vociferous public debate over the merits of outplacement versus institutional care. Ultimately, the critical issue became whether medical control or lay control was appropriate in child-welfare facilities. Embedded in these controversies were larger questions about class, gender, and professional status, but, in this instance, leading personalities – Mary Du Bois and pediatrician Abraham Jacobi – held center stage, and the drama concerned both mortality and mission. Jacobi, the premier pediatric specialist in New York City, took broad aim at the city's congregate care facilities. Armed with statistics from infant asylums throughout the world, he charged that institutional care inevitably caused excess deaths and that "the necessity of distributing abandoned infants among private families, especially in the country, [was] urgent."[80] Du Bois, defending her institution and pointing to the use of wet nurses, argued that her work could not be reduced to simple numbers. For her, the trust of the community and the aid offered to "penitent mother[s]" counted as much as the mortality rate.[81] Holding the upper hand, Du Bois ordered Jacobi dismissed from the medical board of the Nursery and Child's Hospital.

Du Bois bested Jacobi in the short run but later acquiesced to medical judgment, first by opening a country branch on Staten Island and later by permitting a partial separation of medical and social-welfare functions of the Nursery. In 1910, the Nursery and Child's Hospital merged with the New York Infant Asylum, which sent approximately one thousand dependent infants and children to private homes annually. Jacobi would later refer to the bad old days when "ladies with their long trails" visited the infant asylums each week, "always finding fault with the nurses and doctors."[82] In exchanging its goal of aiding wet nurses for a more expansive vision involving medical services for mothers and children, the Nursery and Child's Hospital withdrew from service to private families. New Yorkers seeking wet nurses had to turn to the lying-in homes and found-

80 Abraham Jacobi, "Foundlings and Foundling Institutions," in William J. Robinson, ed., *Collectanea Jacobi: Collected Essays, Addresses, Scientific Papers and Miscellaneous Writings of A. Jacobi*, vol. 4 (New York: Critic & Guide, 1909), p. 317. The disagreements between Du Bois and Jacobi are further analyzed in Quiroga, *Poor Mothers and Babies*, pp. 66–84.
81 In a description of her work for the National Conference of Charities and Corrections Du Bois couched much of what she did in terms of responding to the needs of women. Although the attack by Jacobi fifteen years earlier is not mentioned, it is clear that Du Bois recalls their battles and she points to the support of the state and the city. By the time Du Bois wrote this piece, she had surrendered somewhat and inaugurated a large country branch. Mary A. Du Bois, "Thirty Years' Experience in Hospital Work," Nursery and Child's Hospital, *Thirty-Second Annual Report* (New York, 1886), pp. 12–28.
82 A. Jacobi, "Remarks on 'The Proper Management of Foundlings and Neglected Infants,' " *Medical Record* 79 (1911): 324.

ling hospitals, which, by the twentieth century, had become the premier sites for hiring candidates.

One foundling hospital that actively engaged in wet nurse placement was the Massachusetts Infant Asylum, which opened in Boston in 1868 to serve foundlings and the offspring of parents too poor to care for their babies at home but willing to contribute to their upkeep. Healthy babies went to foster homes. The sick and frail ones remained institutionalized and cared for by wet nurses, who entered with their own infants.

Like the Nursery, the Infant Asylum was a prime source for private families seeking wet nurses. Of thirty-seven families with identifiable occupations who retained wet nurses from the Infant Asylum between 1867 and 1907, thirty were professionals and proprietors, and seven were lower-level white-collar workers. Unlike the Boston City Temporary Home, which several decades earlier had attracted a broader class of employers, the Infant Asylum appeared to be a hunting ground restricted to the wealthy.[83] Perhaps middle- and working-class families were reluctant to seek wet nurses from an institution known to be supported by elite Bostonians. Or perhaps they were turning to bottle-feeding as a cheaper and easier alternative that was becoming ever more reliable. The wet nurse marketplace, after all, responded not only to the creation of new sources of supply but also to the shifting levels of demand.

In mapping the rise and fall of various sectors of the wet nurse marketplace, it is critical to recognize the varied trajectories of each as they responded to customer demand and to burgeoning competition. Newspaper advertisements rose in number in the middle third of the nineteenth century and then experienced a rapid decline. The reasons most likely included the inconvenience of chasing down help only to find that the woman had already accepted a position and the growing competition from other sources, such as intelligence offices. Yet, the portion of intelligence office business devoted to the placement of wet nurses probably remained small, due in part to competition from public and private enterprises and in part because the bulk of intelligence office work involved placing other types of household servants. The trajectory for employment offices likely remained relatively low and flat. Maternity homes probably had a similar profile, with a small but steady place in the wet nursing business. Facilities run by respectable midwives may have received regular inquiries from families and physicians, whereas those with less savory reputations may have ultimately lost clients to institutions with greater prestige or larger

83 Family occupations were traced through city directories. Occupational rankings come from Stephen Thernstrom, *The Other Bostonians*, pp. 289–302. At least two families who hired wet nurses from the Boston Temporary Home later employed wet nurses from the Massachusetts Infant Asylum.

pools of potential workers: lying-in hospitals, infant asylums, and shelters for women.

The expanding sectors of the wet nurse marketplace were the public and private shelters for women and infants. Despite their different goals and leadership, they had one thing in common from the perspective of employers: all of them discharged wet nurses who had been under supervision, in some cases by a matron, in other instances, by physicians. Each, however, had its own trajectory. Public institutions appear to have been eclipsed by medical facilities, whereas private shelters, for the most part, dropped out of the market. The growing use of lying-in hospitals and infant asylums as sources for wet nurses represented several phenomena: convenience, a large number of candidates, and medical supervision.

The segmentation of the marketplace reveals little about the overall level of demand. Clearly, the growing popularity of artificial feeding (discussed in Chapter 5) eroded demand in the late nineteenth century. At the same time, the doctors, who increasingly mediated between wet nurses and employers, came to recognize that wet nursing cost more than money.

4

"Victims of distressing circumstances": The wet nurse labor force and the offspring of wet nurses, 1860–1910

No one described the moral economy of wet nursing more eloquently than the Irish-born, British writer George Moore. In his 1894 novel *Esther Waters,* the heroine confronts a selfish employer who has denied her permission to visit her sick child and rages:

What about them two that died? When you spoke first I thought you meant two of your own children, but the housemaid told me that they was the children of the two wet-nurses you had before me, them whose milk didn't suit your baby. It is our babies that die, it is life for a life; more than that, two lives for a life and now the life of my little boy is asked for.[1]

Moore's heroine, Esther Waters, articulated what physicians had long admitted – that wet nursing often involved trading the life of a poor baby for that of a rich one. Or, as one physician depicted it, "by the sacrifice of the infant of the poor woman, the offspring of the wealthy will be preserved."[2] Luther Emmett Holt, the preeminent pediatrician of the late nineteenth and early twentieth centuries, concurred. "Employment of wet-nurses tends, on the whole," he wrote, "to increase infant mortality rather than reduce it, owing to the excessively high mortality rate of the wet-nurses' infants."[3]

The medical literature makes clear that doctors wrestled with the moral dimensions of wet nursing and, in some cases, tried to mitigate its impact. Holt argued that a family "should be compelled by the physician to see that proper provisions were made for the wet nurse's child in order to give it the best possible chance with artificial feeding."[4] Effa V. Davis agreed,

1 George Moore, *Esther Waters* (London: W. Scott, 1984; Chicago: Academy Press, 1977), p. 142.
2 Charles West, *Lectures on the Diseases of Infancy and Childhood,* 5th Am. ed. from 6th English ed. (Philadelphia: Henry C. Lea, 1874), p. 452. See also Rebecca Crumpler, *A Book of Medical Discourses* (Boston: Cashman, Keating, 1883), p. 45.
3 L. Emmett Holt, "Infant Mortality and Its Reduction, Especially in New York City," *Journal of the American Medical Association* 54 (1910): 689.
4 L. Emmett Holt, *The Care and Feeding of Children: A Catechism for the Use of Mothers and Children's Nurses* (New York: D. Appleton, 1894), p. 159.

arguing that wet nursing "is not demoralizing if the nurse is given sufficient salary to pay for skilled care for her own baby."[5] Doctors knew full well that removing the wet nurse from her baby very often led to the infant's death. They walked a fine line between meeting the expressed need of clients to secure wet nurses and the implied need for poor women to breast-feed their own babies. Physician Samuel Busey objected strenuously to the idea that an institution might "engage in the immoral and criminal business of making wet-nurses, or hold out inducements for them to make themselves."[6] Yet, he certainly knew the practice occurred. The marketplace, after all, evolved to meet the needs of private employers, not those of wet nurses or their infants.

One legacy of the institutionalization of the wet nurse marketplace – the creation of case records – reveals the ramifications that wet nursing had for wet nurses and their offspring. Handwritten accounts from hospitals, municipal shelters, and benevolent homes make it possible to reconstruct the life histories of wet nurses and to answer three questions. First, who were the women who suckled infants in private homes? Second, how did they differ from wet nurses who were employed in public institutions or who worked within their own residences? And third, what were the consequences of wet nursing for the offspring of these women? Were the institutions truly engaged in activities that were "criminal and blame-worthy"?

The circumstances that sent women into the wet nursing business are not difficult to fathom; theirs was a career born of poverty. However, for many of the women working at home, it was also a career of circum-stance: their own infants had died, leaving them free to suckle other women's babies.

Women who wet nursed in their own homes remained a relatively invisible sector of the labor force, appearing only through their notices in the newspapers or on the registries of public and private agencies. In Philadelphia, the Society for the Relief and Employment of the Poor kept wet nurses on their list of people seeking work.[7] Similarly, Boston's City Temporary Home, which placed resident women in service as wet nurses, also maintained registers of wet nurses seeking work, with 122 names appearing between 1862 and 1864. Fifty-one of the women wanted a baby

---

5 Effa V. Davis, "Maternal Feeding," *Pediatrics* 17 (1905): 777.
6 Samuel C. Busey, "The Mortality of Young Children: Its Causes and Preventions," in Elizabeth Garrett-Anderson, et al., eds., *The Sanitary Care and Treatment of Children and Their Diseases* (Boston: Houghton, Mifflin, 1881), p. 133.
7 Society for the Relief and Employment of the Poor, List, 1852–4? Coates Family Papers, 1763–1915. HSP.

to suckle at home, fifty hoped to go out to service, twelve were willing to accept either form of work and nine expressed no preference.[8]

Typical of the married women seeking work at home was Elizabeth Loomis, whose husband visited the Temporary Home to request an infant following the death of their three-day-old child.[9] Another registrant, Jane Walters, had a husband at sea and four children to support. The three oldest were sent to live with their grandmother in New York, while Walters kept custody of her one-month-old infant and registered for work at the Temporary Home. According to the matron's notes, she had "plenty of milk."[10]

The matron screened registrants carefully, acting both as a moral arbitrator and in a quasi-medical capacity. She termed Margaret Kenny, the wife of a foundry worker, a "doubtful case" because Kenny lived on her own and was "intemperate."[11] Catherine Driscoll, the mother of a stillborn child, received good marks, arriving "highly recommended by her physician." Driscoll took in the baby of a former Temporary Home resident, Doris Burns, who left to became a wet nurse in the home of a physician. Ten months later, Driscoll returned to the Temporary Home and asked for another baby. The matron questioned her ability to suckle another child but ultimately placed the baby of another former Temporary Home resident in her care.[12]

As suggested earlier, the registrants comprised two distinct groups: women seeking babies to suckle in their own homes and those looking for jobs in service. Although the data are extremely limited, there is some indication that the registrants wanting a baby to suckle at home were more likely to have support from a male breadwinner and more likely to have lost their infants than the registrants wanting or willing to go out to service. Nine of thirteen seeking home employment and whose marital status was stated in the records were married. Of those seeking to work in service, only nine of twenty-four had husbands. The differences are even more stark in regard to the status of their infants. Of those for whom there is data, only three of the twenty-two women seeking work at home had living infants.

8 Calculated from the records of the Boston, Overseers of the Poor, City Temporary Home Records. Box 16, Folder 1. MHS. Note that the period covered was May 11–December 1862; January 6–July 1863; August 9–March 4, 1864.
9 Boston, Overseers of the Poor, City Temporary Home Records, May-December 1862, p. 82. Box 16, Folder 1. MHS.
10 Boston, Overseers of the Poor, City Temporary Home Records, August 1863–May 1864, p. 121. Box 16, Folder 1. MHS.
11 Boston, Overseers of the Poor, City Temporary Home Records, May-December 1862, p. 53. Box 16, Folder 1. MHS.
12 Ibid., p. 82; and August 1863–May 1864, p. 49. Box 16, Folder 1. MHS.

Table 4.1. *Marital status of Boston City Temporary Home registrants by occupational choice*

	Occupational choice		
Marital status	Live home	Live out	Either
Single	1	5	1
Married	9	9	3
Widowed	1	2	—
Deserted	1	7	—
Other	1	1	—
(Missing cases	38	26	8)

Source: Records of the Boston Overseers of the Poor, City Temporary Home, Box 16, Folder 1, MHS.

By contrast, of those desiring or willing to go out to service, eleven of sixteen were mothers of living infants. As a group, 64 percent of the registrants had lost their babies, and this appears to have been a primary motivation for seeking work.

The demographic characteristics of home-based wet nurses are obscure and their work days invisible. Although they were not the poorest of the poor, not the deserted wives or homeless single mothers often found in institutions, neither were they women who could afford to pass up the chance to earn some money by suckling babies. In this they resembled earlier generations of women who contributed to the family economy by taking in babies and whose acts, for the most part, went unrecorded. In the nineteenth century, however, their invisibility was a function of their structural position in the urban labor force – home workers – and of the clients they typically served – other working women.

The absence of the home-based wet nurses from the historical record also makes it impossible to determine whether women who were wet nursing at home held to the implied contract to breast-feed rather than bottle-feed the infants in their care. Some undoubtedly fulfilled their obligation, whereas others lost their milk or their willingness to suckle and began exposing their charges to a regimen of artificial feeding or a combination of breast milk and other foods. A similar continuum no doubt existed for the emotional bonds between the wet nurse and her infant boarder. Some women presumably were indifferent to the babies, viewing the arrangement strictly as an economic matter, taking the infants to the almshouse if payments ceased to arrive. Others may have become deeply attached to their young boarders. The presence of the woman's own child

Table 4.2. *Infant status of Boston City Temporary Home registrants by occupational choice*

	Request		
Infant status	Live home	Live out	Either
Living	3	11	1
Dead	19	5	3
(Missing cases	29	34	8)

Source: Records of the Boston Overseers of the Poor, City Temporary Home, Box 16, Folder 1, MHS.

may have been the critical variable, not only in terms of the emotional bonding between the wet nurse and her suckling but also in terms of nourishment. A woman's own baby clearly had a stronger claim on her milk and, equally important, her attention.

One factor helping to obscure the work of home-based wet nurses was the notoriety of baby farmers, who cared for but did not suckle large groups of infants. The evidence suggests that some baby farmers earned their ignominy through wholesale neglect or conscious infanticide, whereas others sincerely attempted to aid fellow working women.[13] Nevertheless, newspaper exposés and investigations by local authorities and by private organizations such as the Society for the Prevention of Cruelty to Children vilified baby farmers as a group and spawned efforts at regulation. In 1876, for example, the Massachusetts legislature enacted a law requiring the registration and inspection of maternity hospitals and baby farms. Boston health officials began making annual inspections and licensing local facilities, causing many operators to conceal their ventures.[14] In 1882, the law was extended to include the registration not only of all boarding homes but also of illegitimate children sent out to board.[15] The effects of such regulations may have been to tar honorable wet nurses and less than honorable baby farmers with the same brush. Furthermore, although regulation may

13 Sheri Broder, "Child Care or Child Neglect? Baby Farming in Late-Nineteenth-Century Philadelphia," *Gender and Society* 2 (1988): 128–48; Linda Gordon, *Heroes of Their Own Lives: The Politics and History of Family Violence, Boston, 1880–1960* (New York: Viking, 1988), pp. 27–58; Richard A. Meckel, *"Save the Babies": American Public Health Reform and the Prevention of Infant Mortality, 1850–1929* (Baltimore: Johns Hopkins University Press, 1990), pp. 50–1.
14 Boston Board of Health, *Twenty-seventh Annual Report* (Boston, 1879), p. 20.
15 Acts of 1882, Chapter 270, *Revised Manual of Laws of Massachusetts Concerning Children* (Boston: Massachusetts Society for the Prevention of Cruelty to Children, 1882), p. 24, cited in Gordon, *Heroes of Their Own Lives*, n. 99, p. 324.

have encouraged some women, such as those registering at the Temporary Home, to take a public, regulated route to obtaining a baby, it may have caused others to go underground, making home-based wet nursing a less visible enterprise over the course of the nineteenth century but not necessarily a less extensive one.

Ironically, both abandoned babies and the offspring of the well-to-do shared the same pool of wet nurses, comprised largely of poor, young, institutionalized, foreign-born single mothers. Shut out of home-based wet nursing by their lack of a domicile and their need to care for their own infants, these women entered institutional service hoping it would be a bridge to private employment. In some instances, they found their paths blocked, and they remained trapped in the unremunerative life of an asylum wet nurse. The more fortunate escaped to private service, leaving their infants behind.

The records of numerous foundling homes and lying-in hospitals reveal the backgrounds of both privately employed and institutional wet nurses, demonstrating their similarities. The data include case records of 959 women who worked as wet nurses at the Massachusetts Infant Asylum between 1868 and 1907. For privately employed wet nurses, the records are fewer in number but come from more institutions. Two hundred and sixteen women were discharged to private service from the Boston Lying-In Hospital, the New England Hospital for Women and Children, and the Massachusetts Infant Asylum between 1868 and 1907.[16] In addition, private-duty wet nurses entered service by way of the New York Nursery and Child's Hospital, the Philadelphia Home for Infants, and Boston's City Temporary Home.

The records of the institutions reveal structural similarities in the lives of the wet nurses, but the aggregate data should not be allowed to obscure the individual calamities that led wet nurses to their positions. Just as home-based wet nurses seem to have been women with careers built on the tragic loss of their infants, institutional wet nurses and wet nurses working in private homes appear to have been women whose misfortunes were the result of their pregnancies and their poverty.

The most easily explained characteristic of wet nurses was their age, a reflection of the life course of working women, of patterns of fertility, and of the demands of employers. The vast majority were under thirty years of age. Thirty percent of the wet nurses employed by the Massachusetts

16 The figures are calculated from the maternity records of the New England Hospital for Women and Children and the Boston Lying-In Hospital, FACLM, and the records of the Massachusetts Infant Asylum, HLUMB. In many cases, wet nurses were sent from one of the maternity hospitals to the Massachusetts Infant Asylum before taking a position with a private family. (Records of these women have been matched by hand according to the woman's name and the name and birth date of her child.)

Table 4.3. *Age of wet nurses in the Massachusetts Infant Asylum*

Age	Number	Percentage
Under 21	221	30
21–29	446	61
Over 29	68	9
Total	735	100
(Missing cases	234)	

Source: Records of the Massachusetts Infant
Asylum, HLUMB.

Infant Asylum were under twenty-one. Louisa Green, a native of Canada, entered the facility when she was eighteen. The father of her child, a nineteen-year-old German immigrant, worked as a cigar maker.[17] Another youthful resident was Katie McCall, a sixteen-year-old factory worker married to a nineteen-year-old toll collector on the trolley car. Apparently, her husband's earnings were insufficient to support the family, and thus McCall took up wet nursing. She quickly proved too weak to perform the suckling required of her and left after seventeen days, sending her baby to live with an aunt and returning to work.[18]

Private employers retained somewhat fewer of the younger women, perhaps feeling that a child would be cared for best by a woman of greater maturity. Nevertheless, one-quarter of the wet nurses in service had not reached age twenty-one. At age fifteen, for example, Victoria Colson left the New England Hospital for Women and Children to wet nurse in the family of Boston lawyer and public official, David H. Coolidge.[19] Several years later, the Coolidge family hired Ellen Rodale from the Massachusetts Infant Asylum. Rodale, a native of Ireland, was older than Colson (twenty-two), more typical of the wet nurse population as a whole, and more in keeping with the recommendations of physicians.[20]

A second characteristic of wet nurses, their poverty, reflected the low-wage positions held by the wet nurse's partners and, more profoundly, the number of women who lacked the support of a male breadwinner. Like Green's lover who worked as a cigar maker and McCall's toll collector

17 Case Records, Massachusetts Infant Asylum, 1876, p. 837. HLUMB.
18 Case Records, Massachusetts Infant Asylum, 1880, p. 237. HLUMB.
19 New England Hospital for Women and Children, Maternity Cases, December 8, 1889. FACLM.
20 See, for example, Robert B. Dixon, *What Is To Be Done: A Handbook for the Nursery* . . . (Boston: Lea & Shepard, 1884), p. 63.

Table 4.4. *Age of private-duty wet nurses
discharged from the Massachusetts Infant
Asylum, the Boston Lying-In Hospital, and
the New England Hospital for Women and
Children*

Age	Number	Percentage
Under 21	39	26
21–29	96	63
Over 29	17	11
Total	152	100
(Missing cases	64)	

Source: Records of the Massachusetts Infant
Asylum, HLUMB; records of the New England
Hospital for Women and Children and the
Boston Lying-In Hospital, FACLM.

husband, most of the fathers of the wet nurses' infants labored in low-paying positions. Records of the fathers from the Massachusetts Infant Asylum indicate that 36 percent were skilled workers, another 25 percent were semiskilled and service workers, and 18 percent worked in jobs considered to be lower white-collar occupations. Others were unemployed or, in a few cases, incarcerated. The upper-class "wolf in gentleman's garb" who spoiled innocent young girls was a mythic figure in the minds of many moral reformers but was not responsible for the fate of the women in the infant asylum.[21] The overwhelming majority of wet nurses were pregnant by working men and were victims of shared passions and shared economic insecurity. Most critically, relatively few of the fathers were married to or living with the women who bore their children.

Women pregnant out of wedlock slid down a slippery slope. Their pregnancy and poverty often caused them to be abandoned by their lovers; furthermore, their pregnancy led them to lose work, and soon they found themselves at the almshouse gate or at the door of a private charity, asking for aid. Seventy-nine percent of the institutional wet nurses were single, widowed, or deserted. Maggie McLean, a native of Ireland who had pre-viously worked as a factory girl and a domestic, gave birth in the Tewks-

21 For a discussion of this metaphor and its uses, see Barbara Meil Hobson, *Uneasy Virtue: The Politics of Prostitution and the American Reform Tradition* (New York: Basic Books, 1987), pp. 49–76.

Table 4.5. *Occupation of fathers of wet nurses' babies, Massachusetts Infant Asylum, 1868–1907*

Occupation[a]	Number	Percentage
Skilled workers	285	36
Semiskilled & service workers	203	25
Low White Collar	145	18
Unskilled & menial service workers	101	13
Farmers	51	6
High White Collar	16	2
Total	801	100
(Missing cases	168)	

[a]Occupational categories from Stephen Thernstrom, *The Other Bostonians: Poverty and Progress in the American Metropolis, 1880–1970* (Cambridge: Harvard University Press, 1973), Appendix B, "On the Socioeconomic Rankings of Occupation," pp. 289–302.
Source: Records of the Massachusetts Infant Asylum, HLUMB.

bury Almshouse. The father of her child was a carpenter.[22] Another graduate of the Almshouse, twenty-three-year old Marjorie Grimes, became pregnant by an unskilled factory worker, Charles Grimes, whose name she took and whose name she gave to her son, Wallace Theodore Grimes. The boy lived almost a year before succumbing to croup.[23] Without question, single motherhood – the result of death, desertion, or abandonment by a lover – was a powerful impetus to becoming a wet nurse.

The marital status of wet nurses varied among the institutional settings and in the context of local and historical circumstances. Two-thirds of the 101 wet nurses who lived at the Boston City Temporary Home prior to finding private positions were without a spouse because their husbands had deserted them or died or because they had never married. In addition, many of the women who described themselves as married were without the support of a breadwinner because of the wartime emergency. The Civil War took many men to the front and led others to flee military service. The husband of twenty-one-year-old Mary O'Connor, for example, went to Ireland to avoid the draft.[24] When the situations of the women who entered the Temporary Home are examined not for their marital status but

22 Case records, Massachusetts Infant Asylum, vol. 1880, p. 437. HLUMB.
23 Case records, Massachusetts Infant Asylum, 1880, p. 210. HLUMB.
24 Boston, Overseers of the Poor, City Temporary Home Records, May–December 1862, p. 165. Box 16, Folder 1. MHS.

Table 4.6. *Marital status of wet nurses at the Massachusetts Infant Asylum, 1868–1907*

Status	Number	Percentage
Single	598	63
Married	195	21
Deserted	112	1
Widowed	38	4
Total	943	
(Missing	26)	

Source: Records of the Massachusetts Infant Asylum, HLUMB.

Table 4.7. *Marital status of women discharged as wet nurses from the Boston City Temporary Home, 1862–1864*

Marital status	Number	Percentage
Married	3	4
(husband away at war	7	10)
(husband away	13	19)
Single	22	31.5
Deserted	15	21.5
Widowed	10	14
Total	70	100
(Missing cases	31)	

Source: Records of the Boston Overseers of the Poor, City Temporary Home, Box 16, Folder 1, MHS.

concerning whether or not they had the support of a husband, the reason for their career choice becomes obvious. A startlingly high total of 96 percent lacked support from a spouse. Furthermore, in at least thirteen instances, the women entering the Temporary Home had one or more children to support in addition to their infants.[25]

Similarly, two-thirds of the women who were discharged from Boston's private institutions were also single, widowed, or deserted. Many of those

25 The records indicate that at least thirteen of the residents had other children and that eighteen did not. For the majority of cases this information was unavailable. Boston, Overseers of the Poor, City Temporary Home Records. Box 16, Folder 1. MHS.

Table 4.8. *Marital status of wet nurses from Boston's Private Institutions, 1868–1907*

Marital status	Number	Percentage
Single	108	51
Married	71	34
Deserted	22	10
Widowed	11	5
Total	212	100
(Missing cases	4)	

Source: Records of the Massachusetts Infant Asylum, HLUMB; records of the New England Hospital and the Boston Lying-In Hospital, FACLM.

with husbands found the insecurities of working-class life – periodic unemployment, low wages, seasonal layoffs, and days lost from work due to illness – forcing them into service. In 1885, Eva Flanigan's husband left his job because of illness. Flanigan worked until the time of her confinement and then found a position as a wet nurse. Her earnings paid the rent for her husband's room, the board for her two-year-old, and the costs of placing her baby at the Massachusetts Infant Asylum.[26]

The Civil War encouraged female employment in the 1860s, but the need for married women to work persisted long after the battlefields fell silent. As Flanigan's case illustrated, the presence of a husband could not alone guarantee financial security. Of the twenty-eight women who placed their babies at the Philadelphia Home for Infants from 1873 through 1899 while they worked as private duty wet nurses, thirteen were single, two had been widowed, and the remaining thirteen (nearly half) were married. Their marriages brought them little economic security. Two of the husbands lived in Ireland, where one was a laborer and the other a cabinet-maker; the four others whose occupations were identified had jobs marked by economic uncertainty and periodic unemployment: one was a farmer, another a sailor, a third a waiter, and a fourth a boilermaker.[27]

Desertion also served as a catalyst for a woman's becoming a wet nurse. Esther Tower's husband reportedly shipped out on the steamer *Arcadia*, bound for Rio.[28] Vinnie Dennis's husband, a hotel waiter, left her with

26 Massachusetts Infant Asylum records, June 17, 1885. HLUMB.
27 Calculated from the register of the Philadelphia Home for Infants. HSP.
28 Massachusetts Infant Asylum records, May 7, 1880, p. 877. HLUMB.

Table 4.9. *Birthplace of wet nurses enter-*
ing the Nursery and Child's Hospital,
1859–1860

Birthplace	Number	Percentage
Ireland	87	73
United States	18	15
English	8	7
German States	4	4
Scotland	2	1
Total	119	100

Source: Register #2, Nursery and Child's Hospital, NYHCMC.

four children and an infant to support. She left her baby at the Massachusetts Infant Asylum and her four older children with another family, and
she went to work as a wet nurse for the family of a boot-and-shoe merchant, Alfred S. Foster. Her case was unique; Dennis was an African-
American woman employed in a white household. The Infant Asylum kept
close tabs on Dennis's case, with the records noting that Mrs. Foster had
spoken highly of her and that she was "trying to do all she can for herself
and her four children."[29]

A third characteristic of the wet nursing population was that most were
either foreign born or the daughters of immigrants. The majority came
from Ireland, the Canadian maritime provinces, Britain, Scandinavia, and
Germany. The Irish were heavily overrepresented. Seventy-three percent
of the wet nurses discharged from the Nursery and Child's Hospital in
New York City between February 1859 and May 1860 were of Irish birth;
67 percent gave their religion as Catholic.[30]

A similar pattern prevailed at the Boston City Temporary Home, where
the overwhelming majority of residents, 71 percent, had come from Ireland. The high proportion mirrored the disproportionate representation of
Irish women working in domestic service and the similarly disproportionate number of Irish-born inmates in state- and city-run facilities for the
poor.[31] Although newspapers carried advertisements from wet nurses of

29 Massachusetts Infant Asylum records, March 30, 1890. HLUMB.
30 Twenty-eight percent were Protestant. In five percent of the cases, no religious affiliation
   was listed. Calculated from Register #2 of the Nursery and Child's Hospital. NYHCMC.
31 According to Handlin, Irish paupers filled the state institutions in Massachusetts between
   1845 and 1854 and thereafter predominated in municipal facilities serving the criminal and
   destitute. Oscar Handlin, *Boston's Immigrants: A Study in Acculturation*, rev. ed. enlgd.
   (New York: Atheneum, 1970), p. 118.

Table 4.10. *Birthplace of wet nurses discharged from the Boston City Temporary Home, 1862–1864*

Birthplace	Number	Percentage
Ireland	42	71
Canada	9	15
Britain	4	7
United States	3	5
German States	1	2
Total	59	100
(Missing cases	42)	

Source: Records of the Boston Overseers of the Poor, City Temporary Home, Box 16, Folder 1, MHS.

Table 4.11. *Birthplace of private-duty wet nurses in Boston, 1868–1907*

Birthplace	Number	Percentage
Ireland	60	29
Canada	57	28
United States	50	24
Great Britain	19	9
German States	10	5
Scandinavia	8	4
Other	2	1
Total	206	100
(Missing cases	10)	

Source: Records of the Massachusetts Infant Asylum, HLUMB; records of the New England Hospital for Women and Children and the Boston Lying-In Hospital, FACLM.

"good American stock," the marketplace was unquestionably saturated with Erin's daughters. In later decades, the number of Irish-born wet nurses declined, although many of the native-born women were probably of Irish descent.[32]

32 On the foreign-born population in domestic service, see Daniel E. Sutherland, *Americans and Their Servants: Domestic Service in the United States from 1800 to 1920* (Baton Rouge: Louisiana State University Press, 1981), p. 58.

Table 4.12. *Birthplace of wet nurses in the*
Massachusetts Infant Asylum, 1868–1907

Birthplace	Number	Percentage
United States	334	36
Canadian Maritimes	226	24.5
Ireland	208	22.5
Great Britain	66	7
Scandinavia	52	6
German States	21	2
Other	19	2
Total	926	100
(Missing cases	43)	

Source: Records of the Massachusetts Infant
Asylum, HLUMB.

Surprisingly, a comparison of the ethnic backgrounds of wet nurses who
were privately employed and those who worked in institutions reveals that
the latter were more likely to be native born. Only 24 percent of the
private-duty wet nurses discharged from the New England Hospital for
Women and Children, the Boston Lying-In Hospital, and the Massachusetts Infant Asylum were native born. The most common birthplace of
women working in the Infant Asylum was the United States; 36 percent
were native born. Perhaps employers preferred to stock their houses with
"biddies" (the stereotypical name for Irish-born domestics), or, alternatively, native born women may have shunned service.
    A fourth characteristic of wet nurses was their widespread experience in
domestic labor. The majority of all wage-earning women worked in service; household workers comprised 65.6 percent of nonagricultural employees in 1870 and in 1890 were 44.7 percent of the total.[33] The declining
percentage demonstrates that, as new opportunities became available in the
late nineteenth century, the women who could left domestic work – rejecting the long hours, isolation, and harsh discipline. Wet nurses were not
among the escapees, perhaps marked by their immigrant backgrounds. A
total of 73 percent had worked in service, whereas only 20 percent were
previously employed in hand manufacturing, retail, and factory jobs. In
effect, wet nurses who went out to work from infant asylums and lying-in
hospitals were returning to a familiar life.

33 David M. Katzman, *Seven Days a Week: Women and Domestic Service in Industrializing*
   America (New York: Oxford University Press, 1978), Table 2–2, p. 53.

Table 4.13. *Previous occupation of wet nurses from Boston's Private Institutions, 1868–1907*

Occupation	Number	Percentage
Domestic service	48	73
Hand manufacturing	8	12
Retail trades	3	5
Factory work	2	3
Not working	5	7
Total	66	100
(Missing cases	150)	

Source: Records of the Massachusetts Infant Asylum, HLUMB; records of the New England Hospital for Women and Children and the Boston Lying-In Hospital, FACLM.

Table 4.14. *Previous occupations of wet nurses employed at the Massachusetts Infant Asylum*

Occupation	Number	Percentage
Domestics	604	76
Factory work	63	8
Retail trades	45	6
Not working	38	5
Hand manufacturing	34	4
Student	5	1
Total	789	100
(Missing cases	180)	

Source: Records of the Massachusetts Infant Asylum, HLUMB.

Although the data for privately employed women are relatively sparse, amounting to only 66 cases, the findings are supported by the much larger numbers from the Massachusetts Infant Asylum. The directors of the Asylum argued that institutional employment helped qualify the women for places at service, and they prided themselves on transforming idle, dependent single mothers into workers. Only 5 percent of the women, however, had never been previously employed, whereas 76 percent had done domestic work.

Not only did wet nursing attract women who had previously engaged in domestic service work, it appears to have repelled women who avoided domestic careers. Italians and Jews comprised the largest groups of late nineteenth- and early twentieth-century immigrants, but few of them were in institutions providing wet nurses.[34] Their low rates of domestic employment and illegitimacy militated against the employment of Italian women as private-duty wet nurses and encouraged their work suckling foster babies in their homes.[35] Jewish women also avoided domestic service of all types, probably reflecting a reluctance to live in the homes of gentile employers.[36]

African-American women were an exception within the changing patterns of female employment; a larger percentage of married African-American women were engaged in the paid labor force than was the case for any other group, and the proportion in service occupations was growing.[37] Work as cooks, laundresses, or general servants did not, however, translate into work as wet nurses. With the exception of Vinnie Dennis and a small number of others, few African-American women entered the institutional stream supplying wet nurses to private employers. Their absence from institutional case records reflects the restricted admissions policies of the various facilities and raises the compelling questions of how employer demands influenced the characteristics of the wet nurse labor force and how the supply of wet nurses molded the expectations and opinions of employers.

The demographic profile of wet nurses suggests that employers did not find what they and the experts like Jerome Walker's Dr. Lyons considered to be ideal candidates – respectable married women. The conditions of working-class life, the limited options for women pregnant out of wedlock, and the institutionalization of foundlings shaped the wet nurse labor force far more than did employer preferences. Families may have wanted a

34 Irish and Scandinavian women predominated in domestic service. Katzman, *Seven Days a Week*, p. 67. On the numbers of immigrants and their sources, see Leonard Dinnerstein and David M. Reimers, *Ethnic Americans: A History of Immigration*, 3d ed. (New York: Harper & Row, 1988), pp. 43–62.
35 Virginia Yans-McLaughlin, *Family and Community: Italian Immigrants in Buffalo, 1880–1930* (Ithaca: Cornell University Press, 1977), pp. 53, 90–1, 170, 200–207; Sutherland, *Americans and Their Servants*, p. 53. Another consideration was that both Italian and Jewish women tended to breast-feed more frequently and for longer periods than women from other groups. This tradition may have made them reluctant to forgo nursing their own infants in order to become wet nurses. See Samuel H. Preston and Michael R. Haines, *Fatal Years: Child Mortality in Late Nineteenth-Century America* (Princeton: Princeton University Press, 1991), pp. 28–9.
36 Katzman, *Seven Days a Week*, p. 69; and Sutherland, *Americans and Their Servants*, p. 59.
37 Katzman, *Seven Days a Week*, Table 2–11, p. 73; and Alice Kessler-Harris, *Out to Work: A History of Wage-Earning Women in the United States* (New York: Oxford University Press, 1982), p. 123.

certain kind of wet nurse, but those with knowledge of the labor force understood that they were unlikely to find her. The demand for "just the right kind of woman" had long been part of the popular discussion of wet nurses, with religious, domestic, and medical writers in turn outlining the desired characteristics. Yet, according to all available sources, the ideal woman never appeared.

Of course, infant asylums did not search for the exemplary wet nurse. The women who embarked upon careers as institutional wet nurses did so because they had no other options; they lacked access to private employment or to any other means of supporting themselves and their infants. The jobs they took were created as the result of a transition in urban welfare policy, with the care of foundlings shifting from outplacement in private homes to congregate care in facilities established by religious leaders, lay reformers, and civic authorities. Thus, the rise of the institutional wet nurse marked the decline of her predecessor, the woman who suckled city-supported foundlings in her home. Moreover, as the demographic profile just noted makes clear, this transition brought a new group of women into the work force: poor single mothers who lacked homes of their own.

Americans had long confronted the problem of caring for foundlings, but the problem became even more visible and acute in the growing cities of the nineteenth century. Babies appeared on the steps of police stations, in church doorways, and at the gates of almshouses; they were tossed out of carriages and shoved into alleyways, and their corpses filled public burial grounds.[38] Some of those who survived were sent to live – and die – in the homes of baby farmers. Equally deadly were efforts to rear the infants in public almshouses by coercing inmates to act as caretakers. An 1857 report on the almshouse population in Massachusetts found a death rate of 80 percent for infants, and statistics from other areas proved equally grim. Child-welfare advocate Charles Loring Brace referred to the "treatment of these poor helpless infants by brutal women in our public institutions" as "one of the saddest chapters in the history of human wickedness."[39] Similarly, Dr. J. Lewis Smith, physician to the foundlings of New York City, complained about the wretched conditions at the Blackwell's Island Almshouse, recalling that the superintendent had informed him "it would be an

---

38 Paul A. Gilje, "Infant Abandonment in Early Nineteenth-Century New York City: Three Cases," *Signs: Journal of Women in Culture and Society* 8 (1983): 580–90. Other descriptions of abandoned infants can be found in the records of the Sheltering Arms, described in Chapter 3.

39 Charles Loring Brace, *The Dangerous Classes of New York, and Twenty Years' Work Among Them*, 3d ed. (New York: Wynkoop & Hallenbeck, 1880), pp. 408, 410.

act of humanity if each foundling were given a fatal dose of opium on its arrival."[40] Local authorities were not, however, prepared to sanction infanticide. Instead, they looked to improve the care of foundlings by placing them in special facilities and, whenever possible, providing them with human milk.[41]

Americans came late to the foundling asylum enterprise, which had begun in the Middle Ages to halt the sin of infanticide and save infant souls. Church authorities in the cities opened architecturally distinct houses of reception marked by doors with turning cradles into which a baby could be deposited anonymously and then rotated into the home.[42] Once inside, the infants often failed to survive. The institutions, however, prospered; by the late eighteenth century many cities, particularly in Catholic countries, had foundling hospitals and systems for placing infants in foster homes.[43] A second stage of foundling care developed in the nineteenth century when the state became involved and when the goal shifted from saving souls to saving lives.

Church and state systems of foundling care competed with private families in the effort to hire rural wet nurses. In France, urban working-class families depended upon the economic contributions of women, and thus even the offspring of this group was sent to the countryside to be wet nursed.[44] Of the 54,937 babies born in Paris in 1869, for example, 22,529 (41 percent) were wet nursed commercially. This figure includes foundlings, babies sent to the country by the municipal wet nurse bureau, and babies who had private arrangements made on their behalf.[45] The Russians, consciously emulating the French plan, created an even more extensive system of rural placement of foundlings and faced the same problem of competition from private employers. In the second half of the nineteenth century the annual tally of children sent to the countryside from the Moscow Foundling Home reached seventeen thousand, while in St. Petersburg it totaled approximately nine thousand. Historian David Ransel labeled this urban-to-rural "foundling traffic" a "school for capitalism among the

40 J. Lewis Smith, "Hindrances to the Successful Treatment of the Diseases of Infancy and Childhood," *Transactions of the New York State Medical Association* 13 (1896): 95.
41 Brace thought it would be impossible for asylums to board and employ enough wet nurses; he favored a "placing-out" system. Brace, *Dangerous Classes*, p. 410.
42 John Boswell, *The Kindness of Strangers: The Abandonment of Children in Western Europe from Late Antiquity to the Renaissance* (New York: Pantheon, 1988).
43 Valerie Fildes, *Wet Nursing: A History from Antiquity to the Present* (Oxford: Basil Blackwell, 1988), p. 144. For Spain see Joan Sherwood, *Poverty in Eighteenth-Century Spain: The Women and Children of the Inclusa* (Toronto: University of Toronto Press, 1988).
44 Louise A. Tilly and Joan W. Scott, *Women, Work and Family* (New York: Holt, Rinehart & Winston, 1978), pp. 132–4.
45 Rachel Ginnis Fuchs, *Abandoned Children: Foundlings and Child Welfare in Nineteenth-Century France* (Albany: State University of New York Press, 1984), pp. 185–6; and George D. Sussman, *Selling Mothers' Milk: The Wet-Nursing Business in France, 1715–1914* (Urbana: University of Illinois Press, 1982), pp. 101–29.

peasants." Rural wet nurses soon looked for better-paying positions caring for the infants of the well-to-do. By the end of the century, Moscow and St. Petersburg each had five private wet nursing agencies employing five thousand and ten thousand women, respectively.[46] The problem of competition occurred elsewhere on a smaller scale. A report in the early twentieth century noted that approximately three thousand women gave birth in the state lying-in hospital in Prague, Bohemia (Austria-Hungary), each year and then served as wet nurses in the foundling asylum. Private employers lured many women away, leaving the remaining wet nurses with the task of suckling two or even three infants until they were old enough to go to foster families to be fed from a bottle.[47] One effect of extensive, state-controlled systems of foundling care was to highlight their poor results. In France, the limits of wet nursing spawned increased regulation. By 1874 commercial wet nursing no longer fell under municipal control but was governed nationally by the Rousel Law passed to protect "infants and especially nurslings."[48]

The British briefly and early experimented with national support for foundling care. In 1756 parliament agreed to pay the recently established (1741) London Foundling Hospital to accept all infants brought to its doors. The result was a rise in infant mortality, complaints that the hospital facilitated profligacy, and a drain on the public treasury. In 1760, public funding ceased.[49] Thereafter, care of foundlings was a local responsibility. Articulating what might be termed the Protestant case against state care of foundlings, the Reverend Thomas Malthus charged that foundling asylums "subverted the state by discouraging marriage and encouraging licentiousness."[50] Not surprisingly, similar moral and political objections to state welfare schemes took root in the colonies.

Like the British, Americans eschewed national schemes for infant welfare as they did other forms of social assistance and instead confronted the problem at the local level. At times authorities looked to outplacement plans. In the second half of the nineteenth century, when outplacement became too costly and was too visibly a failure, local leaders turned to asylum care. Following in the wake of efforts to institutionalize the sick, the poor, and the deviant, the infant asylum was a step toward controlling both infant mortality and infant abandonment. The infant asylums offered

46 David L. Ransel, *Mothers of Misery: Child Abandonment in Russia* (Princeton: Princeton University Press, 1988), p. 3.

47 Louis Fischer, *Infant-Feeding: In Its Relation to Health and Disease*, 2d ed. (Philadelphia: F. A. Davis, 1901), p. 82.

48 Sussman, *Selling Mothers' Milk*, pp. 101–35; and Fuchs, *Abandoned Children*, pp. 28–61.

49 Ruth K. McClure, *Coram's Children: The London Foundling Hospital in the Eighteenth Century* (New Haven: Yale University Press, 1981), pp. 108–14.

50 Thomas Robert Malthus, *An Essay on the Principle of Population*, 6th ed. (London: J. Murray, 1826), p. 312.

work to single mothers – suckling foundlings while they cared for their own babies – in the hopes that they would not leave their own babies abandoned on a doorstep.

In conflating the goals of saving infants and saving mothers Americans created a pattern of foundling care that rested on a false assumption. Just as almshouse officials had placed foundlings in the arms of residents and learned that the women had little interest in tending to the babies, their bureaucratic successors were also forced to recognize that care could not be coerced. Despite good intentions, in the words of the reformer Amos Warner, it "can matter but little to the individual infant whether it is murdered outright or is placed in a foundling hospital."[51] Mortality within the largest European foundling homes ranged from 40 to 90 percent, and Americans soon learned they could not do much better.[52]

The lessons of the infant asylum had implications for private families as well as for public officials, supplying evidence supporting many long-held suspicions. First, women employed in the asylums did not always have enough milk for two infants. Some of the women were too malnourished, were too weak from giving birth, or were, for other reasons, unable to perform their dual obligation satisfactorily. This finding supported the practice among private employers and their physicians of making the wet nurse send her own baby away. Second, the women working in infant asylums tended to view their jobs as a means of finding private positions. As in Europe, the women who could escape the institution for higher-paying private service did so. Those who remained behind apparently favored their own babies with attention and milk, and the motherless infants suffered from neglect, from artificial feeding, and from the fatal infections that spread quickly from crib to crib.[53] The death rates in institutions, increasingly measured and reported, supported the growing belief that wet nursing was not necessarily better than carefully managed artificial feeding. The histories of three infant asylums in New York City and two in Boston illustrate the problems of congregate care while also demonstrating how institutions employed wet nurses and the consequences of their employment.

The Randall's Island Infant Hospital, constructed in the late 1860s as an

51 Amos G. Warner, *American Charities*, rev. ed. by Mary Roberts Coolidge (New York: Crowell, 1908), p. 266.
52 For European institutions, see Routh, "On the Mortality of Infants in Foundling Institutions and Generally as Influenced by the Absence of Breast Milk," *Lancet* 2 (1857): 420. For American institutions, Edward Jarvis, "Infant Mortality," *Fourth Annual Report of the Massachusetts State Board of Health* (Boston, 1874), p. 30; and W. L. Richardson, "Infant Mortality," Board of Health, Boston [Appendix,] *Fourth Annual Report* (Boston, 1876), p. 63.
53 When infant hospitals developed in the late nineteenth century they faced many of the same problems. See L. Emmett Holt, "The Scope and Limitations of Hospitals for Infants," *Transactions of the American Pediatric Society* 10 (1898): 147–60.

alternative housing site for foundlings previously sent to the New York City Alms-House, cared for a large proportion of the approximately three thousand infants abandoned in the city each year.[54] The Infant Hospital also sheltered destitute women with babies under two years of age.[55] A comparison of the mortality rates of abandoned babies with those of babies who entered with their mothers demonstrates the importance of maternal care and the value of human milk. Foundlings were three times more likely to die. In 1870, for example, mortality for abandoned babies was 59 percent, whereas for infants accompanied by their mothers, it was 15 percent. A decade later, the figures grew even further apart, 67 percent of the motherless infants died, and only 13 percent of the others perished.[56]

Access to maternal care and to mother's milk explains the variations, with each variable playing a role. Thirty percent of institutionalized babies bottle-fed by their mothers died before their first birthday, whereas 90 percent of the bottle-fed foundlings failed to survive. Access to human milk was a second critical variable. Only 12 percent of the babies wet nursed by their mothers died, whereas 72.5 percent of those wet nursed by women other than their mothers perished.[57] The figures suggest that although artificial feeding was risky, other factors played a role in the loss of infant life, such as the frequency of feedings and less tangible elements subsumed under the heading of care. After the disheartening results at Randall's Island, the Medical Board recommended a "farming-out system" employing wet nurses.[58] Despite the recommendation and subsequent efforts to place out babies, infants continued to live – and to die – in the Randall's Island facility until the end of the century.[59]

Private foundling homes presumably possessed what the public authorities did not: small, well-run facilities, with a dedicated staff and supportive directors and the ability to bargain with prospective wet nurses. Despite

54 The state of New York subsidized the institutional care of infants by private charities, including the New York Infant Asylum and the Foundling Asylum of the Sisters of Charity described in this chapter and the Nursery and Child's Hospital discussed in Chapter 3. For background on the care of dependent infants in New York, see Peter C. English, "Pediatrics and the Unwanted Child in History: Foundling Homes, Disease, and the Origins of Foster Care in New York City, 1860–1920," *Pediatrics* 73 (1984): 699–711; and Peter Romanofsky, "Saving the Lives of the City's Foundlings: The Joint Committee and New York City Child Care Methods, 1860–1907," *New-York Historical Society Quarterly* 61 (1977): 49–68.
55 For a description of the infant hospital, see J. F. Richmond, *New York and Its Institutions, 1609–1872: A Library of Information* . . . (New York: E. B. Treat, 1872), pp. 564–5.
56 For a calculation of the mortality statistics, see English, "Pediatrics and the Unwanted Child," p. 703.
57 Joel Foster, "A Minority Report on Foundlings and Foundling Institutions," *Medical Record* 8 (1873): 423.
58 Abraham Jacobi, "Foundlings and Foundling Institutions," *Collected Essays, Addresses, Scientific Papers, and Miscellaneous Writings of A. Jacobi*, vol. 4, William J. Robinson, ed. (New York: Critic & Guide, 1909), pp. 288–91.
59 Romanofsky, "Saving the Lives of the City's Foundlings," pp. 58–64.

these advantages, they too experienced high death rates linked to the problems of congregate care, maternal favoritism, and feeding difficulties. The New York Infant Asylum, founded in 1865 by Sarah A. Richmond, tried to bargain with its wet nurses. Women who gave birth in the facility were expected to pay for their care by remaining for three months and nursing an abandoned baby along with their own infants.[60] Women who wished to leave their children in the care of the Asylum were expected to remain as wet nurses for a year in order to earn this privilege. By then, of course, they would not be able to find employment as wet nurses. After a rocky start following the death of Mrs. Richmond, the institution closed for several years and then reopened in 1871. Soon thereafter, it added a country home on Long Island to its House of Reception in the city.[61]

The Infant Asylum directors and affiliated physicians discovered almost immediately that most of the wet nurses had only enough milk for their own babies. The foundlings received very little breast milk and as a result, suffered a disproportionate number of deaths. In 1873 the *Annual Report* conceded that whereas 17 percent of the wet-nursed infants had died, the rate for the others was 40 percent. "It becomes a question for some serious consideration whether it would not be expedient to provide wet nurses for all children in the Asylum even if they had to be brought in at the same pay as in private families," the author of the report noted, assessing the economic advantages of such a plan. "Such a course would scarcely be more expensive than to provide medicines, and, finally, for interment."[62] Several years later, J. Lewis Smith, physician to the House of Reception in the city, reviewed the mortality statistics and recommended that in the deadly summer season, when mortality rates peaked, the infants be farmed out.[63] Rather than do so, the directors changed the mission of the institution. They transformed the city House of Reception into a lying-in hospital and sharply limited the number of abandoned infants accepted at the Country Home. In 1876, for example, the Infant Asylum had admitted 942 babies; by 1879, the figure had dropped to 69.[64] Nevertheless, the resident

60 On its dual aims, see New York Infant Asylum, *Annual Report* (New York, 1872), p. 12.
61 On the New York Foundling Asylum, see Charity Organization Society of the City of New York, *A Classified and Descriptive Directory to the Charitable and Beneficent Societies and Institutions of the City of New York* (New York: Charity Organization Society, 1883), p. 96; New York Infant Asylum, *Annual Reports*; and Virginia A. Metaxas Quiroga, *Poor Mothers and Babies: A Social History of Childbirth and Child Care Hospitals in Nineteenth Century New York City* (New York: Garland, 1989), pp. 85–93. Two physicians actively involved in the asylum also analyzed its activities. See Foster, "Minority Report"; and J. Lewis Smith, "Recent Improvements in Infant Feeding," *Archives of Pediatrics* 6 (1889): 848.
62 New York Infant Asylum, *Annual Report* (New York, 1873), p. 24.
63 New York Infant Asylum, *Annual Report* (New York, 1874), pp. 28–9.
64 English, "Pediatrics and the Unwanted Child," p. 702. See also New York Infant Asylum, *Ninth Annual Report* (New York, 1882), p. 11; and idem, *Fourteenth Annual Report* (New York, 1886), p. 40. In 1880 the asylum opened an additional country home in Mt. Vernon, New York, and, shortly thereafter, closed its Flushing facility.

physician from 1888 until 1892 recalled that repeated efforts to induce nursing mothers to suckle foster babies in addition to their own were "rarely a success."[65] However, in changing its mission from one of aiding foundlings to that of helping women during and after their confinement, the Infant Asylum essentially avoided the large-scale failure so visible on Randall's Island.

Even in relatively small institutions, the marriage of saving infants and aiding mothers often yielded very little, as institutional benevolence was undermined by high mortality rates. St. Mary's Infant Asylum and Lying-In Hospital, established by the Daughter's of Charity of St. Vincent De Paul in Dorchester, a section of Boston, took the customary step of requiring free patients to nurse foundlings as well as their own infants whereas the few paying patients were enticed to make a similar agreement in exchange for a reduction in fees.[66] During its first ten years of operation it admitted a total of 550 patients, thus remaining small in size.[67] Nevertheless, it was beset by the same problems as plagued the larger facilities. An investigation by the Boston Board of Health found an infant mortality rate of 68 percent in 1875, and the Asylum faced an investigation by the local Society for the Prevention of Cruelty to Children.[68] Eventually, St. Mary's limited to 15 the number of motherless infants it accepted.[69]

Defining and measuring success in a private infant asylum proved vexing. It could be determined either by the number of infant lives saved or by the number of women who once planned to abandon their babies but, after a period of nursing them, changed their minds. The Foundling Asylum of the Sisters of Charity, a "house of reception for unwanted babies," tried to fulfill both missions. Like the other facilities, it attacked the problem of infant mortality by convincing young mothers to enter the facility voluntarily and suckle abandoned babies along with their own offspring.[70] In 1889, according to social reformer Jacob Riis, 460 women "did voluntary penance for their sin . . . by nursing a strange waif besides their own until both should be strong enough to take their chances in life's battle."[71]

65 Charles G. Kerley, "The New York Infant Asylum," *Archives of Pediatrics* 13 (1896): 22–32.
66 St. Mary's Infant Asylum and Lying-In Hospital Records. Folder 26. DCA. St. Mary's began as part of Carney Hospital and was then called St. Ann's ward. In 1874 it became a separate institution.
67 Benjamin Cushing, "St. Mary's Lying-In Hospital," *Boston Medical and Surgical Journal* 110 (1884): 363.
68 Richardson, "Infant Mortality," p. 65.
69 Board of Health, *Seventh Annual Report* (Boston, 1879), p. 21.
70 J. Lewis Smith, "Recent Improvements in Infant Feeding," *Transactions of the American Pediatric Society* 1 (1889): 87. See also Helen Campbell, *Darkness and Daylight, or, Lights and Shadows of New York Life* (Hartford: Hartford Publishing, 1899), pp. 381–7; and Richmond, *New York and Its Institutions*, pp. 353–5.
71 Jacob A. Riis, *How the Other Half Lives: Studies Among the Tenements of New York* (New York: Charles Scribner's Sons, 1901), p. 190.

Despite their efforts, the death toll remained high; 59 percent in 1870, and 53.9 percent in 1890.[72] Undoubtedly, the death rate for babies suckled by their mothers was far lower than that of the infants nursed as part of a compact with the Sisters. This may have been why the Foundling Asylum eventually turned to a system of outplacement, paying women ten dollars a month to suckle babies in their homes.[73] In taking this step, the Sisters of Charity returned to an older form of wet nursing and brought a different class of women into the business. In the late nineteenth century, many other facilities also began to shift from providing in-house care to out-placement.

The problems experienced at the Massachusetts Infant Asylum illustrate most clearly the difficulty of securing adequate breast milk and maternal attention from wet nurses. By its own account, the Massachusetts Asylum was the most successful institution of its type. Yet, its mortality figures show the same pattern as those of other congregate-care facilities.

The Massachusetts Infant Asylum admitted babies under nine months of age and kept them, if necessary, until their second birthday.[74] Healthy babies went to board in the country; sick babies remained in the Boston facility to be suckled by wet nurses – who also cared for their own infants. The directors, at times, considered the question of whether these women were a labor force or recipients of charity, but they never combined the aims of saving infant lives and mothers' souls. The only test of success was the infant mortality rate.

Prior to the opening of the Infant Asylum, abandoned infants entered the Tewksbury State Almshouse, where inmates were assigned to care for them. In 1866 and 1867, the two years preceding the opening of the Massachusetts Infant Asylum, the infant mortality rate was 87 percent and 70 percent respectively.[75] When the Massachusetts Infant Asylum opened, it arranged for its resident wet nurses to suckle and care for two foundlings in addition to their own babies. It was an ambitious assignment that could

---

72 English, "Pediatrics and the Unwanted Child," pp. 703–4.
73 English, "Pediatrics and the Unwanted Child," p. 705; and Richmond, *New York and Its Institutions*, p. 355.
74 The history of the Massachusetts Infant Asylum is drawn from the *Annual Reports* and the registers. HLUMB.
75 Directors of the Massachusetts Infant Asylum, *First Annual Report* (Boston, 1868), pp. 19–20. Foundlings continued to be admitted to Tewksbury even after the opening of the Massachusetts Infant Asylum. In 1876, the superintendent reported receiving eighty-two babies of whom seventy died; in 1875, all twenty-seven infants admitted had died. The superintendent wanted all of the infants committed to the Massachusetts Infant Asylum. Inspectors of the State Asylum at Tewksbury, "Superintendent's Report," *Twenty-third Annual Report* (Boston, 1877), p. 12. In 1880, the state took responsibility for all found-lings, placing them either in the Massachusetts Infant Asylum or in boarding homes. The result was a drop in the mortality rate of children under three years of age from 97 percent to 50 percent. Several years later, the rate fell further to an average of 14 to 20 percent. H. S. Shurtleff, "State Care of Destitute Infants – The Massachusetts System," *Proceedings of the National Conference of Charities and Corrections* 16 (1889): 1.

not always be fulfilled. The directors conceded that the wet nurses were "destitute women" who frequently lacked sufficient milk to satisfy three infants.[76] Moreover, the often short-staffed institution periodically compromised its program and gave the babies a mixture of bottle- and breast-feedings.[77] Even after the managers recognized that women would not be lured into institutional service by the opportunity to remain with their own infants and tried offering wages equivalent to those offered by private employers (after a two-month probation), the Asylum remained undersupplied with wet nurses.[78] Many of the women did not stay long enough to earn any income; they left on their own, perhaps because they found private employment or were dismissed for lack of milk, strength, or proper character.

The directors of the Asylum believed their efforts yielded enormous success, boasting in 1891 of a mortality rate "lower than had ever been known before in any infant asylum in any country" and crediting wet nurses for the achievement.[79] Two years later, the Asylum mounted a display of its work – including wet nurses and babies – at the World's Columbian Exhibition in Chicago.[80]

Despite its grand displays and boasts, the Infant Asylum's claims of success are undermined by its own statistics. A study of the first one thousand infants to enter the facility (between April 1868 and June 1881) revealed a mortality rate of 35.6 percent. Among the wet nurse's babies, however, the figure was 10 percent. For infants referred by the state, the figure was more than three times higher – 37 percent – and for those admitted by an Asylum committee the figure rose to 53 percent.[81] The results can be partially attributed to the wet nurses' favoring their own infants. But the motherless infants had another disadvantage: only infants too sick to go out to boarding places were admitted to the Asylum, making their survival uncertain from the very beginning. Whatever the cause, the combination of illness and congregate care cut short many lives. Babies entering the Massachusetts Infant Asylum were better off than those admitted to the almshouse, but their survival was far from guaranteed.

A wet nurse's career pattern had an enormous influence on the fate of her baby, and, conversely, the status of a mother's child influenced the kind of wet nursing job she took. The offspring of home-based wet nurses

76 Directors of the Massachusetts Infant Asylum, *Fifth Annual Report* (Boston, 1872), p. 19.
77 Directors of the Massachusetts Infant Asylum, *Second Annual Report* (Boston, 1869), p. 10.
78 Directors of the Massachusetts Infant Asylum, *Third Annual Report* (Boston, 1870), p. 12.
79 Directors of the Massachusetts Infant Asylum, *Twenty-fourth Annual Report* (Boston, 1891), p. 9.
80 Directors of the Massachusetts Infant Asylum, *Twenty-sixth Annual Report* (Boston, 1893), p. 6.
81 Directors of the Massachusetts Infant Asylum, *Seventeenth Annual Report* (Boston, 1884), p. 13.

Table 4.15. *Infant mortality rates for institutionalized infants suckled by their mothers*

Year(s)	Institution	Mortality rate (%)
1868–1881	Massachusetts Infant Asylum	10
1873	Randall's Island Infant Hospital	12
1873	New York Infant Asylum	17
1881–1898	Massachusetts Infant Hospital	14

Sources: Massachusetts Infant Asylum, *Seventeenth Annual Report* (Boston, 1884), p. 13; and *Thirty-First Annual Report* (Boston, 1898), p. 11; Joel Foster, "A Minority Report on Foundlings and Foundling Institutions," *Medical Record* 8 (1873): 423; and New York Infant Asylum, *Annual Report* (New York, 1873), p. 24.

often expired prior to their mother's entry into service. The offspring of privately employed wet nurses often died because their mothers went away. But among women living in institutions, many of whom probably preferred to work in a private home, the effect of their misfortune on their babies was often lifesaving.

Mortality rates for institutionalized infants suckled by their mothers were relatively low compared with the mortality figures for babies institutionalized without their mothers, though they were higher than those for babies reared at home. The figures from the Massachusetts Infant Asylum indicate the gap, and data from other institutions reveal the same pattern. At the Massachusetts Infant Asylum the rate was 10 percent for the wet nurses' babies who were among the first 1,000 infants admitted and 14 percent for those among the second 1,000. At the Randall's Island Hospital, 12 percent of the infants wet-nursed by their mothers perished; at the New York Infant Asylum it was 17 percent. The rates were relatively low given that infants reared in congregate settings had a greater exposure to deadly infectious diseases, and they compared favorably with infant mortality rates recorded among larger noninstitutionalized populations. The infant mortality rate in Suffolk County, Massachusetts, in 1875 ranged from a low of 187.8 per 1,000 for the offspring of native-born parents (approximately 19 percent) to a high of 220.4 per 1,000 (approximately 22 percent) when both parents were foreign born.[82] After the United States established a Death Registration Area in 1900 in order to obtain mortality statistics, the rate of infant mortality for the years 1900 to 1902 was found to be 12

82 Meckel, *Save the Babies*, p. 28, Table I.

Table 4.16. *Outcome of wet nurses' infants placed in the Massachusetts Infant Asylum, 1868–1911*

Status	Number	Percentage
Discharged with mother	50	45
Died	32	29
Adopted	17	15
Referred to other institution	7	7
Taken by family member	4	4
Total	110	100
(Missing cases	76)	

Source: Records of the Massachusetts Infant Asylum, HLUMB.

percent.[83] In sum, institutionalized infants suckled by their mothers suffered some excess mortality, but the rate was not extraordinarily high.

Although the data are not as plentiful, the figures for infants whose mothers worked as private-duty wet nurses show that the babies were handicapped by the absence of maternal care and milk. One hundred eighty-six infants remained in the Massachusetts Infant Asylum while their mothers worked as privately employed wet nurses between 1868 and 1911. Case records reveal the fate of 110 of them. Thirty-two (29 percent) died, typically of gastrointestinal ailments and respiratory diseases common among infants. In other cases, the emotional bonds between mother and infant appear to have been severed by the separation. Seventeen (15 percent) of the infants were given up for adoption, and seven (6 percent) were sent to other institutions for care. Only 50 of the children (45 percent) were reunited with their mothers; another four (4 percent) were taken home by relatives.

Despite the paucity of cases, a similar record appeared for twenty-eight babies at the Philadelphia Home for Infants whose mothers were wet nurses. Fourteen died, twelve went home with their mothers or with other relatives, and two were adopted.

Scholarly studies undertaken in the early twentieth century on the effect of feeding method on infant mortality demonstrated conclusively that breast-fed babies had far lower mortality rates than babies fed by bottle.[84] More recent findings suggest that the reason was the protection that breast-

83 Preston and Haines, *Fatal Years*, p. 52.
84 Robert M. Woodbury, *Causal Factors in Infant Mortality: A Statistical Study Based on Investigations in Eight Cities* (Washington, D.C.: U.S. Government Printing Office, 1925).

Table 4.17. *Outcome of wet nurses' infants
placed at the Philadelphia Home for Infants,
1873–1899*

Status	Number	Percentage
Died	14	50
Discharged to		
mother or relative	12	43
Adopted	2	7
Total	28	100

Source: Register of the Philadelphia Home for
Infants, HSP.

feeding conferred against diarrheal diseases.[85] In the nineteenth century, when milk and water supplies were more likely to be contaminated, the risks of bottle-feeding were enormous. Infants left behind in institutions were particularly vulnerable, given the shortage of wet nurses. Some received only limited quantities of breast milk; others, none at all. Similarly, babies left in private boarding places risked exposure to artificial feeding and, like babies in the infant asylum, probably received care that ranged from excellent to criminal.

Confounding the problem of feeding method was the infant's age at separation; the younger the child, the more vulnerable it was to illness and the more it needed human milk. The leading cause of death among neonates (infants less than one month of age) was premature birth, followed by congenital debility and malformations – conditions that were not heavily influenced by feeding method. The next leading causes, however, diarrheal and respiratory diseases, were more highly correlated with feeding method and exposure to disease.[86] Thus, it can be inferred that babies who ceased receiving their mother's milk at a young age faced a particularly difficult battle to survive. Sadly, this was precisely the problem for infants whose mothers went to work as wet nurses. Women who entered service after being discharged from lying-in hospitals left behind two-week-old infants, women hired from maternity homes probably had infants of the same age, and women retained from asylums were likely to be chosen on the basis of the age of their milk, a selection criterion that put their infants at grave risk.

Figures from a number of institutions indicate that for a significant

85 Harold R. Lentzner, "Seasonal Patterns of Infant and Child Mortality in New York, Chicago, and New Orleans: 1870–1919" (Ph.D. diss., University of Pennsylvania, 1987), cited in Preston and Haines, *Fatal Years*, p. 27.
86 Meckel, *"Save the Babies,"* p. 167.

Table 4.18. *Age of wet nurses'*
infants at the Philadelphia Home
for Infants by outcome

Age	Lives	Dies
Less than 1 month	3	6
1–4 months	5	7
5–9 months	6	1
Total	14	14

Source: Register of the Philadelphia
Home for Infants, HSP.

Table 4.19. *Age of wet nurses' infants at the*
Nursery and Child's Hospital, 1859–1860

Age	Number	Percentage
Less than 1 month	23	20
1–2 months	32	28
3 months	17	15
4 months	14	12
5 months	4	3
6 months	7	6
7 months	8	7
8 months and older	10	9
Total	115	100

Source: Register #2, Nursery and Child's Hospital,
NYHCMC.

portion of infants the separation came during the neonatal period or shortly thereafter. Of the eleven babies who survived their institutionalization at the Philadelphia Home for Infants, two remained for less than two weeks before their removal, substantially limiting their period of risk. Several of the other surviving babies were over six months of age at their time of admission, making them less vulnerable to the gastrointestinal ailments that struck the youngest most ferociously. Indeed, mortality varied by age; the older the infant, the greater the chance of survival.

Twenty percent of the women discharged to service from New York's Nursery and Child's Hospital in 1859 and 1860 had infants less than a month old; by the time the babies were three months old, 63 percent of them had been separated from their mothers. The risk for these infants was

Table 4.20. *Age of wet nurses' infants at the*
Charles Street Temporary Home, 1862–1864

Age	Number	Percentage
Less than 1 month	11	34.5
1–4 months	18	56
5–9 months	3	9.5
Total	32	100
(Missing cases	69)	

Source: Records of the Boston Overseers of the
Poor, City Temporary Home, Box 16, Folder 1,
MHS.

high, and it is unclear whether the wet nursing they received mitigated the effects of separation, or if the Nursery and Child's Hospital, like other congregate facilities, was as Abraham Jacobi charged, a death house for babies.

At the Boston City Temporary Home, there was a similar pattern of early separation. Although some of the residents had entered the facility having already lost their babies, placed them at board, weaned them, or determined to give them up for adoption, others were undoubtedly still nursing. The records although sparse indicate that eleven of thirty-two women had infants less than a month old. Sometimes, a few weeks elapsed between a woman's arrival and her departure to private service, giving her infant more time to enjoy the benefits of its mother's milk. In other instances, a woman's stay was much shorter.

There is no evidence that women who went out to private service intended their infants to die. They placed their children in harm's way because of need. Undoubtedly, they hoped to earn enough money both to pay for proper care for their absent babies and to save so as to support themselves and their offspring after their work ended. But they had made a trade-off; their infants suffered from a lack of breast milk and an absence of what one asylum doctor termed "motherly sympathy and affection."[87] Indeed, the employment of wet nurses in private homes led, often, to the deaths of the women's babies, or what Esther Waters called "a life for a life."

What one novelist's heroine uttered in a moment of dramatic defiance, actual observers perceived on quieter, more individual terms.

87 Inspectors of the State Almshouse at Tewksbury, *Eleventh Annual Report*, "Physician's Report" (Boston, 1865), pp. 22–3.

Physician Oliver Wiggin called wet nurses "victims of distressing circumstances" and "creatures of grief," sympathetically observing the faces etched with "a 'far away and long ago' look painful to behold."[88] The hardships Wiggin observed could have been a reflection of many emotions – grief over separation from their babies, mourning for their loves lost or dead infants, humiliation over their treatment as unwed mothers, or discomfort in their employers' households. Whatever the wet nurses' position in the marketplace, it was earned in part by the women's suffering. Wet nursing, at its core, was a career track paved with misfortune.

Physicians did more than just observe the sad looks and sad lives of wet nurses. They increasingly participated in shaping the work of these women and thus bore ever-greater responsibility for the fate of the wet nurses' babies. In the early nineteenth century, blame for the deaths of the wet nurses' infants fell largely on the wet nurses themselves, who were cast as coldly calculating mercenaries expelling their own offspring in order to take up residence in the homes of the wealthy. Secondary responsibility rested with the "fashionable women" who out of vanity chose not to nurse their babies. In the later decades of the nineteenth century, as physicians were more often called upon to orchestrate the employment of wet nurses, a period of professional self-scrutiny and questioning began. Doctors had to ask whether wet nurses belonged in foundling asylums suckling homeless babies or in the homes of rich women who chose not to engage in the increasingly unpopular act of breast-feeding. As alternative methods of feeding became safer – but not as safe as wet nursing – and as doctors became trusted family advisors, the physicians' dilemma deepened.

88 Oliver C. Wiggin, *Artificial Feeding of Infants* (Providence, 1897), p. 33.

5

Medical oversight and medical dilemmas: The physician and the wet nurse, 1870–1910

The task of locating healthy wet nurses remained a difficult one for late nineteenth- and early twentieth-century physicians, despite the development of institutions housing large numbers of new mothers. New York pediatrician Louis Fischer complained in his 1901 textbook, *Infant-Feeding: In its Relation to Health and Disease,* that there was no easy means for finding acceptable candidates. "As no licensed agencies, exist," he wrote, "a few people having so-called influences procure wet-nurses by friendship, or something similar, from superintendents and house physicians where obstetrical work is done." The procurers bedeviled Fischer by sometimes referring women with only "colostrum-milk" or, in one case, offering a seventeen-year-old who had given birth prematurely, "evidently an abortion," and whose milk was "thin water."[1] Just as a previous generation had found itself at the mercy of the proprietors of intelligence offices and maternity home operators, early twentieth-century physicians believed themselves to be preyed upon by a new kind of entrepreneur, succinctly labeled by Fischer as "people who traffic in wet-nurses for a fee."

Although Fischer's observations regarding the lack of a reliable system echo those of an earlier generation of physicians, his specific allegations suggest that doctors had more resources at hand than in previous decades. The "traffickers" Fischer wrote of mediated between hospital-based physicians and physicians who worked for private families. Their niche was made possible by the rise of obstetric facilities serving poor women, the development of hospital internships, and the growing expectation that physicians, not individual families, would inspect and hire wet nurses. In short, Fischer's complaints reveal that by the dawn of the twentieth century wet nursing had become medicalized.

In terms of wet nursing medicalization means the process by which the practice came under the control of professionals. It refers first to the fact

---

1 Louis Fischer, *Infant-Feeding: In Its Relation to Health and Disease,* 2d ed. (Philadelphia: F. A. Davis, 1901), pp. 83–4.

that wet nurses had begun to be hired from institutions, such as lying-in hospitals and infant asylums, either run by physicians or in which physicians had the opportunity to examine women before they went out to service. Second, medicalization points to the fact that wet nurses had come to be seen not as a class of domestic servants, but, to use Fischer's revealing phrase, as "one of the most valuable forms of adjuncts to our maternal feeding."[2] Third, medicalization alludes to the assessment of wet nurses according to scientific as well as moral standards. Fischer, for example, examined the milk of wet nurses under the microscope, and other physicians had their own protocols for inspecting potential candidates, their infants, and their milk. Finally, medicalization means that physicians had come to exercise greater control not only in selecting wet nurses but also in managing their work in private homes. Indeed, the medicalization of wet nursing was the culmination of the expanding authority of physicians, the development of pediatric medicine, and the growing social value of children.

Of course, wet nursing was never fully medicalized, nor could it be. The inherent moral and managerial problems of wet nursing confounded attempts to place the practice on a fully scientific footing, making it just another form of infant feeding. Significantly, the language used to discuss wet nurses was never entirely purged of emotional and sometimes irrational statements. Even as physicians secured the trust of families and began to demonstrate a modicum of skill in treating childhood ailments, even as infant feeding became the centerpiece of both public health and pediatric medicine, and even as proprietary infant foods and scientific infant formulas offered new alternatives to human milk, perplexing questions about wet nurses remained. When should a wet nurse be hired – when mothers refused to nurse or when bottle-feeding failed? Once employed, what should she be fed? What was to be her daily routine? How could her behavior be controlled and her temper contained? At times, the doctors' answers resonated with scientific certainty; on other occasions they sounded like homilies about managing household help. Physicians confronting wet nurses agonized over moral complexities and became frustrated with mundane details. Predictably, they resented both.

Medical science was the underpinning of the medical profession's expanding power. Manifested in the germ theory, which transformed both diagnosis and treatment, it stimulated the development of the modern general hospital and the growth of university-based and hospital-affiliated medical schools. Scientific advances also encouraged the growth of new medical specialties and transformed public health practices by linking the

2 Ibid., p. 84.

work in the streets with work in the laboratory.[3] Yet, the flowering of modern medicine was also influenced by the soil in which the seeds of science were planted. The public's acceptance of, demand for, and, ultimately, reliance upon doctors occurred in the context of industrialization and urbanization, as towns and cities created new political means for responding to the social disorder brought by disease and as individual men, women, and children sought relief from pain and illness. In short, modern medicine had a social as well as a scientific foundation.

Pediatric medicine, inextricably linked to the growing social value of children as well as to developments in science, exhibited this dual genesis most profoundly. In the late nineteenth century the young, in the words of sociologist Viviana Zelizer, went from being valueless to being "priceless."[4] As children's economic contribution to the family slowly diminished, their sentimental worth grew. This created new demands on and opportunities for middle- and upper-class women, who continued to expand their sphere of civic action in the name of child protection and who simultaneously worked to see that their own children survived.[5]

The public and private commitment to viewing the young as protected future citizens encouraged the development of pediatric institutions, among them children's hospitals, infant asylums, institutions for crippled children, and dispensaries specializing in the treatment of the young.[6] From these establishments, a generation of pediatric practitioners emerged. They, in

3 Charles E. Rosenberg, *The Care of Strangers: The Rise of America's Hospital System* (New York: Basic Books, 1987); Paul Starr, *The Social Transformation of American Medicine* (New York: Basic Books, 1982); Rosemary Stevens, *American Medicine and the Public Interest* (New Haven: Yale University Press, 1971); and John Harley Warner, "Science in Medicine," *Osiris*, 2d ser., 1 (1985): 37–58.
4 Viviana A. Zelizer, *Pricing the Priceless Child: The Changing Social Value of Children* (New York: Basic Books, 1985). Lasch contends that the reformulation of childhood was due in part to an "invasion" of the family by the helping professions. Christopher Lasch, *Haven in a Heartless World: The Family Besieged* (New York: Basic Books, 1977), pp. 12–21 and passim. Daniel T. Rodgers, "Socializing Middle-class Children: Institutions, Fables and Work Values in Nineteenth Century America," *Journal of Social History* 13 (1980): 356–7, sees the authority of physicians growing because of alarm at infant mortality. He believes that the effect of this authority was "to shoulder a new set of public health authorities and hospital doctors into the ranks of experts bearing on middle-class families."
5 The fullest expression of this occurred in the Progressive Era, but it began in the late nineteenth century. Richard A. Meckel, *"Save the Babies": American Public Health Reform and the Prevention of Infant Mortality, 1850–1929* (Baltimore: Johns Hopkins University Press, 1990), pp. 92–197; Robyn Muncy, *Creating a Female Dominion in American Reform, 1890–1935* (New York: Oxford University Press, 1991), pp. 3–65; and Sheila M. Rothman, *Woman's Proper Place: A History of Changing Ideals and Practices, 1870 to the Present* (New York: Basic Books, 1978), pp. 13–174.
6 On children's hospitals, see Mary L. Roger's "Children's Hospitals in America," in John S. Billings and Henry M. Hurd, eds., *Hospitals, Dispensaries and Nursing; Papers and Discussions in the International Congress of Charities, Corrections and Philanthropy* (Baltimore: Johns Hopkins Press, 1894), p. 374; and Samuel X. Radbill, "A History of Children's Hospitals," *American Journal of Diseases of Children* 90 (1955): 411–16. On orthopedic hospitals and

turn, created pediatric societies, pediatric journals, pediatric textbooks, and pediatric medical education – the visible manifestations of a new medical specialty.[7] More critically, the knowledge they produced proved instrumental in changing the ways in which children were cared for both in large institutions and in the nurseries of private homes.

In the private sphere, pediatrics was not medicine practiced by specialists but was specialized medical knowledge applied by family doctors. As families sought advice about feeding babies and rearing children, they turned to physicians who translated the expertise developed on the infant wards and in modern laboratories into practical guidelines for mothers and nurses. Some pediatricians argued that general practitioners were not up to the challenge, particularly in the area of infant feeding. One specialist recalled it was a subject that "took a year or two of study and practice to learn well."[8] Another took a belated swipe at the less proficient general practitioner who "abhorred digestive disturbances, as the death of a baby ruined his standing in the family."[9] Nevertheless, there were too few pediatricians to meet the needs of private families; general practitioners provided the bulk of professional medical care to children. As a 1907 textbook acknowledged, the family doctor treated "more ailing little ones and [saw] more of the pathological conditions which affect immature humanity than all the pediatrists put together."[10]

Infant feeding stood at the core of both pediatric practice and public health concerns in the late nineteenth century as reformers "discovered" the problem of infant mortality, sparking ever more specific measures to save the lives of the young. As historian Richard Meckel has described, broad-ranging campaigns for municipal sanitary reform were followed by efforts to improve the milk supply and, later, by the creation of maternal education programs that stressed breast-feeding but also taught safe artificial-feeding practices. The crusade to save babies engaged public-

children's medicine, see Saul Benison, "An Interpretation of the early Evolution of Care and Treatment of Crippled Children in the United States," *Birth Defects: Original Article Series* 12 (1976): 103–15.

7 Traditional accounts of the development of pediatrics include Isaac A. Abt, "A Survey of Pediatrics during the Past One Hundred Years," *Illinois Medical Journal* 77 (1940): 485–94; Thomas E. Cone, Jr., *History of American Pediatrics* (Boston: Little Brown, 1979); and Sydney A. Halpern, *American Pediatrics: The Social Dynamics of Professionalism, 1880–1980* (Berkeley: University of California Press, 1988). For contemporary accounts see L. Emmett Holt, "American Pediatrics - A Retrospect and A Forecast," *Transactions of the American Pediatric Society* 35 (1923): 9–17; and Abraham Jacobi, "The Relationship of Pediatrics to General Medicine," *Transactions of the American Pediatric Society* 1 (1889): 6–17.

8 Alton Goldboom, "A Twenty-Five Year Retrospect of Infant Feeding," *Journal of the Maine Medical Association* 45 (1954): 263.

9 John Zahorsky, *From the Hills; An Autobiography of a Pediatrician* (St. Louis: C. V. Mosby, 1949), p. 240.

10 George H. Candler, *Every-Day Diseases of Children and Their Rational Treatment* (Chicago: Clinic Publishing, 1907), pp. v–vi.

health professionals, female reformers, and politicians and resulted in a variety of innovations, ranging from clean-milk depots to new local and state regulations. In the twentieth century, more vigorous measures followed, including pasteurization of the urban milk supply, federal legislation establishing the Children's Bureau in 1912, and passage of the Sheppard-Towner Act for the promotion of the welfare and hygiene of maternity and infancy in 1921.[11] One effect of the various programs was to reinforce the belief that infant-feeding practices were among the most significant determinants of infant health and that access to clean milk was vital.

Physicians and reformers identified and addressed numerous problems in the milk supply. At midcentury, they waged a battle against "swill milk," which came from cows fed on brewery slops and was nutritionally incomplete.[12] Following development of the germ theory, concern shifted to problems of milk contamination and adulteration. Well into the twentieth century, physicians detailed the minor illnesses, such as septic sore throat, and the major diseases such as diphtheria, scarlet fever, tuberculosis, and typhoid, transmitted via milk from diseased cows.[13] Even if the animals were healthy, the road from producer to consumer proved treacherous. At worst, milk from unsanitary dairies traveled to the city in contaminated milk cans and, upon arrival, was diluted with polluted water and had chemicals added in order to disguise spoilage. At the next stop, the corner grocery store, the milk sat unrefrigerated in milk cans exposed to flies, dust, and other pollutants. As a professor of hygiene at Harvard Medical School commented, "A city's milk supply is so often richer in bacteria than its sewage."[14] When babies drank from their bottles (which may also have harbored bacteria due to improper cleaning), they risked their lives.

The advent of bacteriology in the late nineteenth century along with the public efforts to lower mortality rates led to reinvigoration of municipal boards of health. The boards took responsibility for identification of individual pathogens and contaminants in milk and enforced newly passed laws

11 Analysis of the infant-welfare movement is based on Meckel, *"Save the Babies."*
12 For the campaign against swill milk in New York, see Norman Shaftel, "A History of the Purification of Milk in New York; or, 'How Now Brown Cow,' " in Judith Walzer Leavitt and Ronald L. Numbers, eds., *Sickness and Health in America: Readings in the History of Medicine and Public Health* (Madison: University of Wisconsin Press, 1978), pp. 275–91. For a contemporary view, see Robert M. Hartley, *An Historical, Scientific and Practical Essay on Milk as an Article of Human Sustenance . . .* (New York: J. Leavitt, 1842).
13 According to one account, fifty-three outbreaks of typhoid, twenty-six of scarlet fever, and eleven of diphtheria occurred between 1880 and 1896, with numerous other incidents going unreported. Rowland Godfrey Freeman, "Milk as an Agency in the Conveyance of Disease," *Medical Record* 49 (1896): 433.
14 Charles Harrington, "Infantile Mortality and Its Principal Cause – Dirty Milk," *American Journal of the Medical Sciences* 132 (1906): 829.

outlawing the watering or adulteration of milk.[15] Although such measures helped improve the quality of the urban milk supply, they did not solve all of the problems related to infant feeding. The poor often lacked the means to purchase clean milk and the ability to store it properly. Their particular problems stimulated reformers and municipalities to open milk stations that supplied pasteurized milk at little or no cost. At the same time, the milk stations often served as public-health centers, providing well-baby care and home visits by public-health nurses as part of a general effort to lower the infant mortality rate. Much of the stations' work, despite their provision of milk, involved efforts to convince poor women to breast-feed their babies.[16]

Wealthy families obtained safe milk by purchasing it from certified dairies that provided milk guaranteed to be free of bacteria. Developed in the mid-1890s, certification involved physicians in overseeing the production of milk. They established strict standards of hygiene at every step of the production process, from the care of the cow to the sale of the final product.[17] Such oversight was rather expensive. One physician recalled that certified milk cost twenty-five cents a quart, whereas a quart of uncertified milk sold for between six and nine cents; he also remembered that, at the time, "the day labourer earned a dollar a day and the office clerk from twelve to twenty dollars a week."[18]

Middle- and working-class families, unwelcome at the milk depots and unable to afford certified milk, had to purchase milk sold locally. Although municipalities attempted to control the milk's quality through inspection and regulation, the task proved too massive and complex for them to be entirely successful until the pasteurization laws in the twentieth century. Before the laws were passed, doctors and public-health workers often taught mothers to boil their children's milk, although there was some debate among specialists about the advisability of this measure. Some physicians suggested that raw milk remained the superior choice because boiling milk limited its digestibility and diminished its nutritive value.

15 Ernest Christopher Meyer, *Infant Mortality in New York City: A Study of the Results Accomplished by Infant-Life Saving Agencies, 1855–1920* (New York: Rockefeller Foundation International Health Board, 1921), pp. 22–3; and Edward T. Morman, "Scientific Medicine Comes to Philadelphia: Public Health Transformed, 1854–1899," (Ph.D. diss., University of Pennsylvania, 1986), pp. 148–91.

16 Meckel, "Save the Babies," pp. 62–91; and Patricia Mooney Melvin, *The Organic City: Urban Definition and Community Organization, 1880–1920* (Lexington: University Press of Kentucky, 1987), pp. 26–56.

17 Rima D. Apple, *Mothers and Medicine: A Social History of Infant Feeding, 1890–1950* (Madison: University of Wisconsin Press, 1987), pp. 59–60; Meckel, "Save the Babies," pp. 80–4; and Manfred J. Wasserman, "Henry L. Coit and the Certified Milk Movement in the Development of Modern Pediatrics," *Bulletin of the History of Medicine* 42 (1972): 359–90.

18 Alton Goldbloom, "The Evolution of the Concepts of Infant Feeding," *Archives of Disease in Childhood* 29 (1954): 390.

Similarly, as the movement for pasteurization grew, there were physicians who opposed it, believing that the process would be used to disguise an inferior product.[19]

Regardless of the bacteriological content of cow's milk, most doctors believed that cow's milk was not a food for babies. Before it could be poured into feeding bottles, it had to be modified to resemble human milk. Research into artificial feeding paralleled the movement for milk hygiene. Just as the latter depended upon a scientific understanding of bacteriology, the former was also built upon a bedrock of science, specifically upon milk chemistry and nutrition. Working in their laboratories, physicians and chemists developed formulas that called for the dilution of cow's milk with water, the enhancement of its fat content by the addition of cream, and the augmentation of its carbohydrate level through the addition of sugars and starches.[20] The new milk science led in two directions: toward the creation of proprietary infant foods and toward the creation of scientific infant feeding – a set of formulas for modifying milk mixtures in the home.

Developed by European chemists, proprietary food mixtures typically consisted of milk, flours, and other substances that were to be diluted, either with water or with a combination of milk and water. At first, foreign brands dominated the market, but by the 1870s and 1880s American manufacturers entered what would prove to be a lucrative business and the number of domestic brands proliferated. Advertisements for infant foods became a standard feature of women's magazines, and the foods' burgeoning sales suggested that they were rapidly becoming a standard feature of middle-class life. If the volume of advertisements was one sign of success, then the content of the advertisements was another. The first American notices for an infant food, Leibig's, appeared in *Hearth and Home* in 1869 under the banner headline: "No More Wet Nurses" – a clear indication of what the manufacturer viewed to be the food's rival.[21] However, the emphasis among marketers quickly shifted to positioning individual brands to outsell their competitors. The wet nurse was no longer mentioned. Although there are no sales data for these artificial infant foods, by all indicators business was booming. As a result, doctors encountered ever-increasing numbers of bottle-fed babies.[22]

19 J. Scott MacNutt, *The Modern Milk Problem in Sanitation, Economics, and Agriculture* (New York: MacMillan, 1917); and Meckel, *"Save the Babies,"* pp. 88–9.
20 On the mixing of formulas, see Grover F. Powers, "Infant Feeding," *Journal of the American Medical Association* 105 (1935): 753–61. For recollections of those involved in the creation of infant feeding, see Goldbloom, "The Evolution of the Concepts of Infant Feeding"; and John Lovett Morse, "Recollections and Reflections on Forty-Five Years of Artificial Feeding," *Journal of Pediatrics* 7 (1935): 303–24.
21 Apple, *Mothers and Medicine*, p. 9.
22 Ibid., pp. 138–9.

Many physicians resented both the usurpation of their role as infant-feeding experts and the economic rivalry of manufacturers. As Harvard Medical School pediatrician Thomas Morgan Rotch declared, "The proper authority for establishing the rules for substitute feeding should emanate from the medical profession, and not from non-medical capitalists."[23] Despite his objections, and those of his fellow specialists, many doctors began recommending their favorite brands of infant foods, and many families purchased them on their own without medical advice. In the end, the medical profession capitulated to the "capitalists," settling for agreements that restricted advertising and urged that products be used under medical supervision.[24]

Concurrently, pediatricians developed formulas that mothers could use to make their own artificial foods. Rotch developed the most elaborate scientific infant formula: the "percentage system." A calculation of the proper mix of milk and other substances that presumed to duplicate precisely the proportions of fat, sugar, and protein found in human milk, Rotch's system was so mathematically complex that it baffled many physicians and was incomprehensible to mothers. Pediatrician L. Emmett Holt, who later developed the more popular "caloric system," recalled percentage feeding as "a system that could never be put into the hands of the public."[25] Holt's own formulas were designed to be easily understood. His best-selling infant-care book, *Care and Feeding of Children: A Catechism for the Use of Mothers and Children's Nurses* (1894), provided mothers with several easy-to-mix formulas. Published in numerous editions, it became one of the most influential publications of the twentieth century, earning the popular moniker "Dr. Holt's Bible."[26]

Scientific infant feeding gave pediatricians four essential elements of specialty practice: a laboratory science, a body of special knowledge, a method of attacking the practical problem of how to feed the baby, and a way of answering the marketing skills of infant-food manufacturers. Recalling the bad old days before scientific infant feeding, Rotch awkwardly described the mothers and nurses who "dominated the physicians" and the doctors who "by culpable neglect in their study of the subject . . . took

23 Thomas Morgan Rotch, "The General Principles Underlying All Good Methods of Infant Feeding," *Boston Medical and Surgical Journal* 129 (1893): 506, cited in Apple, *Mothers and Medicine*, p. 24.
24 Apple, *Mothers and Medicine*, pp. 72–94.
25 R. L. Duffus and L. Emmett Holt, Jr., *L. Emmett Holt: Pioneer of a Children's Century* (New York: Appleton-Century, 1940), p. 117. On the theories and contents underlying specific formulas and patented foods, see Apple, *Mothers and Medicine*, pp. 8–11, 23–34.
26 Holt's book remained in print until 1946, long after his death. His son, L. Emmett Holt, Jr., made the revisions. On Holt's influence, see Kathleen Jones, "Sentiment and Science: The Late Nineteenth Century Pediatrician as Mother's Advisor," *Journal of Social History* 17 (1983): 79–96.

136   *A social history of wet nursing*

refuge with still a third barrier to scientific feeding, namely with the commercial venders of patent and proprietary foods innumerable."[27] Yet the victory of scientific infant feeding was not absolute. Despite the enormous strides that had been made in the development of a healthy food for babies, mother's milk could not be fully duplicated in the laboratory. Wet nurses therefore remained a significant and sometimes lifesaving resource.

Medical case reports from leading pediatricians contained numerous accounts of babies who suckled wet nurses after bottle-feeding or even maternal breast-feeding had failed. Rotch published several cases in which nursing mothers were replaced by wet nurses because of problems with the mothers' milk.[28] When he asked the mothers of sick babies what they were feeding their children, Isaac Abt recounted, they "showed me a can containing one of the many proprietary foods that were then extensively advertised." The babies had a "starch injury" caused by the formula, and he "usually advised the mother to get a wet nurse."[29]

Little wonder, then, given the problems with the milk supply, with artificial foods, and even with "scientific" formulas, that infant feeding remained a bread-and-butter issue for doctors.[30] The growing cultural and scientific authority of physicians and the shifting expectations of families meant that many women no longer handled infant-feeding problems on their own or relied exclusively on friends, relatives, and home guidebooks for advice. Instead, they turned to doctors, who became the arbiters of wet nurse selection and management.

The same force propelling sales of artificial infant foods and the prescription of scientific infant formulas also stimulated demand for wet nurses: many women were not breast-feeding their babies. Their failure to do so elicited both criticism and guidelines on how to manage the alternatives.

In the years following the Civil War, the discourse on maternal nursing began to encompass a critique of modern society and its effects on women. Although similar to earlier arguments about flighty women being unfit for nursing, the new analysis blamed vaguely defined social pressures as well as individual mothers. Late nineteenth-century life came to be seen as inherently enervating, with single young women from well-off families

27 Thomas Morgan Rotch, "An Historical Sketch of the Development of Percentage Feeding," *New York Medical Journal* 85 (1907): 532.
28 Thomas Morgan Rotch, *Pediatrics: The Hygiene and Medical Treatment of Children* (Philadelphia: Lippincott, 1895), pp. 209–12.
29 Isaac A. Abt, *Baby Doctor* (New York: McGraw Hill, 1944), pp. 110–11.
30 John M. Keating, "A Few Practical Notes," *Archives of Pediatrics* 10 (1893): 842–3; cited in Apple, *Mothers and Medicine*, p. 55.

falling prey to bouts of neurasthenia brought on by overexcitement.[31] Married women with children also suffered the ills of modern society. As the leading neurologist of the day, William A. Hammond, explained to the readers of the *Ladies Home Journal* in 1888, "causes incident to civilization" were responsible for their difficulty in suckling babies. He recommended to readers that if necessary they delegate the responsibility to another woman.[32] Nativists also expressed alarm over the decline in breast-feeding, linking it to the problem of "race suicide." They complained that Americans of "good stock" were giving birth to fewer children than in past generations and that these few infants were being nursed at the breasts of immigrants. Why, wondered Nathan Allen, were "foreign born wet nurses" summoned to families "whose ancestresses had never failed to furnish enough milk?"[33] Why, pondered another physician, were American women "less likely than Irish or German women to have a sufficient supply of milk?"[34] Even the well-known pediatrician Abraham Jacobi, himself an immigrant, alleged that the refusal of women to nurse "depopulated the child-world" and reduced "original Americans to a small minority." This, he believed, left "the creation of the future American in the hands of twentieth-century foreigners."[35]

Warnings of "race suicide" provoked neither an upswing in the birthrate of native-born white Americans nor, the evidence suggests, a mania to nurse babies. By 1900, the average number of children born to a white native-born American woman was only 3.56, and the rate continued to fall

31 Barbara Sicherman, "The Uses of a Diagnosis: Doctors, Patients, and Neurasthenia," in Leavitt and Numbers, *Sickness and Health in America*, pp. 25–38.
32 William A. Hammond, "The Hygiene of Infancy," *Ladies Home Journal* 5 (1888): 7. For an analysis of Hammond's view of women, see Bonnie Ellen Blustein, *Preserve Your Love for Science: Life of William A. Hammond, American Neurologist* (New York: Cambridge University Press, 1991).
33 Nathan Allen, "The Decline of Suckling Power Among American Women," *Babyhood* 19 (1902): 6. Allen linked the problem of suckling power to the larger question of race suicide. The essay clearly was reprinted from another source, as Allen died in 1891. On race suicide and medical ideology, see Anita Clair Fellman and Michael Fellman, *Making Sense of Self: Medical Advice Literature in Late Nineteenth-Century America* (Philadelphia: University of Pennsylvania Press, 1981), pp. 75–87; and Linda Gordon, *Woman's Body, Woman's Right: A Social History of Birth Control in America* (New York: Penguin, 1976), pp. 136–58.
34 Charles E. Buckingham, "The Treatment of Children," *Medical Communication* 11 (1874): 295; and idem, "Wet Nursing," *Boston Medical and Surgical Journal* 16 (1875): 268. Others noted this particular limitation of "American women of higher walks of life." See R. P. Harris, "Milk as a Diet During Lactation," *Boston Medical and Surgical Journal* [reprinted from the *Richmond and Louisville Medical Journal* 86 (1872): 395.
35 Abraham Jacobi, "The History of Pediatrics in Relation to Other Sciences and Arts," *American Medicine* 8 (1904): 801. Jacobi did acknowledge, however, that rickets was more common among the poor, who breast-fed, than the rich, who used artificial feeding. Abraham Jacobi, *Infant Diet*, rev. ed. enlgd. and adapted to public use by Mary Putnam Jacobi (New York: J. B. Putnam's Sons, 1874), p. 33.

rapidly in the first third of the twentieth century. In addition, births were more closely spaced, and women ceased having children at an earlier age than they had previously.[36] Infant-feeding practices, though more difficult to document, clearly changed as well. Upper- and middle-class mothers turned to either the bottle or the wet nurse, despite the admonitions of social critics and the recommendations of physicians. In doing so, they rejected a biological definition of motherhood in favor of a social definition. Well-off families understood that their obligation was not to produce large numbers of children, but to prepare the few they did produce to assume a responsible and economically comfortable place in society.

Despite the allegation that "civilization" left some women unable to nurse their babies, the bulk of observers believed that personal preference, rather than weakened physiological capacity, dictated most women's choices. Mary Terhune, author of the popular domestic book *Eve's Daughters* (written under the pseudonym Marion Harland), described a scene in which a doctor congratulated a woman for her "bountiful supply furnished by nature." He was icily rebuffed. "You cannot," the woman replied, "expect me to injure my figure, ruin my complexion and spoil the fit of my dresses by nursing my baby as a common washerwoman might." Calling nursing "slavery," another mother reportedly asserted that it reduced a "refined intellectual being to the rank of mammal female."[37] Terhune's anecdotes contain several revealing elements. Breast-feeding had come to be seen as coarse. It was also viewed as confining.

Public nursing, acceptable in colonial times, had no place in Victorian America. Rather than accept an arrangement that, in the words of one mother, "confines us closely at home," women preferred the freedom of the bottle.[38] In recognition of this preference, one doctor proposed a compromise in the pages of the magazine *Home Comfort:* mothers could give their infants one bottle a day and otherwise nurse them.[39] In attempting to strike such bargains, doctors were tacitly admitting that breast-feeding may not have been their patients' first choice. In recounting, in the same magazines, their skills at managing bottle-fed babies, they gave further evidence of this fact.

Indeed, everywhere they looked, doctors found proof for their suspicions. In the mid-1880s, Joseph Edcil Winters surveyed his fellow practitioners to discover precisely how many of their well-to-do patients did not breast-feed. Five respondents gave estimates ranging from 10 to 50

36 Steven Mintz and Susan Kellogg, *Domestic Revolutions: A Social History of American Family Life* (New York: Free Press, 1988), pp. 109–10.
37 Mary Virginia (Hawes) Terhune [pseud. Marion Harland], *Eve's Daughters; or, Common Sense for Maid, Wife, and Mother* (New York: J. R. Anderson & H. S. Allen, 1882), p. 23.
38 "How to Keep Up the Milk Supply," *Mother's Magazine* 2 (1906): 15.
39 Jas. T. Osborne, "The Baby's Food," *Home Comfort* 1 (1898): 12.

percent, and a sixth, described as a well-known obstetrician, claimed an astonishingly high rate of 95 percent.[40] A more extensive but equally unscientific study of 1,000 women reported in 1908 that 90 percent of the 500 women described as poor and living in tenements were able to nurse their babies for nine months, whereas only 17 percent of the 500 prosperous women living in better parts of the city were able to do so.[41] Clearly, an element of choice was at work among the latter group. Neither survey indicated whether women who did not breast-feed turned to wet nurses or the bottle, but the swelling sales of commercially marketed foods strongly suggest that a growing proportion chose the latter, perhaps seeing it as a more scientifically progressive and domestically manageable choice. Still, a market for wet nurses remained. As the Chicago physician Alfred Cleveland Cotton noted in 1900, the "dictum of some eminent teachers – that artificial feeding can be conducted successfully in ninety percent of these cases" was a "tacit admission that the remaining ten percent may only survive upon the breast."[42]

The effects of the reduced demand for wet nurses were paradoxical. On the one hand, wet nurses moved to the margins of medical practice, becoming a "last resort" when bottle-feeding failed. On the other hand, the wet nurse hired out of desperation was in a strong bargaining position. She could make many demands on the family and the doctor and, under the desperate circumstances, was likely to have them met.

The trouble with a wet nurse, one doctor explained dispassionately, was the "discrepancy between her theoretical value and actual efficiency."[43] In theory, of course, human milk was better for babies than any substance concocted in laboratory or factory. The American Medical Association took this position, but it gave its stamp of approval to wet nurses only when bottle-feeding was clearly becoming the most popular choice.[44] Others too believed it was safer to endorse wet nurses when they

40 Joseph Edcil Winters, "The Relative Influences of Maternal and Wet Nursing on Mother and Child," *Medical Record* 30 (1886): 507.
41 J. Ross Snyder, "The Breast Milk Problem," *Journal of the American Medical Association* 51 (1908): 1213.
42 Alfred C. Cotton, *Lessons on the Anatomy, Physiology, and Hygiene of Infancy and Childhood for Junior Students* (Chicago: Chicago Medical Book, 1900), p. 126.
43 Nathan Oppenheim, *The Medical Diseases of Childhood* (New York: MacMillan, 1900), p. 78.
44 Among the many physicians who declared wet nurses "next best" to mother's milk were George Cooper, *Healthy Children. How to Get Them* . . . (Brooklyn: Institute for the Treatment of Chronic Disease, 1875), p. 27; Cotton, *Lessons*, p. 126; Edward P. Davis and John M. Keating, *Mother and Child* (Philadelphia: J. B. Lippincott, 1893), p. 75; John DeWar, *What Ails the Baby* (New York: Brentano, 1890), p. 11; Augustus K. Gardner, *Our Children: Their Physical and Mental Development* (Hartford: Belknap & Bliss, 1872), p. 72; Thomas N. Gray, *Common Sense and the Baby; A Book for Mothers* (New York: Bewick, 1907), p. 48; John Price Crozer Griffith, *The Care of Baby: A Manual for Mothers and Nurses*

seemed, increasingly, an anachronism. Thus, in a statement of supreme ambivalence published in the *Archives of Pediatrics,* Charles Warrington Earle acknowledged that "very frequently we know that it is impossible for a mother to nurse a child, and then the question comes to us what its nutrition shall be. I believe more and more every year that a wet nurse should be provided." Yet, in the next breath, he cautioned, "in the majority of cases, either from the expense or our inability to procure them, this cannot be accomplished."[45] Warnings followed nearly every endorsement of wet nursing, as doctors alerted the public and their fellow practitioners to potential difficulties. Each step taken to improve commercial infant foods or to simplify the rules for mixing "scientific" formulas at home tipped the balance away from wet nurses.

Among the factors weighed against wet nurses were their cost, the managerial hardships they imposed, the problems in hiring them, and the threat of hidden diseases. Outside of the urban northeast, with its numerous institutional sources, finding acceptable candidates was a challenge. Texas practitioner Charles L. Gwyn lamented that the "difficulty in securing a suitable wet-nurse almost amounts to an impossibility."[46] Oliver C. Wiggin of Rhode Island, and F. L. S. Aldrich, a female physician in Minnesota, made similar complaints, and a physician from Grand Rapids, Michigan, reported in 1912 that he had to get wet nurses from Chicago.[47] Exacerbating the problem, one physician charged, was the custom in some families of hiring wet nurses unnecessarily, which ultimately deprived those who truly required their services.[48]

In many cases, of course, those who needed wet nurses simply could not afford them, whatever their availability. Anecdotal reports show that the wages of wet nurses remained consistently higher than those of other domestic workers and, equally important, beyond the range of the vast

(Philadelphia: Saunders, 1896), p. 119; Amie M. Hale, *The Management of Children: In Sickness and in Health,* 2d ed. (Philadelphia: Blakiston, 1881), p. 21; and Lawrence T. Royster, *A Handbook of Infant Feeding* (St. Louis: C. V. Mosby, 1916), p. 35.

45 Charles Warrington Earle, "Summer Diseases of Children and Infant Diet," *Archives of Pediatrics* 1 (1884): 559. See also Charles P. Putnum, "On Artificial Food for Young Infants," *Boston Medical and Surgical Journal* 16 (1872): 77.

46 Charles L. Gwyn, "Babies and Their Troubles" [pamphlet reprint], *Transactions of the Texas State Medical Association* (1886), p. 6.

47 F. L. S. Aldrich, *My Child and I, In Sickness and Health, from Pre-Natal Life until Sixteen* (Philadelphia: P. W. Ziegler, 1903), p. 120; Oliver C. Wiggin, *Artificial Feeding of Infants* (Providence, 1897), p. 33; and idem, "Discussion," *Journal of the American Medical Association* 59 (1912): 1881. See also Henry B. Hemenway, *Healthful Womanhood and Childhood: Plain Talks to Non-Professional Readers* (Evanston: V. T. Hemenway, 1894), p. 222; and J. O. Webster, "Children's Diseases in Massachusetts," *Boston Medical and Surgical Journal* 39 (1874): 153. By contrast, Buckingham wrote about "examining the numerous applicants for the place." Buckingham, "Wet Nursing," p. 273.

48 J. Lewis Smith, "Hindrances to the Successful Treatment of the Diseases of Infancy and Childhood," *Transactions of the New York State Medical Association* 13 (1896): 95.

majority of families. An 1870 guidebook, *How Women Can Make Money,* stated that children's nurses earned between $1.00 and $1.25 per week, with wet nurses doing even better.[49] Jerome Walker reported paying a wet nurse $25 per month in New York City in the novel *The First Baby;* in 1885, Grace Peckham related that wet nurses earned between $20 and $30 per month.[50] Luther Emmett Holt provided figures of $20 to $35 per month in his 1897 textbook.[51] By contrast, the family purchasing even forty-five quarts of certified milk each month spent only $11.25.

When the value of their room and board is considered, wet nurses seem to have been better off than most working women. The average weekly wage earned by women working in large cities was $5.24 as reported by the U.S. Department of Labor in 1889. In many cases, working women had housing and living expenses that exceeded their pay.[52] When wet nurses are compared to other domestic workers who also received room and board, the advantages of wet nursing come into sharper focus. The highest-paying domestic occupation, that of a cook, paid an average weekly wage of $3.80 in the years 1889–90, less than half what a wet nurse made.[53] Moreover, in addition to receiving pay, room, and board, wet nurses sometimes were able to arrange for their employers to assume the costs of boarding their babies.

Other expenses borne by families hiring wet nurses included the cost of new clothes for the women. Clara Penniston, a regular columnist for *Motherhood* magazine, who in 1910 had estimated the cost of wet nurses to be less than thirty dollars per month, also revealed that the wet nurses usually "must be clothed from top to toe."[54] Fanny B. Workman, in a letter to *Babyhood* magazine, recalled that she had purchased a new set of clothes for a wet nurse who was soon replaced, presumably by a woman who also required new garments.[55] Servants too sometimes received new clothes, with the cost being deducted from their pay. Purchasing clothes

---

49 Virginia Penny, *How Women Can Make Money; Married or Single* . . . (Springfield, Mass.: D. E. Fisk, 1870), p. 430.
50 G[race] Peckham, "Infancy in the City," *Popular Science Monthly* 28 (1885): 686; and Jerome Walker, *The First Baby: His Trials and the Trials of His Parents* (New York: Brown & Derby, 1881), p. 78.
51 L[uther] Emmett Holt, *Diseases of Infancy and Childhood for the Use of Students and Practitioners of Medicine* (New York: Appleton, 1897), p. 159.
52 U.S. Department of Labor, *Women Working in Large Cities,* cited in Lynn Y. Weiner, *From Working Girl to Working Mother: The Female Labor Force in the United States, 1820–1980* (Chapel Hill: University of North Carolina Press, 1985), p. 25.
53 See David M. Katzman, *Seven Days a Week: Women and Domestic Service in Industrializing America* (New York: Oxford University Press, 1978), p. 306, Table A-20; and U.S. Industrial Commission, *Report of the Industrial Commission on the Relations and Conditions of Capital and Labor Employed in Manufactures and General Business. . . . and a Special Report on Domestic Service,* (Washington D.C.: U.S. Government Printing Office, 1901), p. 751.
54 Clara A. Penniston, "The Feeding of Infants," *Motherhood* 8 (1901): 142.
55 Fanny B. Workman, "The Wet-Nurse in the Household," *Babyhood* 2 (1885–6): 142–3.

for wet nurses, especially those hired from institutions, had a specific rationale – nursery hygiene – and families may have been forced to bear the expense rather than pass it on to the wet nurse.[56]

The cost of wet nurses sometimes caused a dilemma for physicians. They wanted to discourage the unnecessary use of wet nurses but had to be prepared, under certain circumstances, to convince some families that a wet nurse, however expensive, was necessary to their child's survival. At least one doctor saw it as a matter of arguing for short-term costs against long-term savings. Wet-nursed infants, he explained, developed better digestion than those fed on the bottle and, as a result, spared the family future medical expenses.[57] Or, as a twentieth- century practitioner argued, "After the wet nurse comes the trained nurse disappears and the doctor makes very few visits."[58] This was quite a concession. Physicians had made scientific infant feeding the backbone of infant care, and yet they knew that with a wet nurse in the house, their services would not be quite so necessary.

In selecting wet nurses, physicians applied the same standards as their antebellum predecessors: good health, healthy babies, high quality milk, and acceptable personal habits. What had changed was the language in which physicians elaborated on these requirements; they used an increasingly scientific prose, which was sometimes interrupted by more personal asides. These short remarks revealed the conundrums of trying to meld modern science into the art of household management.

The question of the wet nurse's baby, for example, brought medical reasoning into conflict with management logic and medical ethics. Sound management suggested that a woman who had lost her own baby would have no reason to resent the suckling she was paid to care for nor have any outside distraction.[59] Furthermore, if doctors accepted wet nurses whose infants had died, they could not be held responsible for the consequences of sending a baby out to board. Yet, sound scientific practice demanded that a wet nurse's baby be examined in order to assess its health and the quality of its mother's milk. One doctor, understandably eager to skirt the inherent conflicts, recommended that if the wet nurse had no baby to display, the causes of the infant's death needed careful investigation.[60] But

56 Another aspect of nursery hygiene was the demand that the wet nurse take a bath upon entering the house. See Rowland Godfrey Freeman, *Elements of Pediatrics for Medical Students* (New York: MacMillan, 1917), p. 140.
57 On the expense of wet nurses, see Gray, *Common Sense and the Baby*, p. 48; and J. O. Webster, "Children's Diseases in Massachusetts," *Boston Medical and Surgical Journal* 39 (1874): 153. On the economic advantages, see Hale, *Management of Children*, p. 43.
58 John Lovett Morse, *Clinical Pediatrics* (Philadelphia: W. B. Saunders, 1926), p. 140.
59 Cotton, *Lessons*, p. 127.
60 Alvarado Middleditch, *The Doctor's Advice; or, How, When and What to Eat and Drink . . .* (Philadelphia: Ziegler, 1898), p. 200.

most practitioners took no chances, and popular opinion held that a wet nurse must prove her value by showing off her fat and healthy baby. A popular portrayal of the situation appeared in the novel *Helen Brent, M.D.* (1892). The doctor-heroine rejected a wet nurse without a baby, and the woman complained of having received the same treatment on three other occasions.[61]

According to the medical literature, savvy wet nurses knew the rules and circumvented them when necessary. Women borrowed healthy babies to show to prospective employers and the physicians working on their behalf.[62] In one reported case, a woman with scrofula spent over two years working as a wet nurse, disguising her condition by wearing high-necked dresses and by displaying to each prospective employer a healthy young baby lent by a friend. During the course of her career, three, and possibly four, of her sucklings died.[63]

The specter of women with hidden diseases haunted practitioners – and with good reason. Wet nurses could and did spread tuberculosis, the deadliest killer of the nineteenth century, and families unknowingly took risks. Sophie Crane left the Massachusetts Infant Asylum to suckle young Stephen Perkins Cabot, scion of an elite Boston family. Her own infant later died of scrofula – making it likely that she was infected with tuberculosis. Young Cabot, fortunately, survived the encounter.[64] George B. Drake, a Boston commission merchant, also retained a wet nurse from the Massachusetts Infant Asylum to feed his child. The woman eventually gave up her position to enter the Consumptives Home "hopeless ill." Even more ominous, her own baby later died of syphilis.[65]

Although bottle-fed babies could and did die quickly of infections caused by bacteria-laden milk, the slow and elusive venereal infections were even more dreaded, not least because of the social stigma attached to them. Most syphilis was latent but contagious. The best that physicians could hope to do was to inspect the wet nurse for a chancre or for a rash indicating secondary syphilis. Evidence of other venereal diseases – such as large lymph nodes, ulceration, or swollen fallopian tubes – had to be discovered by pelvic examination. Just as it is difficult to believe that antebellum physicians followed the medical advice to taste the wet nurse's milk, it is equally unlikely that their successors thoroughly screened

61 Annie (Nathan) Meyer, *Helen Brent, M.D.: A Social Study* (New York: Cassell, 1892), pp. 70–1.
62 On the borrowed baby problem, see Buckingham, "Wet Nursing," p. 273; and Peckham, "Infancy in the City," p. 687.
63 Winters, "Relative Influences," p. 511.
64 Admission Records, Massachusetts Infant Asylum, October 15, 1869, p. 100; November 18, 1872, p. 269. HLUMB.
65 The records do not reveal the fate of the Drake child. Admission Records, Massachusetts Infant Asylum, January 29, 1868, p. 22. HLUMB.

women for venereal infections. But even when they did, latent infections went undiagnosed. Physicians lacked effective diagnostic techniques as well as therapeutic interventions until the diffusion of the Wassermann test, developed in 1906, and the creation of salvarsan – an effective but dangerous therapy for syphilis – in 1909.[66] Even with these medical breakthroughs, doctors remained uncertain as to whether women with latent syphilis secreted infected milk, or, if they did not, whether milk from infected women was nutritionally deficient.[67] In this light, their reluctance to hire wet nurses seems quite understandable.

The avenue of venereal infection ran both ways, however, and reports began to appear in the medical literature of women infected with syphilis by their nurslings.[68] An extensive and chilling account of a woman who unknowingly nursed two syphilitic infants in a hospital and then went out to service appeared in the *American Journal of Obstetrics and Diseases of Children* in 1875.[69] In 1906 the *Journal of the American Medical Association* detailed another frightening episode involving a baby farmed out by the Baltimore Board of Supervision of City Charities to a woman who had lost twins. Not only did the wet nurse become infected, her nine-year-old daughter reportedly developed a chancre on her lip from kissing the baby. It was not an isolated case. After making inquiries, the author learned that some babies sent out by New York City institutions had given infections to their wet nurses and that the problem occurred overseas as well.[70]

The case reports sympathetically described the working-class wet nurses who, struggling to support their families, became infected by foundlings. Missing from the medical literature were cases of wet nurses blighted while in the employ of the well-to-do. Class and morals mapped the social geography of venereal disease; infections were understood to spread from the vicious to the innocent. Popular and medical discussions of venereal infection typically centered around the "vice problem," with accounts por-

---

66 Laboratory and technical facilities necessary for conducting Wassermann tests took several years to develop, and the tests were not always accurate. The widespread use of neosalvarsan, a safer though still toxic treatment, did not begin until the 1920s. See Allan M. Brandt, *No Magic Bullet: A Social History of Venereal Disease in the United States since 1880* (New York: Oxford University Press, 1985), pp. 40–1.

67 David Nabarro, *Congenital Syphilis* (London: Edward Arnold, 1954), p. 57.

68 Nabarro, *Congenital Syphilis*, pp. 442, 445. As Nabarro notes, the problem of infection of and by wet nurses was well known for centuries (p. 10).

69 R. W. Taylor, "The Dangers of the Transmission of Syphilis Between Nursing Children and Nurses in Infant Asylums and in Private Practice," *American Journal of Obstetrics and Diseases of Women and Children* 8 (1875–6): 436–53.

70 William T. Watson, "A Square Deal for the Wet Nurse," *Journal of the American Medical Association* (1906): 1909–11. See also James H. McKee and William H. Wells, *Practical Pediatrics; A Modern Clinical Guide in the Diseases of Infants and Children for the Family Physician*, vol. 1 (Philadelphia: P. Blakiston's Sons, 1914), p. 115. McKee and Wells describe a case in which the municipal "Poor-board" gave a syphilitic infant to a wet nurse, causing the wet nurse's entire family to become infected.

traying the horrors of middle-class wives infected by husbands who had visited prostitutes or children born with a congenital taint.[71] Nevertheless, with estimates of infection among the "better classes" ranging from 6 percent to 18 percent in the early twentieth century, wet nurses had reason to worry.[72]

Dividing the afflicted into innocent and guilty parties did little to control the spread of venereal disease, but the prevailing ideology permitted no alternative models. For the practice of wet nursing this meant that physicians could take precautions against retaining an infected wet nurse, but that they could take few steps to protect the wet nurses from infected babies. Unless the doctor had knowledge of an infection in the family or saw evidence of congenital infection in the child, the disease would almost certainly remain undetected. In an era in which physicians treated venereal diseases in secret, protecting their own reputations as well as those of their patients, few risked probing the personal histories of the families that employed them.[73]

Still, professionals raised the issue among themselves. "Should a Wet Nurse Be Employed for the Child of a Cured Syphilitic?" read the title of one article translated from the French and published in the *Journal of the American Medical Association*. The consensus among doctors was No.[74] Yet, physicians were not without recourse in these situations; they simply had to find an infected wet nurse. According to the medical understanding of syphilitic immunity known as Colles's law, a syphilitic child could be nursed by a syphilitic wet nurse without further danger to either party.[75]

71 Brandt, *No Magic Bullet*, pp. 7–51.
72 Philip C. Jeans, "A Review of the Literature on Syphilis in Infancy and Childhood," Part I, *American Journal of Diseases of Children* 20 (1920): 55.
73 D. W. Cathell, *The Physician Himself and What He Should Add to His Scientific Acquirements*, 3d ed. (Baltimore: Cushings & Bailey, 1883), pp. 71, 186.
74 Louis Fischer, "The Management of Infant Feeding," *Pediatrics* 21 (1890): 64; and John Zahorsky, *Golden Rules of Pediatrics: Aphorisms, Observations, and Perceptions on the Science and Art of Pediatrics* . . . 2d ed. (St. Louis: Mosby, 1911), p. 147. For an earlier, contrasting view that "a healthy wet nurse may probably correct the taint a child inherits from a diseased parent," see Henry Belinaye, *The Sources of Health and Disease in Communities; or, Elementary Views of "Hygiene"* . . . , Am. ed. (Boston: Allen & Ticknor, 1833), p. 35. In his 1876 lectures on obstetrics and diseases of women, Professor R. A. F. Penrose of the University of Pennsylvania was said to have recommended a wet nurse if the mother had no milk or was "tainted by scrofula, syphillis . . . " Copy of Notes taken in shorthand by Dr. William L. Taylor, class of 1876 of lectures on obstetrics and diseases of women by Professor R. A. F. Penrose, p. 126. CPP.
75 Walter Lester Carr, ed., *The Practice of Pediatrics in Original Contributions by American and English Authors* (Philadelphia: Lea Brothers, 1906), pp. 104–5. One study of beliefs regarding infantile syphilis found that many misunderstood and misquoted Colles's law. More importantly, the notion of maternal transmission of syphilis (as spirochetes crossed the placental barrier in the later months of pregnancy), did not become accepted in the medical community until the 1930s. Elizabeth Lomax, "Infantile Syphilis as an Example of Nineteenth Century Belief in the Inheritance of Acquired Characteristics," *Journal of the History of Medicine and Allied Sciences* 34 (1979): 23–39.

Undoubtedly, the hiring of wet nurses with venereal infections constituted one of the most idiosyncratic and heavily camouflaged of labor market transactions.

One complicating factor in the effort to avoid infection of wet nurses was that syphilitic infections were a major cause of prematurity. According to one historian of pediatrics, syphilis accounted for 50 to 80 percent of all cases of prematurity.[76] Although there were no medical protocols for treating the premature until the twentieth century, families and physicians typically tried to procure human milk for them. The result was an increased likelihood of exposure to syphilis for the wet nurses who were hired to suckle premature or frail infants. Physicians often had no way of making an accurate diagnosis, as the babies often showed no signs of infection until they were six to eight weeks old and as diagnosis by Wassermann reaction was unreliable for infants under three months of age.[77] Even when babies exhibited the most common signs of infection, rhinitis and rash, diagnosis remained difficult because these were symptoms of many other conditions as well. A further complication was that the infected parents often showed no signs and reported no symptoms because of the long asymptomatic period that characterized the disease. Physicians might assume parents either were healthy or had taken some type of treatment and been cured.[78] One practitioner reassured his colleagues that they could put "a healthy newborn babe of a formerly syphilitic father to the breast of a wet nurse without fear." Still, he hedged by suggesting that if a wet nurse did become infected on the job, it was the duty of the family to have her undergo treatment.[79] Whether such families actually paid for treatment upon discovering that their infant had infected a wet nurse cannot be

76 Thomas E. Cone, Jr., *History of the Care and Feeding of the Premature Infant* (Boston: Little, Brown, 1985).
77 Abraham Colles, *Practical Observations on the Venereal Disease and on the Use of Mercury* (Philadelphia: A. Waldie, 1837), pp. 163–4; Nabarro, *Congenital Syphilis,* pp. 5, 95, 97.
78 Jeans stated that 75 percent of all offspring in a syphilitic family were infected, implying that he believed that those without symptoms, 25 percent, were free of disease, when, in fact, they were simply asymptomatic. Part of the problem of diagnosis had to do with three prevailing beliefs that were false. First, that women who were asymptomatic (in a latency phase of the disease) were not infected. Second, that a fetus could be "paternally infected" and that by exchanging antibodies with the mother, the fetus gave the mother immunity. Third, that there was a diminishing virulence of infection. In other words, children born early in the course of infection would be infected, but those born later would be free of diseases. For discussion of these ideas, see Adrien Delahaye, "Syphilis: Its Relation to Marriage" [trans. from the French], *American Journal of Syphilography and Dermatology* 4 (1873): 318; C. Hochsinger, "Syphilis," in M. Pfaundler and A. Schlossmann, eds., *The Diseases of Children; A Work for the Practising Physician,* vol. 2, English trans. Henry L. K. Shaw and Linnaeus La Fetra (Philadelphia: Lippincott, 1912), pp. 514–74; and Jeans, "Review of the Literature," pp. 57–8. For examples of how asymptomatic cases were misunderstood, see Graham, *Diseases of Children,* p. 164.
79 Hochsinger, "Syphilis," p. 574.

determined, although they might have had an interest in buying the wet nurse's silence.

The opening of Eugene Brieux's play, *Damaged Goods,* in 1913 tore off the veil, bringing the largely taboo subject of venereal disease into public discussion. Furthering popular awareness was publication of Upton Sinclair's translation of the play, which was released as a novel. In this laboriously didactic morality tale, a young man becomes infected with syphilis after visiting a prostitute and in turn infects his new bride. She then conveys the infection to their infant. Hoping to preserve the baby's life, the scheming mother-in-law searches for a wet nurse. Only the intervention of a brave physician prevents the infection of the young peasant woman hired for the job.[80] *Damaged Goods* heralded the shift from a "Victorian" to a "Progressive" attitude towards sexuality and disease control.[81] Whether it encouraged any protection for wet nurses or for infants sent out to wet nurses remains unknown. On the stage, the doctor stood as the solitary defender against the corruption of the innocent wet nurse; in real life, this proved a more difficult role to play.

Physicians were the directors, not the stars. Not infrequently they settled disputes about who, in fact, would play the lead – the mother or the wet nurse. Physician Isaac Abt, recalling some of the imperious wet nurses he had encountered, remarked, "Their price was more than rubies, and they made the family pay for it in submission to their whims, accession to their demands and forbearance with their bad habits."[82] Other doctors reached the same conclusions, finding that wet nurses ruled households "with a rod of iron."[83] The social order gave way when an infant's life hung in the balance. Families and physicians alike capitulated, or so they believed, to women who under ordinary circumstances would never be allowed into the servants' quarters, much less the nursery. Being neither servants, and compelled to follow the rules of the household, nor trained

---

80 Upton Sinclair, *Damaged Goods, The Great Play, "Les Avaries" of Brieux* . . . (Philadelphia: John C. Winston, 1913). There is no mention of the source of Brieux's inspiration. However, Sturgis cites a case in France in 1885 in which a wet nurse who insisted she had been infected by her nursling sued for 10,000 francs. The father of the child had passed on the disease to his wife, who then conveyed it to the child at birth. The wet nurse lost her case; apparently, it was determined that she had been infected prior to employment. F. R. Sturgis, "On the Venereal and Genito-Urinary Diseases of Children, Part 8: Medico-Legal Aspects of Venereal Disease in Children," *Archives of Pediatrics* 5 (1888): 457–70.
81 Brandt, *No Magic Bullet,* pp. 47–9
82 Abt, *Baby Doctor,* p. 111.
83 Peckham, "Infancy in the City," p. 686. Similar sentiments were expressed by Louis Starr, *Hygiene of the Nursery* (Philadelphia: Blakiston, 1888), p. 125. It was not just the elite physician who recognized the problem of the self-important wet nurse. See Gwyn, "Babies and Their Troubles," p. 6.

nurses, and bound to honor the dictates of the doctor, wet nurses defied the existing hierarchy.

Settling disputes between wet nurses and employers thrust doctors into the role of domestic advisors, a situation that threatened to crack the facade of expertise. In responding to concerns about the wet nurse's daily regimen, for example, physicians could offer little more than common sense. F. H. Getchell recommended that the family require their wet nurse to "exercise in open air each day and to take an entire bath as often as twice a week."[84] Other seemingly trivial matters soon confronted them. Should the wet nurse undertake household chores in addition to tending to the infant, or would exertion vitiate her milk? Theron Kilmer equivocated, suggesting that "she should not be overworked by other duties," but also warning, "she should not be kept in a state of idleness."[85] Compared to the assurances of formula advertisers and to the physicians' own precise instructions about mixing infant foods, such indecision reveals the difficulty doctors faced with managerial problems that had no scientific solutions.

Moreover, questions that seemed petty on the surface often had serious consequences. Medical experts stepped into a morass when confronted with the question of the wet nurse's diet. Most urged that the women consume wholesome, "peasant food" as befitted their station in life and their alimentary needs. Much to their chagrin, the doctors lacked a means of enforcing the restrictions they attempted to impose. Thus, kitchens became combat zones. Wet nurses reportedly demanded food in great quantity and of a quality usually withheld from the household staff.[86] Doctors could barely disguise their contempt for poor women who wanted to dine like their social superiors, although they wrapped their analyses in medical terms. John Price Crozer Griffith argued that "a woman from the lower walks of life given unrestrained opportunity to indulge freely in food to which she has not been accustomed" was "liable to indigestion."[87] Another doctor, rejecting the American dream of upward mobility, stated authoritatively that the shift from poverty to luxury would be difficult for the wet nurse to bear.[88] A third alleged that kitchen social climbing led to "digestive derangement which interferes with lactation."[89] Physicians made few references to the physical demands of breast-feeding or to the way in

84 F. H. Getchell, *The Maternal Management of Infancy* (Philadelphia: J. B. Lippincott, 1868), p. 25.
85 Theron W. Kilmer, *The Practical Care of the Baby* (Philadelphia: F. A. Davis, 1903), p. 146.
86 See, for example, Davis and Keating, *Mother and Child*, p. 91.
87 Griffith, *Care of Baby*, p. 186.
88 Oppenheim, *Medical Diseases of Childhood*, p. 78. See also Clement Cleveland, "Some Observations Upon the Feeding of Infants," *Medical Record* 25 (1884): 485; Getchell, *Maternal Management of Infancy*, p. 25; and Zahorsky, *Golden Rules of Pediatrics*, p. 107.
89 Freeman, *Elements of Pediatrics*, p. 139.

which breast-feeding stimulated the appetite. Nor did the doctors suspect that the wet nurses' demands may well have exceeded those of other servants because the latter had greater access to the kitchen and thus more frequent opportunities to indulge without being observed.[90] Although one doctor acknowledged that nursing women were "eating for two," most preferred to take the family's side in what they perceived as sublimated class warfare.[91]

The problem of the wet nurse's diet loomed large because it subsumed both the conflict over authority within the home and the medical question of how food influenced milk. Physicians and patients alike believed that nursing women needed to avoid certain foods and select others in order to cure an infant's complaints. An annoyed Boston practitioner complained of the "idea prevalent among women, that fish is an article of food fatal in its effect upon recent nurses." The actual cause of digestive upset, he explained, lay in the wet nurse's indulgence in a "mixture of ice cream, oysters, fruit cake and lobster salad, after the sweating of last night's polka."[92]

When wet nurses indulged in ice cream and oysters it provoked an outburst; when nursing mothers disobeyed dietary orders, physicians may not have learned of their transgressions, or, if they knew about them, felt free to act upon them. Charlotte Perkins Gilman, the feminist writer, described in her journal how she took ginger and gave up cocoa when her nursing infant suffered from indigestion. In another passage, she confessed a momentary disdain for the rules, writing that she had eaten a banana "defiantly."[93] Physicians who confronted such defiance had little recourse. Thomas Morgan Rotch, treating an infant suffering from colic and a failure to gain weight, demanded that the mother reduce the amount of protein in her diet. When she resisted, he ordered a wet nurse. The colic disappeared, but weight remained a problem and Rotch prescribed moderate exercise and a diet richer in fat. The wet nurse obeyed, and the problem was solved.[94] Mothers had the power to defy physicians, to threaten the health of babies, and to frustrate attempts to bring order to the nursery. In the end, physicians could do little to bring them in line. The criticisms doctors

90 Daniel E. Sutherland, *Americans and Their Servants: Domestic Service in the United States from 1800 to 1920* (Baton Rouge: Louisiana State University Press, 1981), p. 113; and "Domestic Service," *Harpers Bazaar* 8 (1874): 284.
91 On eating for two, see Buckingham, "Wet Nursing," p. 274; and the popular guidebook by David Wark, *The Practical Home Doctor for Women* (New York: Gay Brothers, 1882), p. 425. Wark recommended hiring wet nurses with "good appetites and vigorous digestion."
92 Buckingham, "The Proper Treatment of Children," p. 303.
93 Journal of Charlotte Perkins Gilman, April 17 and May 5, 1885. SLRC. Charlotte Perkins Gilman, *The Living of Charlotte Perkins Gilman: An Autobiography by Charlotte Perkins Gilman* [reprint] (New York: Appleton-Century, 1935; New York: Harper & Row, 1975), pp. 88–9.
94 Rotch, *Pediatrics*, p. 211.

voiced about wet nurses undoubtedly carried an undertone of frustration with the families who hired them. Wet nurses, after all, could be and were dismissed when their transgressions were serious.

More threatening to an infant's health than a mother's indulgence in a banana or a wet nurse's dangerous choice of fruit cake and lobster salad was the use of drugs and alcohol. In the eighteenth and early nineteenth centuries, both physicians and families believed that spirits stimulated the supply and flow of milk. As temperance agitation increased, so did opposition to "poison" in the nursery.[95] In some instances, families retained a belief in the advantages of alcohol for nursing mothers (as well as for other members of the household) while doctors struggled to persuade them of their error. One nursing mother wrote to *Babyhood* magazine asking whether beer would improve her milk supply. No, she was assured, it would not. The wet nurse who drank, the respondent reminded her, would be dismissed.[96] In another discussion in the medical literature, Effa Davis accused employers of forcing wet nurses "to drink beer and take hearty foods."[97]

The greatest danger came not from the woman who drank beer to increase her own milk supply or who encouraged her wet nurse to do so, but from the secret tippler. In another letter to *Babyhood* a doctor detailed the misfortunes of a young infant intoxicated with "milk punch" by its wet nurse, who imbibed periodically from a hidden bottle of whiskey.[98] In this case, the stench of cheap alcohol made investigation of a clandestine drinker easy work. Similar tales appeared in other magazines. An anonymous correspondent to *Baby* recalled reading of an infant put in a "drunken stupor by drawing liquor-poisoned milk from the breast of a supposedly trustworthy wet nurse."[99] Notably, doctors understood the use of alcohol partly as a means of quieting a baby. When mothers drank, it was because they were ill advised. For wet nurses, drinking was a character flaw.

A similar double standard appeared in descriptions of women who used soothing syrups made of laudanum, paregoric, or other narcotics to ease the nursling's pain from teething or colic. The syrups stupefied the infants

95 T. D. Crothers, "Alcoholic Heredity in Diseases of Children," *Journal of the American Medical Association* 15 (1890): 531–3.

96 C. E. W., "Beer for the Nursing Mother," *Babyhood* 21 (1905): 174. Belief in the lactogenic value of beer may have been more important than any physiological property. Psychoanalyst Helene Deutsch reported on a case in 1945 in which a Polish wet nurse was unable to produce milk unless she received a full quart of beer. Helene Deutsch, *The Psychology of Women: A Psychoanalytic Interpretation*, vol. 2 (New York: Grune & Stratton, 1944–5), p. 280.

97 Davis, "Maternal Feeding," p. 774.

98 Will H. Wall, "A Young Doctor's Report on a Case of 'Milk Punch' at Three Months," *Babyhood* 2 (1885–6): 177. See also "Shall I Keep a Nurse-Maid?" *Baby* 3 (1905): 55; and Winters, "Relative Influences," p. 510.

99 "Shall I Keep a Nurse-Maid?" p. 55.

and, unlike alcohol, left no telltale scent on a woman's breath. As they did in the case of mothers who failed to follow dietary orders or who drank, physicians restrained their criticisms, viewing the use of the nostrums by mothers as misguided efforts to help an infant in pain. Infant nurses and wet nurses, by comparison, came under heavy criticism when they dispensed the same drugs. After all, they were assumed to lack any maternal attachment to the infants. "All sorts of deceptions are practiced by the wet nurse," wrote F. H. Getchell, who, in a sop to his fellow practitioners, added that it was "common for physicians to extract confessions about the administration of drugs when the mother had no suspicions."[100] Getchell's account underscores that it was no longer the vigilant mother who was assigned to watch over the wet nurse, it was the doctor.

Beyond the understandable concerns about diet, drink, and drugs that troubled doctors lay murky questions regarding the influence of passion, heredity, and character on milk. Many antebellum physicians believed that strong emotions made milk toxic. Legends passed among professionals telling of mothers and wet nurses who had witnessed acts of violence, engaged in sexual intercourse, or otherwise become excited. When the babies began to nurse, they fell into convulsions and died shortly thereafter. George Napheys provided a dramatic account in 1864 of a woman who "came out from a ball-room" and nursed her three-month-old baby. He was "taken with spasms two hours after and since is a confirmed idiot and epileptic."[101] Viewed from a distance, such accounts can be interpreted as efforts to decipher otherwise inexplicable seizures. As physician Annie Hale succinctly noted, "Fatal convulsions in the infant, which could not be traced to any other cause, have been known to follow a period of intense excitement in the nurse."[102] Another doctor warned that "thin, bloodless, nervous, peevish, fretful, irritable women never make good nurses," adding, "infants who are fed from the breasts of such women never thrive, and they are especially liable to convulsive disorders."[103] Using more melodramatic language, J. Lewis Smith described how a "night in debauchery" ended in death.[104] Belief in emotion-poisoned

100 Getchell, *Maternal Management of Infancy*, p. 24. See also Griffith, *Care of Baby*, p. 177.
101 George H. Napheys, *The Physical Life of Women: Advice to the Maiden, Wife, and Mother* (New York: G. Maclean, 1864), pp. 215–16.
102 Hale, *Management of Children*, p. 22.
103 Wark, *Practical Home Doctor for Women and Children*, p. 424.
104 J. Lewis Smith, "Recent Improvements in Infant Feeding," *Transactions of the American Pediatric Society* 1 (1889): 89, quoted a "recent western medical journal" article about a wet nurse who "spent the night in debauchery and returned haggard and fatigued the following day. The baby took her breast, but was immediately seized with vomiting and purging, which ended fatally in a few hours." For a homeopathic text endorsing the view of emotion influencing milk, see Tullio Suzzara Verdi, *Maternity: A Popular Treatise for Young Wives and Mothers* (New York: J. B. Ford, 1878), p. 187.

milk left physicians in a quandary. Cautious professionals had to excuse flighty women and those predisposed to passion from suckling. This, in turn, made it necessary to resort either to artificial feeding or to a wet nurse with a placid temperament. If the wet nurse was chosen, she had to be kept from becoming agitated or sexually aroused. And policing her private behavior proved to be a difficult task.

Late nineteenth-century explanations of disease and disability incorporated complex, fluid, and overlapping notions of heredity, constitution, and environment. Thus, it was easy to attribute defects in an infant's character or health to the wet nurse. With no precise dichotomies of nature and nurture, similar problems suffered by wet-nursed children could be ascribed by one doctor to the wet nurse's influence on the nursery environment and by another to the fact that her milk had become "effervesced" and denatured by emotion. Retrospective diagnosis also allowed attribution of adult character flaws to childhood exposure to a dissolute wet nurse.

Physicians and families viewed heredity as a dynamic force, influencing development from the time of conception through weaning.[105] Some believed that children literally drank up their wet nurses' moral and physical imperfections and that their "temper and disposition" were "molded in great measure by the state of the nurse's mind."[106] In addition to their faith in the inheritability of acquired characteristics, many subscribed to gendered theories of endowment with women bequeathing their emotions and men their analytical capabilities.[107] A child's character, accordingly, might be created by the milk of the wet nurse. Mary Terhune narrated the story of a girl said to be "remarkably dissimilar" from other members of her family, with "rough skin, corpulent frame, harsh voice, and loud laugh," and vulgar traits, such as "a liking for tobacco and spirits and a relish for broad wit and low company." Her relatives and acquaintances whispered that as an infant she had been "put to nurse by a fat Irish woman."[108] In a similar vein, physician Joseph Edcil Winters explained the "secretive disposition" of one youngster with reference to an Italian wet nurse. He

---

105 Charles E. Rosenberg, "The Bitter Fruit: Heredity, Disease and Social Thought," in Charles E. Rosenberg, ed., *No Other Gods: On Science and American Social Thought* (Baltimore: Johns Hopkins University Press, 1976), p. 27. See also T. W. Glenister, "Fantasies, Facts, and Faetuses," *Medical History* 8 (1964): 15–30; and Napheys, *Physical Life of Women*, p. 216.

106 Cooper, *Healthy Children*, p. 27.

107 Charles E. Rosenberg, "Factors in the Development of Genetics in the United States: Some Suggestions," *Journal of the History of Medicine and Allied Sciences* 22 (1967): 33; and Carroll Smith-Rosenberg and Charles Rosenberg, "The Female Animal: Medical and Biological Views of Women and Her Role in Nineteenth Century America," *Journal of American History* 60 (1973): 337.

108 Terhune, *Eve's Daughters*, pp. 30–2. For a general discussion of the problem, see John S. Haller, Jr., and Robin M. Haller, *The Physician and Sexuality in Victorian America* (New York: Norton, 1977), p. 134.

also told of twins with diametrically opposed traits. As the reader would easily anticipate, the twin with "evil habits" had been wet nursed. Finally, Winters reported that a medical student had told him that one of his brothers had been nursed by an Irish woman and exhibited "very decided Irish traits, which are so marked that they are noticed by all the friends of the family."[109] Needless to say, only problem personalities betrayed the influence of wet nurses. The medical literature remained silent about the wet-nursed children who grew to adulthood as the most pious, industrious, charitable, or financially successful members of their families.

Theories of lactational heredity meshed easily with the nativist sentiment of the urban North. Apprehensive over the likelihood of training new Americans to adopt Anglo-Saxon traits, many critics expressed deep concern that foreigners, including foreign-born wet nurses, were corrupting society.[110] In the South, with its history of cross-race wet nursing, a more restricted view of heredity prevailed. Southern families believed that a child's personality was inherited from its parents. Thus, the wet nurse could neither endow a child's character with her milk nor influence its development simply through her close and constant contact. Caught in the trap of racial thinking, Southerners eschewed both environmental explanations and those of lactational endowment, adopting a more circumscribed notion of heredity.

One did not have to be a white Southerner, however, to see the logical limitations of lactational heredity. If the milk of a wet nurse could give a child a loud laugh or a secretive disposition, what kind of influence would be derived from the milk of a goat or a cow? In attempting to put to rest older notions of heredity, pediatrician John Price Crozer Griffith argued by analogy, even as he recognized the persistence of old suspicions:

There is no more possibility of a baby imbibing the character of the nurse through the milk which she gives, much as we hear this talked about, than there is a danger of the child learning to "moo" because it is fed on cow's milk.[111]

By admitting that the subject was still much discussed, Griffith demonstrated that the diffusion of new scientific explanations of disease had failed to eradicate old beliefs regarding milk-borne heredity and the threat of emotion-poisoned milk.

109 Winters, "Relative Influences," p. 513. A more general explanation appeared in Verdi, *Maternity,* p. 187.
110 Mark H. Haller, *Eugenics: Hereditarian Attitudes in American Thought* (New Brunswick: Rutgers University Press, 1963), p. 53.
111 J. P. Crozer Griffith, *The Care of the Baby,* 2d ed. rev. (Philadelphia: W. B. Saunders, 1899), p. 186. Griffith was, perhaps, the most pragmatic of the physicians who wrote about wet nursing. On the question of morality, for example, he noted in his first edition, "We are not seeking examples of morality or instrumenting rewards for virtue or punishment for crimes, simply trying to obtain a suitable manufacturer of milk." Ibid., p. 178.

Even as medical professionals and members of the public began to diverge in their respective beliefs about heredity, they continued to share a faith in moral contamination – the belief that wet nurses could and did harm an infant or family merely by their presence. As immoral women drawn from the ranks of the destitute, wet nurses posed problems in the household as well as in the nursery. Thus some doctors portrayed them as invaders in the nursery, destined to destroy the moral universe of the families they served. The most vehement expression of this attitude came from Dr. I. N. Love, who, in 1889, proclaimed it better for an infant to die than for its family to be corrupted:

I recall an experience in my own family – a danger to which my little daughter of seven would have been exposed to by contact with a moral leper, recommended to us as a healthy wet-nurse for our infant boy. Better by far for the latter to have been wafted to the angels than for our first-born to have breathed the same air for a day with the moral monster in the shape of a wet nurse.[112]

Despite his colorful name, Love was neither a religious crusader nor a marginal sectarian. A vice-president of the American Medical Association, he held the chair of clinical medicine and diseases of children at Marion-Sims College of Medicine in St. Louis, and his statement appeared in an article published in the prestigious *Archives of Pediatrics*. Known as a speaker who "held his classes in rapt attention," Love's writing, at least in this instance, was equally engaging.[113] He articulated what many physicians felt about the wet nurses they encountered in the course of their work, and he spoke as well for others of the upper classes who feared those beneath them. In public life, the well-off could erect barriers between themselves and the lower orders. At home, masters and servants had to sleep under the same roof, albeit with the latter living in garret rooms. More ominously, wet nurses often shared a bed with their sucklings.

Other customs and needs differentiated domestic workers from wet nurses. Servants traditionally provided character references and, so long as they remained employed, were considered to be of the "worthy poor." Wet nurses typically had no one to attest to their character other than the matrons of rescue homes or other private charities. Furthermore, their residence in such facilities – and in municipal homes for the destitute – marked them as members of the "vicious poor." In attempting to sift out the most dangerous, physicians employed the same crude measure as moral reformers. A woman with one illegitimate child could be hired; she had made a "mistake." Two or more such children signaled depravity.[114] Still,

112 I. N. Love, "The Problem of Infant Feeding – Intestinal Diseases of Children and Cholera Infantum," *Archives of Pediatrics* 6 (1889): 585.
113 On Love see "Retirement of Dr. I. N. Love from Marion-Sims College, St. Louis," *Journal of the American Medical Association* 27 (1896): 393.
114 See, for example Griffith, *Care of the Baby*, p. 178.

in the eyes of some observers, the family that accepted an unmarried mother into the home made a compromise. According to the standards of Love and others, even wet nurses who willingly fulfilled their duties, who brought their sucklings back from the brink of death, and who followed faithfully the regimen laid down by the doctors nevertheless soiled the homes in which they resided.

Denunciations of wet nurses, heavily laden with the rhetoric of moral pollution, contrasted vividly with the measured scientific descriptions of artificial feeding. Underlying the doctors' invective was no doubt the recognition that physicians could mediate but not fully control relations in the household. Even with the careful selection of the wet nurse and the creation of a strict work regimen there remained too many possibilities for dietary anarchy, nights of debauchery, or secret indulgence in drugs or drink. In describing wet nurses, doctors turned again and again to the metaphors of the cow and the devil. Frank S. Churchill, editor-in-chief of the *American Journal of Diseases of Children,* labeled wet nurses "one quarter cow and three quarters devil."[115] John Lovett Morse, professor of pediatrics at Harvard Medical School, recalled a colleague who referred to them as "one part cow and nine parts devil."[116] The ratios seem unconscious reflections of professional confidence in scientific infant feeding – the more reliable the bottle became, the more satanic the wet nurse appeared.[117]

On the surface, late nineteenth-century complaints about wet nurses had much in common with those voiced many decades earlier. But the actual situation was far different. Infant nurseries had been medicalized, infant feeding had been scientized, and the wet nurse marketplace had been modernized. Both Churchill and Morse acknowledged as much, aware that the wet nurse was needed in fewer and fewer situations. When Morse granted that "a mother should be willing to submit to any amount of annoyance and inconvenience in order to save the life of her child," he did so because "it is usually possible to dispense with a wet nurse."[118]

Usually, but not always. Physicians, struggling to gain the trust of patients and manage difficult infant-feeding problems, found they could not entirely dispense with wet nurses. And wet nurses, hired because of a family's desperate situation, found they had enormous opportunities to save lives or destroy households.

115 Frank S. Churchill, "Infant Feeding," *Chicago Medical Record* 10 (1896): 104.
116 John Lovett Morse, "The Feeding of Infants," *American Journal of Nursing* [reprint] (1901): 3.
117 Or, as Mrs. Dr. Gleason, who wrote for a popular audience, remarked, "We prefer to treat our babies to a good cow rather than a bad woman." Mrs. Dr. Gleason, "How to Treat the Sick: Feeding of Infants," *Herald of Health* 49 (1870): 136–7.
118 Churchill, "Infant Feeding," p. 104; and Morse, "The Feeding of Infants," p. 3.

6

"Obliged to have wet nurses": Relations in the private household, 1870–1925

The decline of wet nursing in the late nineteenth century reflected advances in artificial feeding, shifting cultural beliefs regarding motherhood, and new employment opportunities for women previously hired as wet nurses. Artificial feeding became the first choice of many middle-class women, as Rima Apple has explained, not only because it was easier, safer, and cheaper than wet nursing but also because it was promoted and used in the context of the maternal ideology known as scientific motherhood.[1]

As America industrialized, child rearing became a home industry for middle-class women. Even as the percentage of single women who participated in the labor force soared and the number of women professionals expanded in occupations such as teaching and nursing, motherhood continued to be judged women's most vital career.[2] The cultural significance of motherhood gained strength from women's collective action. Female reform organizations stressed improving society to make a better world for children – an ideology that historians would call "domestic feminism."[3] The Women's Christian Temperance Union, founded in 1873 and one of the most visible and successful women's organizations of the nineteenth century, used the slogan "home protection" in its battle against the evils of alcohol. Other women's groups sailed in the same direction: making better

---

1 Rima D. Apple, *Mothers and Medicine: A Social History of Infant Feeding, 1890–1950* (Madison: University of Wisconsin Press, 1987), p. 97 and passim.
2 By 1900, 21 percent of women over sixteen were in the paid labor force, comprising 18 percent of the entire labor force. Lynn Y. Weiner, *From Working Girl to Working Mother: The Female Labor Force in the United States, 1820–1920* (Chapel Hill: University of North Carolina Press, 1985), p. 5 and passim. See also Alice Kessler-Harris, *Out to Work: A History of Wage-Earning Women in the United States* (New York: Oxford University Press, 1982), pp. 108–41.
3 On domestic feminism see Catherine Clinton, *The Other Civil War: American Women in the Nineteenth Century* (New York: Hill & Wang, 1984), pp. 40–53. Whereas most scholars link domestic feminism to female reform organizations active in the late nineteenth century, particularly the temperance movement, a few link it to Progressive Era movements of the early twentieth century. See Glenda Riley, *Inventing the American Woman: A Perspective on Women's History* (Arlington Heights, Ill.: Harlan Davidson, 1986), p. 160.

children and better homes their collective destination. Among the largest organizations with this goal were the General Federation of Women's Clubs, an umbrella group organized in 1890, whose numerous constituent members engaged in programs of domestic welfare, and the National Congress of Mothers, which was founded in 1897 to support the education of mothers and to expand the relationship between the child and the state. Other women who joined the domestic feminism movement did so not by participating in organizations but simply through their efforts to rear their children and run their households according to scientific precepts. Surveying the myriad attempts to make motherhood a profession, Hannah Whitall Smith, author of *The Science of Motherhood* (1894) encapsulated the ideology of scientific motherhood as well as revealed its class and racial biases when she wrote that nothing was "more important for the improvement of the Anglo-Saxon race than the fact that in all English-speaking countries the science of motherhood is being studied and taught as never before."[4]

Scientific motherhood encompasses both the material condition and the ideological construction of women's domestic roles in the late nineteenth and early twentieth centuries. In practice, it linked the home and the marketplace as well as public reform and private action. In material terms, it referred to the use of new products and technologies, from ready-made clothing and preserved foodstuffs to modern appliances and indoor plumbing. As a value system, it referenced the belief that science and technology could be applied by women to the rearing of children, just as they were being applied in the factory and large organizations.

Science entered the private domain not only through the efforts of women and the actions of the marketplace but also via expert advice. In child rearing this meant, of course, the advice of physicians. Scientific mothers were expected to follow the recommendations of doctors, to rear their children according to modern rules of hygiene, and to supervise nurseries rationally and effectively. At home, in the nursery, women worked hard to banish germs and to prepare formulas according to precise specifications.[5]

Although explicit, the demands of scientific motherhood were also illusive. Even as scientific motherhood offered women new options, it burdened them with new responsibilities and expectations, some of which they could not meet. Careful attention to hygiene and health could not prevent infants and children from becoming sick and dying. Despite public and private health measures to lower mortality rates, nearly one-fifth of all

4 Hannah Whitall Smith, *The Science of Motherhood* [microfilm] (New York: Revell, 1894), pp. 8–9.
5 Andrew McClary, "Germs are Everywhere: The Germ Threat as Seen in Magazine Articles, 1890–1920," *Journal of American Culture* 3 (1980): 33–46; and Nancy Tomes, "The Private Side of Public Health: Sanitary Science, Domestic Hygiene, and the Germ Theory, 1870–1900," *Bulletin of the History of Medicine* 64 (1990): 509–39.

American infants born in 1900 died before their first birthdays.[6] Among the middle and upper classes, falling birthrates seemed to intensify the pressure to ensure that children survived. Thus, in the domestic arena, scientific motherhood was often a struggle against death.[7]

One who waged battle and lost was Julia Carpenter. Her efforts to feed her infant son illustrate both the range and the limits of the options available in the late nineteenth century. In 1888, Carpenter moved from her home in rural South Dakota into Aberdeen seeking a wet nurse for her boy.[8] She had tried a variety of infant foods, including cow's milk, condensed milk, and various formulas, before relocating to town. There, she arranged for her son to be wet-nursed during the day and fed him condensed milk at night. Following a cardinal principle of scientific motherhood, Carpenter made her decisions about infant feeding in consultation with experts. She sought help first from a nurse and later from three physicians, each of whom offered a different piece of advice. None of them had the solution to her son's feeding problems. James Carpenter was buried at the age of eight months.

Many women experienced situations similar to Carpenter's and hired wet nurses in the wake of problems with the artificial feeding of their children. In doing so, they were forced to reconcile their desire to be a scientific mother with their need to rely on an arrangement that, by its very nature, seemed to defy all that was meant by science.

The language with which women described their encounters with wet nurses differed substantially from the medical narratives. Physicians' discussions were typically laced with judgments about the class and character of women who earned their livelihood as wet nurses. Their case reports often described acts of venality that had been cleverly ferreted out by the doctor just in the nick of time. In these accounts, the doctors acted as critical intermediaries, conveying their scientific expertise into the domestic arena. Essentially, the medical literature valorized doctors, demonized wet nurses, and marginalized families. In popular narratives, however, a different story was told. Women saw themselves as the lead actors. Although

---

6 Samuel H. Preston and Michael R. Haines, *Fatal Years: Child Mortality in Late Nineteenth-Century America* (Princeton: Princeton University Press, 1991), p. 3.
7 On infant mortality, the infant welfare movement, and the growth of scientific motherhood, see Nancy Schrom Dye and Daniel Blake Smith, "Mother Love and Infant Death, 1750–1920," *Journal of American History* 73 (1986): 329–53.
8 "Prairie Croquet," *To All Inquiring Friends: Letters, Diaries and Essays in North Dakota, 1880–1910,* Elizabeth Hampsten, comp., (Grand Forks: Department of English, University of North Dakota, 1980), p. 244. See also Elizabeth Hampsten, *Read This Only to Yourself: The Private Writings of Midwestern Women, 1880–1910* (Bloomington: Indiana University Press, 1982), pp. 205–7.

they consulted with medical experts, they judged their own actions and reactions as the pivotal events.

Vital discussions of wet nurses appeared in the pages of popular magazines and did so in two distinct forms: articles on child rearing and infant care and letters to advice columnists. The former were similar in content and style to the medical literature. A typical example, a piece entitled "Pertinent Questions," appeared in *Baby* magazine in 1905. On the subject of wet nursing, the anonymous author supplied the standard medical line:

> Unfortunately for all concerned, it is not easy to procure a satisfactory wet nurse. Women who go out in this capacity often are of low moral status; others unhealthy, and some intemperate. If, however, we can find a perfectly healthy woman who is moral we have, indeed, a wet nurse who is a veritable jewel.[9]

Following this backhanded acknowledgment of the usefulness of wet nurses was a detailed description of cow's milk and its modification for use in the nursery.

Letters from mothers as well as other popular accounts revealed similar sentiments but diverged from the medical accounts in three ways. First, employers focused on their immediate situation. Unlike physicians, who judged wet nurses collectively and weighed their presumptive value against that of artificial infant foods, women forced to hire wet nurses cared only that their children survived. Second, as had been the case in the eighteenth and early nineteenth centuries, employers' expectations of wet nurses were informed by ideas about domestic service as well as by medical science. Once the wet nurse came on duty she was judged not only against the usefulness of artificial foods but also against the standard of the ideal servant. That is, she had both to save the life of the infant and to fit satisfactorily into the domestic environment – her good health and good milk were not enough to mark her as ideal. Third, women questioned how well wet nurses treated their charges and discovered in a few instances what doctors did not: that a genuine affection could develop between a woman and her suckling.

A detailed account of a woman struggling to master her wet nurses appeared in a letter from Fanny Bullock Workman to *Babyhood* magazine in 1886. In it, Workman described her experiences with two wet nurses whom she judged largely in terms of their skill as servants.[10] A resident of Worcester, Massachusetts, Workman was the wife of a physician and the daughter of a former governor. She would become an accomplished author, explorer, and mountain climber who set world records for ascents

9 "Pertinent Questions," *Baby* 3 (1905): 45.
10 Fanny B. Workman, "The Wet-Nurse in the Household," *Babyhood* 2 (1886): 142–4.

and won acclaim for her conquest of glaciers.[11] Thus her description of how she was almost brought to her knees by two wet nurses seems particularly compelling. Her letter demonstrates the temporary power held by wet nurses and why women might judge artificial feeding a better choice. Moreover, Workman's account displays the circumscribed role of physicians in the household.

Workman employed a wet nurse reluctantly. Evidently unable to breast-feed, she tried artificial feeding for three weeks but her infant daughter lost weight and suffered from indigestion. Two physicians, an "older very experienced" doctor and a younger one, recommended a wet nurse. Although both offered the same suggestion, only the younger doctor had some sympathy for the trepidation she felt, whereas the elder merely "smiled blandly as upon a spoiled child" and attempted to calm her fears with stories of faithful wet nurses, including a tale of one woman who became a close friend of her employer. It was an unusual statement. Standard medical opinion held wet nurses in low esteem, hardly qualified by class or character to become confederates of their mistresses.

Employers typically viewed wet nurses as they did all servants – as potentially malevolent influences on their children.[12] Writing to *Babyhood* about child nurses, correspondent Alice P. Carter articulated the problem succinctly:

Why then should they be especially fitted to bring up the children of the upper-class of this country? We do not consider that the best of them are exactly proper social companions for ourselves and husbands. Why then should they be the sole companions of our little children?

The answer, which Carter clearly knew, was that mothers of means could not or would not rear their children entirely on their own. Even she conceded that a mother with several children "will of course need help."[13] Nevertheless, families remained leery of individuals who came from the lower orders.

Help in the nursery could take several forms: nursery maids, trained

11 Elizabeth Knowlton, "Fanny Bullock Workman," Edward T. James, ed., *Notable American Women*, vol. 3 (Cambridge: Belknap Press, 1971), pp. 672–4. Examples of Workman's books, which were written with her husband, William Hunter Workman, M.D., are *In the Ice World of Himalaya: Among the Peaks and Passes of Ladakh, Nubra, Suru, and Baltistan* (London: Unwin, 1900); *Ice-Bound Heights of the Mustagh: An Account of Two Seasons of Pioneer Exploration and High Climbing in the Baltistan Himalaya* (New York: C. Scribner's, 1908); *Peaks and Glaciers of Nun Kun: A Record of Pioneer-Exploration and Mountaineering in the Punjab Himalaya* (London: Constable, 1909); and *Two Summers in the Ice-Wilds of Eastern Karakoram: The Exploration of Nineteen Hundred Square Miles of Mountain and Glacier* (London: Unwin, 1917).
12 Faye E. Dudden, *Serving Women: Household Service in Nineteenth-Century America* (Middletown, Conn.: Wesleyan University Press, 1983), pp. 147–54.
13 Alice P. Carter, "Mothers and Nurses," *Babyhood* 13 (1897): 114.

nurses, and wet nurses. Nursery maids, functioning essentially as domestics assigned to care for children, received little respect from employers or physicians and little pay when their lengthy workday was taken into account.[14] Doctors complained about them as they did about wet nurses, writing of rescuing babies from their ignorance and cautioning that they could convey infectious diseases.[15] Heading the list of maladies were tuberculosis and syphilis.[16]

Trained nurses were, by contrast, the most highly regarded nursery workers because of their education – they were graduates of hospital nursing schools – and because they had been taught to follow the rules laid down by doctors. In many situations physicians viewed them as allies, open to instruction, capable of making the family obey medical direction, and adept at artificial feeding. Physicians sometimes helped place their favorite nurses into positions or referred families to the local nurse registry.[17] Formal medical recognition also came as the authors of advice manuals acknowledged their expanding role. Luther Emmett Holt's catechism on the care and feeding of children, for example, explicitly addressed both mothers and children's nurses.[18]

As skilled, typically native-born professionals, trained nurses rejected the role of servant. Yet they entered the home in an ambiguous position, unsuited to eat in the kitchen with other household help but unwelcome at the family table.[19] One form of compensation for this slight was their pay; they received much higher wages than wet nurses. Nevertheless, their annual income remained relatively low because of the long stretches between jobs. Wages for trained nurses in Philadelphia in the late 1890s

14 One study of domestic workers found that nurses had the longest working day, with 22 percent employed in excess of twelve hours a day. Lucy Maynard Salmon, *Domestic Service* (New York, MacMillan, 1897; New York: Arno Press, 1972), Table XII – "Average Weekly and Daily Wages By Occupations," p. 96; Table XIII – "Classified Weekly Wages By Occupation," p. 97; Table XIV – "Average Weekly Wages By Occupation," p. 97; and Table XIX – "Actual Daily Working Hours," p. 144.

15 See, for example, Thomas Morgan Rotch, "The Value of Milk Laboratories for the Advancement of Our Knowledge of Artificial Feeding," *Journal of the American Medical Association* 18 (1897): 56.

16 Louis Fischer, *Diseases of Infancy and Childhood, Their Dietetic, Hygienic, and Medical Treatment: A Text-book Designed for Practitioners and Students in Medicine*, 2d ed. (Philadelphia: F. A. Davis, 1908), p. 21.

17 Vern L. Bullough and Bonnie Bullough, *The Care of the Sick: The Emergence of Modern Nursing* (New York: Prodist, 1978), pp. 149–52; and Susan M. Reverby, *Ordered to Care: The Dilemma of American Nursing, 1850–1945* (New York: Cambridge University Press, 1987), pp. 95–117.

18 L. Emmett Holt, *The Care and Feeding of Children: A Catechism for the Use of Mothers and Children's Nurses* (New York: D. Appleton, 1894).

19 On nativity see Carroll D. Wright, *The Working Girls of Boston* (Boston: Wright & Potter, 1889; New York: Arno, 1969), Table I, pp. 6–11. On dining see Susan M. Reverby, "'Neither for the Drawing Room nor for the Kitchen': Private Duty Nursing in Boston, 1873–1920," in Judith Walzer Leavitt, ed., *Women and Health in America: Historical Readings* (Madison: University of Wisconsin Press, 1984), pp. 454–66.

ranged from fifteen to twenty dollars per week; in Boston they were twenty to twenty-five dollars, and in New York, five dollars higher.[20] Compared to wet nurses, who earned twenty to thirty dollars per month, trained nurses were an enormous expense, and one that few families could afford.

Families did not, of course, hire wet nurses for reasons of economy but because they provided something no other employee could: human milk. Nonetheless, their work was structurally similar to that of a nursery maid or a trained nurse: they cared for babies, and they oversaw their feeding. This dual demand made perfect sense, but set up standards of judgment that were inherently in conflict. An employer had to fire a woman whose milk was insufficient or unsuitable even if she satisfactorily cared for an infant and would have made a perfectly good nursery maid. At the same time she had to keep on her payroll the woman with good milk but bad work habits.

This was the situation in the Workman home, where the wet nurse, dubbed "Irish Mary," retained her position in spite of serious problems. According to Workman, Mary never learned how to care for her suckling and, on one occasion, put the child in mortal danger. Workman had observed her standing in the middle of the street, holding the baby, and staring at a rapidly oncoming carriage. Workman's complaint about Mary's lack of knowledge echoed that of many physicians. Conflating immorality with ignorance, pediatrician Rowland Godfrey Freeman alleged that "unmarried mothers are women of a low grade of intelligences," and, as a result, they "cannot be trusted to care for the baby on account of ignorance or unreliability."[21]

Although intellectually limited in Workman's eyes, Mary apparently made up for this shortcoming with a charismatic personality. She manipulated the cook into providing her with forbidden foods – tea, ice water, and pickles – and she also, in Workman's word, "contaminated" the other servants. Workman fired her cook for disobedience, but kept Mary on in a classic case of the employers' nightmare: the wet nurse disobeyed but went unpunished because the infant needed her milk.

Mary, it seemed, could make Workman dance to any tune she played. After only six weeks in the Workman home, she announced her intention to resign, throwing the household into a frenzy. According to domestic

20 Reverby, *Ordered to Care,* p. 98; and Nancy Tomes, " 'Little World of Our Own': The Pennsylvania Hospital Training School for Nurses, 1895–1907," in Leavitt, *Women and Health,* p. 474. On p. 102 Reverby notes that untrained nurses earned five to ten dollars a week less. A study of working women in Boston found the average weekly earnings for nurses was $9.50, compared to $4.96 for domestic servants. Wright, *Working Girls of Boston,* pp. 76–7.
21 Roland Godfrey Freeman, *Elements of Pediatrics for Medical Students,* (New York: MacMillan, 1917), pp. 138–9.

advisors, threatening to leave was a favorite ploy among servants to gain the upper hand.[22] In this case, however, it was not a blackmail attempt to secure a wage increase but a necessity: Mary's baby had fallen ill and she wished to be with her child. Workman successfully dissuaded her from leaving and arranged for the child to be brought to her. Subsequently, a place in the countryside was found for the infant, and Mary was permitted to go and visit. Unfortunately, after only two weeks the caretaker declared she could no longer assume responsibility for the baby. After learning of this, Mary became distraught and insisted on having the child with her. This was not to be; Mary's excessive worries about her baby soon spoiled her milk and she lost her job. In the end, it was the quantity and quality of her milk that determined her status in the household.

A week after Mary's departure Workman found a replacement, a wet nurse she never referred to by name, but who might well have been called Irish Mary the Second. The woman resembled her predecessor in a number of ways, including her background, her adjudged lack of intelligence, and her concern for her own baby. The new employee claimed to be an Englishwoman but soon revealed her true origins when she opened her mouth and spoke in "broad Irish." Although the wet nurse was healthy, Workman found her appearance unattractive and referred to her face as having a "most heavy, unintelligent mould." Consequently, the wet nurse required constant observation.

Particularly troublesome for Workman was the woman's abiding concern for the well-being of her own child. Informed that she could not bring her baby with her, she had turned a deaf ear to that declaration and shown up for work with her infant. Workman stood her ground, and apparently the woman arranged to have her child boarded. Two weeks later her infant died. Workman, ever mindful of the needs of her own infant, feared that the death would upset the wet nurse and spoil her milk. She therefore prevailed upon her to forgo the funeral. In an attempt to console her, Workman sent the woman to the seashore.

Though she had been a participant in the exchange of infant lives, Workman remained immune from either guilt or gratitude. The wet nurse, however, clearly understood her own sacrifice – as her subsequent behavior demonstrated. The brief vacation marked a turning point; rather than ease her heartache, her day at the seashore marked the beginning of an extended rebellion. The opening salvo was a simple indulgence in some forbidden pleasures: cucumbers and ice cream. From that day forward, Workman could not control the wet nurse's diet. When the Workman family went to the seashore for several months of vacation, tensions height-

---

22 See, for example, Harriet Prescott Spofford, *The Servant Girl Question* (Boston: Houghton, Mifflin, 1881; New York: Arno Press, 1977), pp. 34–5.

ened. Workman ordered the woman "substantial, nourishing meals," but she left them untouched and gratified her hunger with peanuts, cake, and ice cream.

Physicians assumed kitchen clashes represented the wet nurse's attempt to climb the social ladder, but Workman's experience reveals something far different. Her wet nurse did not want to eat as her employers did; she preferred to eat what she chose for herself. It was a form of self-assertion that emerged in the wake of her child's death and seemed to be about loss, not class. Whatever its source, the mealtime contest quickly escalated into a larger battle, as the wet nurse tested the limits of Workman's tolerance by nursing her suckling irregularly. When the baby lost weight, the wet nurse lost her job.

Workman never associated the wet nurse's rebellious behavior with the death of the woman's child, even though the defiance began the day she missed the funeral. Indeed, Workman seems to have assumed that the matter was of little consequence. Perhaps, like Harriet Smith of Rockdale, Workman thought that poor women lacked the capacity to grieve for their children. It was a theory given some credence by doctors, but for a seemingly different reason. Charles E. Buckingham argued that the wet nurse's suckling "very soon becomes more dear than her own" and that, as a result, "the death of her own child, which frequently happens as a consequence, disturbs her but very little."[23] It is unclear whether Buckingham was reporting his actual observations or attempting to rationalize the all-too-frequent exchange of infant lives that wet nursing entailed. In the Workman case, the felicitous substitution of affections did not take place. The wet nurse clearly resented the cost of her employment.

To preserve the health of the Workman baby, one woman had sacrificed her child and another had nearly done so. Yet Workman had not an ounce of gratitude for either one. Instead, she reserved her accolades for Mellin's Food, which she used after the departure of the second wet nurse. She had apparently forgotten that in the earliest weeks of her daughter's life artificial food had been the problem, not the solution; she saw Mellin's Food as a triumph of artificial feeding over the vagaries of human milk and the difficulties of wet nurse management. Essentially, Workman's judgment rested on her own needs as well as those of her child. The wet nurses had required her "hourly superintendence" to insure that "the food the child received was not impure." Like her medical contemporaries, she ultimately compared the wet nurse to the cow and quickly saw the virtues of the latter: "It is not," she wrote, "affected by indulgence in peanuts, cucumbers and ice-cream."

A letter to *Trained Motherhood* in 1898 told a tale similar to Workman's

---

23 Charles E. Buckingham, "Wet Nursing," *Boston Medical and Surgical Journal* 16 (1875): 244.

and with a similar emphasis on the role of the mother rather than the doctor as the defender of a baby's health.[24] The correspondent, anonymously identified as Interested Reader, reported hiring a wet nurse after her own milk had given out and after she had tried three different artificial mixtures: Just's Food, Mellin's Food, and Fairchild's Peptogenic Powder. The young German wet nurse she retained helped her baby regain its health and strength but failed at her job as a loyal and effective servant. She had a "violent and unmanageable temper," experienced "fits of ugliness," and, in addition, knew little about child care. Interested Reader reported that the woman worried about her own child, whom she was permitted to visit. She also claimed to have learned from another servant that the wet nurse did not want her own child to live. Still, the employer's main complaint concerned neither the wet nurse's motherly feelings nor her temper; instead, it was the wet nurse's wages that were "very hard for us to stand." Interested Reader's forbearance stemmed from the fact that she had already lost one baby and knew that the infant being wet-nursed had "nearly slipped away." Her question to the magazine's medical expert concerned weaning.

It is clear from the accounts of Workman and Interested Reader that both women desired medical advice yet viewed the doctor's role very narrowly. They and other women saw themselves as nursery administrators with ultimate responsibility for the welfare of their children. Part of their duty was to consult the proper advice givers, which included soliciting advice by writing to magazines. In such a forum, women heard from the medical experts and also from their peers. In some cases the letters columns in the magazines became informal mothers' clubs in which women could answer each other's queries and voice their own opinions along with the magazine's chosen experts.

Workman's letter, for example, touched a nerve in one *Babyhood* reader, who referred to it specifically when she wrote to ask for advice. Louise J., a resident of San Francisco, reported that she had fed her second child on artificial food, which she termed a "makeshift" solution, and that she had vowed that as long as she could afford to pay for a wet nurse and stand the "inevitable annoyances" she would do so.[25] Mellin's Food would not be, as it had been for Workman, the solution to her infant-feeding problems. Her query concerned the selection of wet nurses. She complained that professional guidance could not always be obtained and that popular books and periodicals yielded no useful information.

In reply, an unidentified respondent, obviously a physician, sought first to calm her fears, observing that Workman had experienced "exceptional

24 Interested Reader, "To the Doctor of *Trained Motherhood*," *Trained Motherhood* 3 (1898): 168–9.
25 Louise J. "The Selection of a Wet-Nurse," *Babyhood* 2 (1886): 245.

ill-luck."[26] The reply then summarized current medical thinking, reiterated old saws about mothers' obligation to breast-feed, and concluded with a few comments that might have been drawn from a textbook on household management. The author suggested that the wet nurse be forcefully disciplined, kept in the dark as to her importance, and made to feel in constant danger of losing her position if she neglected her duties. The woman who failed to take this hard line and made a "pet" of her wet nurse would soon reap "the harvest of her own folly." Only in conclusion did the anonymous expert address the question of wet nurse selection, rejecting the idea that women could do the job themselves. The "burden of the examination," the reply stated, could not "be properly assumed without professional knowledge."

What concerned Louise J. were obvious defects, not hidden diseases. She suspected that wet nurses lacked even "average mental or moral qualifications"; and the response she received supported her assumption. Wet nurses did not come from "the highly-intelligent classes" the expert attested, but added that few were "distinctly vicious." They were, however, women who had given birth out of wedlock. The reference to this fact by Louise J., who admitted at the outset that she intended to use wet nurses in the future, suggested that morality remained an intractable complaint – one that did not prevent a wet nurse from being hired, but one that also never ceased to cause concern. Like the drone of employers who complained about their lazy servants but could not live without them, the frequent references to the moral limits of wet nurses were overshadowed by the reality of their effectiveness. Both Louise J. and her respondent knew this.

The most active forum for scientific mothers, *Babyhood* magazine, was "Devoted Exclusively to the Care of Infants and Young Children, and the General Interests of the Nursery." It began publication in 1884, supplying expert advice to women who viewed child rearing as a highly demanding discipline. The magazine employed leading pediatricians to write articles and answer questions from readers. By 1885 it had earned an endorsement from the American Medical Association.[27] One of its editors, Leroy M. Yale, was a physician and at one time, a lecturer on diseases of children at Bellevue Hospital Medical College in New York City. The other editor was the domestic writer Mary Terhune, who had denounced wet nurses in her book *Eve's Daughters*. The prolific author of twenty-five

26 "The Selection of a Wet-Nurse," *Babyhood* 2 (1886): 245.
27 Daniel Beekman, *The Mechanical Baby: A Popular History of the Theory and Practice of Child Raising* (Westport, Conn.: L. Hill, 1977), p. 88. Physician J. P. Crozer Griffith, author of the popular guidebook for mothers, *Care of the Baby,*, thanked the editors of *Babyhood* for allowing him to use their files. It is possible that he used the queries sent to the magazine as a way of determining what mothers wanted to know. John Price Crozer Griffith, *Care of the Baby* 3d ed. rev. (Philadelphia: W. B. Saunders, 1904), p. 12. On the endorsement see [Book Review,] *Journal of the American Medical Association* 4 (1885): 472–3.

popular books on domestic matters, as well as twenty-five novels, Terhune (who published under the name Marion Harland) believed strongly in artificial feeding.[28] Not unexpectedly, when subscribers opened the pages of *Babyhood* or similar publications, they found a plethora of advertisements for commercially manufactured infant foods bordering the many articles about infant feeding. Terhune herself penned the advertising booklet for Carnrick's Soluble Food.[29]

Babyhood was one of many popular women's journals providing advice about child rearing in columns written by experts. The practice began with Edward Bok, editor of the *Ladies Home Journal*, who hired Elisabeth Robinson Scovil, a nurse, to answer questions posed by readers.[30] Other journals quickly followed suit. *Good Housekeeping* had an advice column, as did magazines aimed at mothers, such as *Trained Motherhood*, which began publication in 1897, and *Baby: A Monthly Magazine Devoted to the Care of Babies and Children: Medical, Moral, Mental and Physical*, which was inaugurated in 1904. When the subject of wet nurses arose in letters to the experts, the reply could easily be anticipated: a half-hearted endorsement that served as a prelude to an extended discussion of the alternatives. Anna M. Fullerton, the medical columnist for *Household News*, advised that when a "mother's milk utterly fails and a good wet nurse cannot be had, some substitute must be found."[31] A Professor Hartshorne wrote in *Housekeeper* that the healthy wet nurse was the "next best thing to mother's milk," but he devoted most of his discussion to bottle-feeding.[32] Similarly, an article in *Trained Motherhood* ignored the old-fashioned and unscientific wet nurse entirely, suggesting a substitute that was "as near as mother's milk as science can offer."[33] The columnists preached to the converted. Women who read popular mothercraft magazines and wrote to their resident experts stood in the vanguard of scientific motherhood.

Letters to magazines provide a way of appraising how employers viewed their wet nurses and a way of contrasting employers' assessments with those made by physicians. On the subject of wet nurse management, as the letters from Workman, Interested Reader, and Louise J. suggest, women and doctors were largely in agreement as to the problems but were divided on the issue of who bore responsibility for solving them. On medical questions, they were again divided, this time on the matter of what constituted the most substantive threats. Doctors focused on the diseases of wet

28 On Terhune see Merrit Cross, "Mary Virginia Hawes Terhune," James, *Notable American Women*, vol. 3, pp. 439–41.
29 Apple, *Mothers and Medicine*, p. 107.
30 James Playsted Wood, *Magazines in the United States*, 2d ed. (New York: Ronald Press, 1956), p. 110. Scovil published a book based on her responses to letters about infant care. Elisabeth Robinson Scovil, *A Baby's Requirements* (Philadelphia: 1892).
31 Anna M. Fullerton, "Artificial Feeding of Infants," *Household News* 4 (1896): 230.
32 Professor Hartshorne, "Infantile Diet," *Housekeeper* 1 (1875): 63.
33 "Infant Feeding," *Trained Motherhood* 7 (1900): 55.

nurses, whereas employers paid close attention to the quality of their milk. Letters evinced concerns that the wet nurse's emotional volatility either would be conveyed through her milk as a hereditary taint or would transform the milk into a lethal substance. Even as medical experts urged women to abandon such outmoded ideas, the letters suggest that many clung to them tenaciously.

Women's accounts were, overwhelmingly, distinguished by personalism: Women viewed wet nursing in terms of their own particular experiences, even as they listened to the collective judgments of others. This helps explain why wet nurses remained in private households even as the occupation of wet nursing came under increasing fire for being dangerous, anachronistic, and unscientific. Women who had successfully employed one wet nurse might see themselves as capable of employing others in the future. Women who had had disastrous experiences hiring wet nurses might be quite leery of doing so again but willing to take the risk if it proved necessary, believing that each experience was bound to be unique. Whereas doctors viewed wet nurses according to their collective characteristics, employers had double vision – seeing wet nurses both as a class and as a collection of individuals.

Personalism becomes visible in women's letters about morality. In general, the writers expressed concern about hiring women known to be unwed mothers. Writing in a time of growing fear of illegitimacy because of its public expense and in a context of the expanding reform efforts to protect single working girls and promote social purity, the correspondents could not overlook the status of most wet nurses.[34] Yet these wet nurses' out-of-wedlock pregnancies hardly tipped the scale when infants' lives hung in the balance. In these cases, mothers reached far different judgments than did mere observers.

Three methods of moral accounting appeared in a letter from N. N. to *Babyhood* magazine in 1887 – her own, that of her doctor, and that of her community. N. N. told readers how, after her milk had failed, she turned to her family physician for advice about hiring a wet nurse, only to meet with vehement opposition.[35] The doctor insistently recommended artificial feeding, a course she had tried before and found inadequate. N. N. protested that the doctor's objections to wet nurses were moral rather than medical. Here was a man "whose character we highly respect" but who "was swayed by prejudice." She acknowledged that many in her commu-

---

34 See Marian J. Morton, *And Sin No More: Social Policy and Unwed Mothers in Cleveland, 1855–1990* (Columbus: Ohio State University Press, 1993), p. 24 and passim; and Sheila M. Rothman, *Woman's Proper Place: A History of Changing Ideals and Practices, 1870 to the Present* (New York: Basic Books, 1978), pp. 74–85.
35 N. N., "The Moral Objections to Wet-Nurses," *Babyhood* 3 (1887): 314–15.

nity shared his antipathy to employing unmarried mothers, but she asked whether the doctor had misjudged his own role and the duty of a mother: "is it not the parents' first duty to preserve the life of the frail being that looks to them for protection and is it not the physician's first duty to offer them the best means of doing so?" Perhaps hoping to find others who shared her misgivings about the doctor's stance, she concluded by inviting "the opinions of *Babyhood*'s readers concerning the prevalence of these objections."

N. N.'s plea that the best interests of the child be the test for hiring a wet nurse evoked no response; the only replies came from women eager to contribute to the morals debate. Four letters appeared in the following issue, three of them in opposition to wet nurses. Although not a valid sample by any measure, the replies demonstrate how women grounded their perceptions in personal judgments rather than scientific findings, how they offered analysis of infant feeding steeped in moral rectitude as well as scientific motherhood, and how they conflated moral and medical concerns. More critically, the women who opposed wet nurses had never had a reason to use them.

One opponent, A. M. B. of Brooklyn, focused almost exclusively on the risk of giving the child a hereditary taint, which she saw as linked to the issue of illegitimacy.[36] She feared "a wet-nurse in whose family some terrible disease may be hereditary or, what is worse than disease or death, who is an immoral woman." What "Christian parents" she asked would imperil their offspring by placing them with a woman "who in nursing the child doubtless conveys to it a tendency to vulgarity and sin?" "Mater" of New Brighton, New York, shared A. M. B.'s fear of hereditary defects, but she viewed the question of illegitimacy with more sympathy.[37] Although she argued that "vicious tendencies" might be communicated by the milk of a wet nurse, she recognized that most of the women employed in the position were "more sinned against than sinning." However, Mater shared with the other correspondents the belief that wet nurses posed too great a risk; she declared herself appalled by the people who accepted wet nurses "almost without a murmur." Having been told that their unborn child was a "citizen in embryo" and that with modern knowledge they could "make of maternity a noble profession," many mothers stated they would never hand over their child to a woman who had betrayed their principles by bearing a child out of wedlock.[38]

36 A. M. B., "The Moral Objections to Wet-Nurses," *Babyhood* 3 (1887): 384.
37 The following discussion is based on Mater, "The Moral Objections to Wet-Nurses," *Babyhood* 3 (1887): 383.
38 James H. McKee and William H. Wells, *Practical Pediatrics: A Modern Clinical Guide in the Diseases of Infants and Children for the Family Physician*, vol. 1 (Philadelphia: P. Blakiston's Sons, 1914), p. 105.

Despite the efforts of physicians to refute theories of milkborne heredity and emotionally toxic milk, many women clung to both. A letter in *Trained Motherhood* from Mrs. Lanta Wilson Smith of Phoenix, Rhode Island, relayed the familiar nursery legend of an infant killed by excited milk.[39] The story she told came from "the Dakotas" and involved a wet nurse who went home for a visit, had a fight with her husband, and proceeded to nurse her own child as well as her suckling. Both babies died soon afterwards of convulsions.

Faith in lactational heredity also remained strong. A third *Babyhood* correspondent, "Materfamilias," of New York, shared with the readers the story of a child who grew

so like the nurse in expression and in little ways and mannerisms, that there could be no doubt that the milk she drank, being nothing less than the veritable blood of the wet nurse undoubtedly changed the character as well as the expression of the face.[40]

Her cautionary tale was not intended as an endorsement of artificial feeding. Instead, Materfamilias suggested that mothers endure any suffering necessary to breast-feed their offspring. She herself had done so and boasted proudly of not having "handed down to my poor innocent children, faults bred in a stranger's blood." In replying to N. N., Materfamilias, like other respondents, evaded the issue of whether the needs of the child counted more heavily than the sins of the wet nurse.

Whereas the vast majority of correspondents, as well physicians, assumed that wet nurses had borne children out of wedlock, one letter made clear that this was not necessarily the case. K. H., of Marshall, Michigan, reported that she had helped a married friend find work as a wet nurse after her friend's child had died.[41] Eager to earn money to pay the doctor's bills and with her husband earning very little as a journeyman shoemaker, the friend had K. H. answer an advertisement in the *New York Times*. The situation, K. H. asserted, was not uncommon. As a former resident of New York and Brooklyn, she claimed to have known many families who employed wet nurses in preference to the feeding bottle, and she attested that all had been respectable married women whose babies had died. Her letter opened a window into the largely invisible world of working-class wet nursing, in which married women continued, as they had in past decades, to turn their misfortune into opportunity.

Acknowledging the controversy stimulated by N. N.'s letter and the replies to it, *Babyhood* ran an unsigned article refuting a number of the ideas

39 Mrs. Lanta Wilson Smith, "To the Doctor of *Trained Motherhood*," *Trained Motherhood* 4 (1899): 37.
40 Materfamilias, "On the Moral Objections to Wet-Nurses," *Babyhood* 3 (1887): 384.
41 K. H., "The Moral Objections to Wet-Nurses," *Babyhood* 3 (1887): 383.

voiced by the opponents. Inadvertently siding with N. N., the author suggested that a strict morals test might prevent wet nurses from being employed under circumstances that absolutely required them. Thus, the writer strove to explain the wet nurses' out-of-wedlock pregnancies in terms of cultural relativity. Among the lower classes in some countries, the argument went, marriage began with the engagement. "In these people," it continued, "unchastity does not suppose the same laxity of principle as among us." The author also attempted to discredit popular beliefs in lactational heredity. "The same tendency that now puts the blame upon the wet-nurse formerly put it upon the witch or the fairy," the piece noted, in an off-hand dismissal of a "scientific truth" held by many readers.[42] Of course, women who worried about "faults bred in a stranger's blood" and the duties of Christian parents might not have been prepared to accept flexible standards of sexual behavior or to adopt modern precepts of heredity.

The editors of *Babyhood* evidently believed that the letters about wet nurses raised significant and timely issues. Editor Leroy M. Yale included several of them in the child-rearing books that he edited.[43] Moreover, in 1902–3 *Babyhood* reprinted, under different names, the letters from Fanny Workman and N. N.[44] Also given a second life was an earlier editorial "The Influence of the Milk of Wet Nurses."[45] The reprinted letters provoked several new replies. One woman, in a letter the editors titled "The Blessed Bottle," wrote that wet nurses were difficult to find and that she favored Mellin's Food and cow's milk.[46] Another reader raised the age-old questions of whether hiring immoral women gave "impetus to evil" and whether the baby could "drink in strong passions capable in some form of changing to evil its whole future life."[47]

The letters, offering glimpses into the experience of wet nursing in the waning decades of the profession, reveal four general responses. Women such as Fanny B. Workman and Interested Reader reported managerial problems with wet nurses, validating the claims of doctors who saw them as only marginally better than artificial feeding. Other women, such as A. M. B., Mater, and Materfamilias, wrote not from experience but simply in opposition to wet nurses on moral and medical grounds. They

42 "The Influence of the Milk of Wet-Nurses," *Babyhood* 3 (1887): 372–3.
43 Leroy Milton Yale, *Nursery Problems* (New York and Philadelphia: Contemporary Publications, 1893), pp. 239–42; and Leroy Milton Yale and Gustav Pollack, *The Century Book for Mothers: A Practical Guide in the Rearing of Healthy Children* (New York: Century, 1901), pp. 408–16. Pollack succeeded Yale as editor of *Babyhood*.
44 W. D., "The Wet Nurse in the Household," *Babyhood* 19 (1902): 32–5; and O. R., "The Moral Objections to Wet-Nurses," *Babyhood* 19 (1903): 138–9.
45 "The Influence of the Milk of Wet-Nurses," *Babyhood* 16 (1900): 132–3.
46 G. D., "The Blessed Bottle," *Babyhood* 19 (1903): 177–8.
47 A. B. S., "The Wet-Nurse," *Babyhood* 19 (1903): 177.

shared with physicians a moral aversion to unwed mothers but disagreed with them about such things as heredity, milk, and character. A third group of women, represented by N. N. and K. H., offered a weak defense of wet nurses based on personal experience – in N. N.'s case with ineffective artificial feeding, in K. H.'s with married wet nurses. A fourth type of response came from women reporting great success with wet nurses and consequently, enormous gratitude toward them.

Generally absent from the medical literature and the domestic advice books and magazines were the cases in which wet nurses earned the lasting gratitude of their employers. Doctors clearly recognized that wet nurses conserved or saved the lives of infants, especially when they were hired after artificial feeding had failed, but the physicians did not report on the aftermath of these heroic encounters. Employers' letters and diaries, however, reveal the psychological complexity of the wet nursing relationship, which evoked many emotions, including a sense of indebtedness. One case that illustrates this involved Jenny, a wet nurse; Fanny, a motherless infant; and Aristeen Pixley Munn, Fanny's grandmother.

In January 1873, after the death of her twenty-nine-year-old daughter, Munn assumed responsibility for her eight-day-old granddaughter Fanny. She quickly sought medical guidance from Edward Mott Moore, a leading surgeon and educator who would later serve as president of the American Medical Association.[48] Moore encouraged Munn to hire a wet nurse, stating that "one fourth of all the children . . . are fed from the bottle and three-fourths of these die."[49] While searching for a suitable candidate, Moore fed Fanny on cow's milk, always feeling uncertain of its quality and preparation.[50] To Munn's relief, she found Jenny with the aid of another local physician, Dr. Will Ely.[51] In a letter to her son more than a month after her daughter's death, she explained how Jenny had come from Buffalo to the Munn home in Gates, New York (outside of Rochester), after obtaining her "husband's" permission to accept the job. Munn expected to be forced to accept Jenny's baby into her home, but the issue never arose as Mr. White, Jenny's so-called husband, arranged for the baby to be placed at board.[52]

Jenny soon earned the respect and gratitude of Munn not simply for her success in feeding Fanny but also because of the mutual affection that

48 Martin Kaufman, "Edward Mott Moore," in Martin Kaufman, Stuart Galishoff, and Todd L. Savitt, eds., *Dictionary of American Medical Biography*, vol. 2, (Westport, Conn.: Greenwood Press, 1984), pp. 534–5.
49 Letter of Aristeen (Pixley) Munn, January 23, 1873. Munn-Pixley Family Papers, 1817–1935. URL.
50 Ibid.
51 Munn letter, February 6, 1873. URL.
52 Ibid.

developed between them. Munn wrote to her son that Jenny was "a great comfort . . . which you could more fully realize if you had been here through the reign of feeding bottles."[53] Baby Fanny's evident attachment to her wet nurse also endeared the woman to Munn, whose own feelings for Jenny became obvious when it was time for her to leave.

White, who as it turned out had not married Jenny, called at the Munn home in November 1873, eleven months after she began her service, and demanded that she return home with him. Munn persuaded him to postpone the departure and allow time for Fanny to be weaned. White agreed. Still, Munn became unsettled about what Jenny's departure would mean for the woman's future. On the day Jenny planned to leave, Munn turned on White and demanded that he marry Jenny in her home or in nearby Rochester. He responded with an "evil, heartless, leering laugh."[54] Munn described the confrontation in two detailed letters to her son. The first began, "That dreadful man came yesterday and took baby's nurse away."[55] Munn wanted to protect Jenny from the stigma of single motherhood and Jenny's child from the stain of illegitimacy. At the same time, she rejected what would have been the standard judgment of Jenny, declaring that she was "not a depraved low girl" and protesting that she "deported herself with utmost propriety," being "too good" for the man who had seduced her.[56] Clearly, Munn never understood Jenny's attachment to her lover or her willingness to return to him.[57]

Munn planned to maintain her ties with Jenny, hoping to give Fanny an opportunity to get to know her wet nurse one day. She asked White where she could write to Jenny and was given what she believed was a false address. She also inquired as to the fate of Jenny's baby, who had suffered an episode of illness while Jenny had been in the Munn household, but she received no reply.[58] Munn's comportment during Jenny's tenure and after her departure betrayed an uncommon attachment. Undoubtedly, very few women moved to intervene in the lives of their wet nurses as she had dared. Her eagerness to do so may have been a displaced longing for her own daughter, but it also reflected her pleasure over Jenny's loving attention to Fanny.

Munn's account of her relationship with Jenny differs greatly from that of many other women. Munn, like other women, had turned to physicians for advice. The wet nurse she had hired exemplified those described in the medical and domestic literature: Jenny was a young, unmarried mother

53 Munn letter, March 13, 1873. URL.
54 Munn letter, December 10, 1873. URL.
55 Ibid.
56 Munn letter, December 11, 1873. URL.
57 Jenny expressed her desire to be reunited with Mr. White earlier. Munn letter, November 12, 1873. URL.
58 Munn letter, December 11, 1873. URL.

who sent her own child to board. The situation in the Munn household had been ripe for the kinds of antagonisms expressed by others. Jenny might have missed her baby and expressed her resentment through callous treatment of Fanny. Once she had established herself she might have demanded more pay, privileges, or both. Yet, the relationship described by Munn was one in which accommodation and respect had developed and had even survived the separation. Although Munn despaired of ever hearing from Jenny again, a few months after her departure she received a letter and a package. Jenny sent Fanny two pairs of shoes, a blue flannel hood and jacket, and a pair of white mittens; the letter was signed "your nurse, Jenny."[59] Evidently, some of the money Jenny had earned by nursing Fanny she had spent on gifts for her. Munn responded with a long letter about Fanny.

Wet nurses had other defenders. Women wrote to magazines trying to shield them from attack, not by defending the occupation but by making reference to their own successful experiences. Unlike opponents of wet nurses, who tended to generalize from their own experiences or who based their objections on moral principles, supporters never directly contested the stereotype of wet nurses. They sensed, perhaps, that it would be unconvincing. Instead, they used their own cases as a way of convincing others that good wet nurses were as plentiful as bad ones.

One of the *Babyhood* correspondents who championed wet nurses, M. M., of Massachusetts, explained that wet nurses could be both successful servants and effective in nursing babies.[60] In her words, she had "never had in my house a servant for whom I entertained a warmer feeling than my wet nurse," noting how quickly the woman had learned the household routine. Grateful for the care her child had received, M. M. defended the woman against the charge of immorality, arguing for Christian charity and an understanding of the wet nurse as victim rather than sinner. Uniquely, M. M. self-consciously examined her own actions. Doctors made frequent reference to the exchange of lives involved in wet nursing; employers typically avoided the subject. M. M., however, faced it head on, asking herself if she had bought her child's health at the expense of another infant life. She could not ignore the fact that a "boarded-out baby in midsummer has a poor chance."

Desperation allowed M. M. to rationalize her decision; the high wages she paid further salved her conscience. She wrote that the money earned by the wet nurse allowed her to lay something aside, and the knowledge she had gained on the job prepared her to "take a place at service." Like the managers of temporary homes and infant asylums, M. M. considered wet nursing a stepping stone to domestic service, overlooking the work histor-

59 Munn letter, February 3, 1874. URL.
60 M. M., "A Warm Defender of the Wet-Nurse," *Babyhood* 4 (1888): 92–3.

ies of most wet nurses. She further recognized the monetary advantages of a wet nursing job, believing that if the woman had not taken work as a wet nurse she would have ended up in a low-paying domestic position earning only $3.00 or $3.50 a week. Most of that, M. M. believed, would have been surrendered to a baby farmer. By becoming a wet nurse, M. M. argued, the woman had helped herself and her child. Her statement implied that the high wages of wet nurses functioned as unspoken compensation for the harm done to the wet nurses' children.

By ignoring the possibilities of deepening ties among wet nurses, infants, and employers, doctors overlooked an aspect of wet nursing that troubled one woman: jealousy. Watching a stranger fulfill a task she had hoped to accomplish, E. B. L., another *Babyhood* correspondent, recalled the bitterness and resentment she had felt and also her gratitude toward her "ignorant yet warm-hearted wet nurse."[61] Like Workman's nemesis "Irish Mary," E. B. L.'s wet nurse was an Irish woman, but, unlike the typical wet nurse, she was a "lawfully-wedded wife." She also appeared unusually sensitive to E. B. L.'s disappointment at being unable to breast-feed. The woman reportedly tried to spare her employer from jealousy by refraining from caressing the child in E. B. L.'s presence and by encouraging him to show affection toward his mother. E. B. L. felt envy nonetheless and ordered the wet nurse to wean the baby. Several weeks later, the infant fell ill and died, leaving E. B. L. to blame herself for her loss. The baby's strength, she judged, had been diminished by his removal from the breast. In later years, E. B. L. turned to her former wet nurse to care for two daughters she nursed herself. Describing the wet nurse to the magazine's readers, E. B. L. concluded "a more unselfish, gentle, kind woman I have never known."

E. B. L.'s account, like that of M. M., reinforced statements made by other correspondents. Both women hired wet nurses after bottle-feeding had failed. M. M. had tried changing the infant's food but saw no improvement, and she turned, like many of her friends, to a wet nurse. She implored readers to make the same choice. E. B. L. had a more trenchant conclusion about any woman who refused to hire a wet nurse: "to be convinced," she wrote, "she has only to pass through the bitter waters as I have done."

Other women had passed through those waters and found an island of salvation in the form of a wet nurse. Temperance advocate and physician Mary Wood Allen described in her book *Ideal Married Life* (1901) a sickly woman who had nursed and lost ten children. She gave her eleventh child to a wet nurse and it survived.[62] Without becoming an advocate of wet

61 E. B. L., "A Plea for the Employment of the Wet-Nurse," *Babyhood* 6 (1889–90): 255–6.
62 Mary Wood Allen, *Ideal Married Life: A Book for All Husbands and Wives* (Chicago: F. H. Revell, 1901; New York, Dabour Social Science Publications, 1978), pp. 137–8.

nursing, Allen admitted its usefulness. The case she cited was, to be sure, extreme, but her point only underscored what physicians and women already knew. Wet nurses were sometimes indispensable, and their personal defects had to be overlooked.

The rare defenders of wet nurses had little success in convincing others. In many instances, bottle-feeding worked, saving the family money and allowing them to avoid many potential management problems. In addition, bombarded with advertisements from infant-food manufacturers and advice from doctors touting the bottle as modern, safe, and scientific, many families actively embraced this alternative. At the same time, wet nurses became less plentiful. The lack of institutional sources in many areas coupled with the new emphasis on keeping unwed mothers united with their babies probably led to the wet nurse scarcities reported by physicians. Moreover, as employment opportunities for women expanded, the lure of wet nursing must have diminished. Its high wages notwithstanding, the job had many drawbacks.

Only one letter from a wet nurse appeared in *Babyhood* although the writer never referred to herself by that term.[63] In 1901, M. S. wrote to ask for advice about nursing a four-month-old baby along with her own newborn. The advice columnist replied that nursing both infants was acceptable as long as she suckled the newborn first and took good care of her nipples. Whether M. S. was wet nursing for money – taking in a foundling or assisting a family needing a wet nurse – or for love – in aid of a close friend or relative – she did not say in her letter. That she even wrote to *Babyhood* for advice suggests she was not a typical wet nurse. The reply intimates that doctors understood that informal wet nursing still occurred and that the act encompassed far more than a domestic occupation.

Sadly, wet nurses left no direct testimony about their experiences on the job. Perhaps, had they written to *Babyhood* in large numbers, they would have described the intrusive employers, officious physicians, and colicky babies that plagued them while at work. Perhaps they would have lamented their separation from their own families and the deaths of the children they had left behind. But wet nurses remain historically silent. They spoke only through their rebelliousness and their loyalty.

Mining the reports of employers and physicians to excavate information about working conditions for wet nurses proves illuminating. The accounts demonstrate that the actions of wet nurses often reflected their immediate experiences on the job rather than a calculated effort to exploit their positions as best they could. In the minds of many employers and doctors, wet nurses were one-dimensional women who capitalized on the

---

63 M. S., "Nursing Another Baby in Addition to One's Own," *Babyhood* 17 (1901): 75.

one commodity they possessed to sell – their milk – for one reason alone – money. Yet the descriptions from these biased observers reveal that the lives, work experiences, and motivations of wet nurses signified far more than unambiguous economic calculations.

Exhaustion and constant scrutiny emerge as two essential experiences for many wet nurses. Although domestic servants of all types faced long workdays, arduous duties, and quarters that were less than ideal, at least they slept at night in separate quarters and escaped from their employers for perhaps half a day on Sundays. Wet nurses had no such respite. Women employed in very wealthy families probably confined their work to the nursery, but in most instances wet nurses had to assume a variety of household tasks along with the job of round-the-clock suckling. Lack of sleep and the recent experience of childbirth undoubtedly worsened their fatigue.

Depending on the doctor's recommendation, the baby's needs, and the preference of employers, wet nurses might be called to the nursery every few hours or might even live in the room and share a bed with the infant. Physician Effa V. Davis described the case of a wet nurse hired into the family of a physician only three weeks after the birth of her own child. Her employers demanded that she nurse the baby "every two hours day and night, sitting one-half hour with him at each feeding." Sleeping only an hour and a half at a stretch in a bed beside the baby's, she quickly became exhausted and drained of her milk. Dismissal soon followed. She returned home, allowed herself more rest, and successfully nursed her own baby.[64]

The practice of housing the wet nurse with the baby may have reflected a belief that she was to be on call at all times or may simply have resulted from a lack of alternative quarters. In 1895 a wet nurse accompanied by her baby entered the Pittsburgh home of merchant Charles Spencer in order to nurse twins. Mr. Spencer moved to the spare room, Mrs. Spencer to a room adjoining her former bedroom, and the wet nurse slept with the twins and her own baby in what had once been the master bedroom.[65] Sympathy for women in such situations was rare. Unlike Davis, who saw exhaustion as the result of employer demands, other doctors failed to make the connection. One medical case report described a woman hired to wet nurse twins. In what was judged a display of power, she began demanding unbroken rest at night.[66] However, it is likely that exhaustion rather than malice fueled her insistence on sleep.

Difficult working conditions extended beyond the bedroom, most often

64 Effa V. Davis, "Maternal Feeding," *Pediatrics* 17 (1905): 774.
65 Ethel Spencer, *The Spencers of Amberson Avenue: A Turn-of-the-Century Memoir*, Michael P. Weber and Peter N. Sterns, eds. (Pittsburgh: University of Pittsburgh Press, 1983), pp. 10–11.
66 McKee and Wells, *Practical Pediatrics*, vol. 1, p. 116.

into the kitchen. Overzealous employers such as Workman took medical recommendations to heart and watched their wet nurse's every move, denying them privacy and strictly controlling their diet and personal hygiene. By scientifically managing their homes as if they were factories, these women put heavy burdens on their wet nurses. Workman seems to have made a mental record of every item her wet nurse consumed. Other employers probably were less scrupulous in their accounting procedures but were still careful to note their wet nurse's daily regimen. Ironically, the women who escaped the regulated life of the foundling asylum or the temporary home, with its daily chores, institutional meals, and prayer meetings, may have found that private service was just as rigidly managed. Moreover, privately employed wet nurses labored in isolation, whereas wet nurses living in institutions enjoyed the companionship of others like themselves. Even in households with other servants, wet nurses could be isolated because of their status as unwed mothers, because of their religion or background, or because of resentment over their high wages. And, once the child left the breast, families could send the wet nurse packing. If the relationship had been particularly acrimonious, the family could deny her the character reference she needed to secure a good position as a domestic. Families and doctors complained bitterly about the power held by wet nurses during their brief reign in the nursery. They clearly regained the upper hand at the conclusion of the relationship.

Neither an army of tyrants nor a band of angels, wet nurses worked on the margins of domestic service and medical practice, negotiating the conditions of work and remuneration as best they could. It was not an accident that the chorus of opposition grew louder as the use of wet nurses declined. As a "last resort," hired after artificial feeding failed, wet nurses had the perceived ability to dominate the household. The family, lacking other options, relied on them as they did on no other servant. Depending on the outcome of the relationship, the employer's resentment or gratitude could be enormous.

As the letters from employers demonstrate, their experiences varied across a broad spectrum of possibilities. What was narrowing were the opportunities for employment. Scientific infant feeding eroded demand for wet nurses, and scientific mothering undermined women's faith in such a recourse. For many reasons, from cost to convenience, from the cultural ideology of motherhood to the related rise of the medical expert, bottle-feeding came to be the first choice of women who could not or would not breast-feed, and wet nursing was increasingly marginalized. Still, wet nurses remained a vital resource for one group of infants: the premature.

7

"Therapeutic merchandise": Human milk in the twentieth century

The steady decline of wet nursing that began in the nineteenth century concluded in the twentieth century with the transformation of human milk into a commodity. In 1900 wet nurses occupied several small niches – suckling foundlings in institutions or working for well-to-do private families. By the 1910s and 1920s the number of wet nurses in these venues had decreased, although new opportunities arose for women willing to suckle abandoned babies in their homes or premature infants in hospitals. At the same time, a new career opened for lactating mothers: expressing and selling their breast milk for use in homes and hospitals. This procedure proved so successful that by the 1930s wet nurses had almost entirely vanished, replaced by bottled human milk. As one physician described it, human milk had become "therapeutic merchandise."[1]

In the case of human milk, commodification – the process by which things come to have economic value – was configured by the long history of wet nursing.[2] Not surprisingly, traditional ideas about milk and character uncoupled slowly. The personal characteristics of wet nurses – their health, morals, willingness to obey authority, emotional ties to their own children – had long been crucial measures of their worth. So too were women who sold their milk judged by more than just the product that they made. In the end, however, commodification transformed the meaning of breast milk. It became a therapy, identified by its value to those who received it rather than by the character of its producers.

1 James A. Tobey, "A New Foster-Mother," *Hygeia* 7 (1929): 1110.
2 My analysis of commodification is drawn from Arjun Appadurai, "Introduction: Commodities and the Politics of Value," pp. 3–63, and Igor Kopytoff, "The Cultural Biography of Things: Commoditization as Process," pp. 64–91, in Arjun Appadurai, ed., *The Social Life of Things: Commodities in Cultural Perspective* (Cambridge: Cambridge University Press, 1986). I begin, however, with Marx's analysis of commodities and their use and exchange values. Karl Marx, *Capital: A Critique of Political Economy*, vol. 1, trans. Ben Fowkes (New York: Vintage Books, 1977), pp. 126–280.

Together twentieth-century physicians and reformers "discovered" the problem of prematurity. In the nineteenth century, the birth of a premature infant was a private, family tragedy; physicians saw no effective means of aiding these babies in their doomed struggle to survive. Writing in 1887, William H. Taylor observed that "an examination of many of the standard works on midwifery shows almost no suggestions as to the care of the child thus prematurely born."[3] As late as 1900 one specialist admitted that most premature and feeble babies were "quietly laid away with but little if any effort being made for their rescue."[4] Even as this statement was made, the sense of impotence that it reflected started giving way to the perception that medical intervention might prove constructive.

Interest in the treatment of prematurity coincided with growing public awareness of the condition's magnitude and with the development of programs aimed at its prevention. According to one estimate, 15 percent of American infants born in 1900 – a total of 420,000 babies – were feeble or premature.[5] The figure probably overstated the actual number, reflecting the lack of a precise definition of either prematurity or feebleness. Yet the quantification itself signified a new understanding that prematurity was a problem to be counted and confronted.[6]

The attack on prematurity followed a long and increasingly focused effort to lower infant mortality rates. Large-scale efforts to sanitize the urban environment opened the public-health crusade of the nineteenth century. The goal then shifted to improving conditions for those commu-

3 William H. Taylor, "Some Points in Relation to Premature Infants," *American Journal of Obstetrics* 20 (1887): 1022.
4 S. W. Ransom, "The Care of Premature and Feeble Infants," *Pediatrics* 9 (1900): 322.
5 Ibid. Ransom's figure was cited by Crandall the following year. See Floyd M. Crandall, "Feeble and Premature Infants," *International Medical Magazine* (1901): 397. The German physician O. Rommel, estimating from evidence supplied by European institutions, arrived at a rate of prematurity of 5 to 25 percent. O. Rommel, "Prematurity and Congenital Debility," in M. Pfaundler and A. Schlossmann, eds., *The Diseases of Children*, 2d ed., vol. 2, trans. Henry L. K. Shaw and Linnaeus LaFetra (Philadelphia: J. B. Lippincott, 1912–14), p. 82. Later figures were much lower. A study of a New York outdoor clinic published in 1921 reported a rate of 2.5 percent. Herman Schwarz and Jerome L. Kohn, "The Infant of Low Birth Weight: Its Growth and Development," *American Journal of Diseases of Children* 21 (1921): 296. According to Cone, Robert Morse Woodbury's study of infant mortality conducted for the Children's Bureau found the rate to be 5 percent. Others placed it between 6 and 7 percent. See Thomas E. Cone, Jr., *History of the Care and Feeding of the Premature Infant* (Boston: Little, Brown, 1985), p. 47.
6 Cone suggests that birth weight did not become a critical assessment of prematurity until the 1870s. Many physicians did not make their assessments of prematurity or feebleness based on weight, but on the appearance of the baby – with weight being one of the factors considered along with other clinical signs of prematurity. Whether the term "feeble" referred to babies who would today be termed "small for date" or to some other constellation of conditions is unclear. Doctors understood the association between multiple births and prematurity, and they also, probably correctly, attributed many of the cases of prematurity to syphilis and chronic diseases in the mother. Cone, *Care and Feeding of the Premature Infant*, p. 14.

nities, families, and individuals judged most vulnerable, with the young becoming the targeted group. In the twentieth century the aim continued to narrow. First infants and then neonates (babies under one month of age) became the subjects of primary concern, with special attention given to the problem of infant mortality and then its major cause: prematurity. Voluntary, municipal, and state efforts to lower infant-mortality rates were enhanced by the establishment in 1912 of the Children's Bureau, which sponsored programs to educate mothers. A second federal effort to reduce these rates began with passage in 1921 of the Sheppard-Towner Act for the promotion of the welfare and health of maternity and infancy, which extended federal aid to the states. (The act lapsed in 1929.)[7]

As the major predisposing cause of death among neonates, premature birth captured the interest of doctors as well as of public officials and reformers. Whereas the latter concentrated on prevention via the provision of prenatal care and the instruction of new mothers, pediatricians created new protocols for treating the premature in homes and institutions. By the second decade of the twentieth century, the profound despair that prematurity once provoked was slowly replaced by the sense that at least some of the babies could be treated and saved.[8]

The early medical reports were largely anecdotal and provide no evidence that the new methods of care actually improved an infant's chance for survival. In much of the literature mortality rates were not broken down by the birth weight or size of the baby – key elements in survival. Nor do the records tell whether the infants died shortly after birth or survived for a few days or weeks. For example, the New York physician Linnaeus LaFetra reported in 1917 on 200 premature infants treated at Bellevue Hospital. Thirty babies survived, but of the 170 who died, 90 did so on their first day. Whether medical intervention helped to save or extend any lives is unclear.[9] Later medical investigations proved far more sophisticated as pediatric specialists issued studies of nutrition, metabolism,

---

7 Richard A. Meckel, *"Save the Babies": American Public Health Reform and the Prevention of Infant Mortality, 1850–1929* (Baltimore: Johns Hopkins University Press, 1990); and Robyn Muncy, *Creating a Female Dominion in American Reform, 1890–1935* (New York: Oxford, 1991), pp. 38–65, 93–123.
8 The late nineteenth-century literature on care of the premature includes R. B. Gilbert, "The Care of Premature Infants After Induced and Accidental Labors," *Transactions of the Kentucky State Medical Society*, new ser. 5 (1896): 189–95; W. Byford Ryan, "The Treatment of Infants Born Prematurely," *Indiana Medical Journal* 8 (1889–90): 246–51; and G. R. Southwick, "The Care of Weak or Prematurely Born Infants," *New England Medical Gazette* 25 (1890): 310–13. For the early twentieth century, see Vanerpoel Adriance, "Premature Infants," *American Journal of the Medical Sciences* 121 (1901): 410–12; Crandall, "Feeble and Premature Infants," pp. 397–9; Ransom, "The Care of Premature and Feeble Infants," pp. 322–6; and James D. Voorhees, "The Care of Premature Babies in Incubators," *Archives of Pediatrics* 17 (1900): 331–46. For a general overview, see Cone, *Care and Feeding of the Premature Infant.*
9 L. E. LaFetra, "Hospital Care of Premature Infants," *Archives of Pediatrics* 34 (1917): 27.

and disease as they related to prematurity.[10] By the 1920s, enough research and knowledge existed to be assembled in the first textbook on prematurity, Julius H. Hess's *Premature and Congenitally Diseased Infants* (1922).[11] Another sign of the maturing scientific interest in the subject was the vigorous debate among specialists over such matters as the best designs for incubators and the temperature at which premature babies should be kept.[12]

Only one subject related to the care of premature babies stood outside the debate. Nearly all pediatricians believed that human milk was a sine qua non in their treatment.[13] As pediatrician Henry Dwight Chapin remarked in 1921 regarding his experiences with several hundred "incubator babies," he had "never been able to raise one without breast milk."[14] Often this meant giving the babies milk from wet nurses rather than from their mothers. Many physicians considered the mother's colostrum to be an unsatisfactory food for the premature infant. Others found that the mothers of premature babies did not have enough milk.[15]

Physicians developed a number of arrangements for securing the human milk needed by premature babies. They continued to hire wet nurses to live and work in the homes of private employers; they arranged for wet nurses to live in hospital "incubator wards"; and, in some cases, they sent feeble babies to infant asylums to be suckled by the resident wet nurses. The Massachusetts Babies Hospital (formerly the Massachusetts Infant Asylum) noted in its annual report that "desperately sick babies are

10 Thomas E. Cone, Jr., *History of American Pediatrics* (Boston: Little Brown, 1979), pp. 187–91; idem, *Care and Feeding of the Premature Infant*, pp. 44–57; and Tom Mitchell, "Some of the Literature Which Has Influenced Present Premature Care," in Solomon R. Kagan, ed., *Abraham Levinson Anniversary Volume: Studies in Pediatrics and Medical History in Honor of Dr. Abraham Levinson on His Sixtieth Birthday* (New York: Froben Press, 1949), pp. 205–10.

11 Julius H. Hess, *Premature and Congenitally Diseased Infants* (Philadelphia: Lea & Febiger, 1922).

12 See, for example, "Discussion of Care of Delicate and Premature Children in the Home. Proceedings of the American Medical Association, Section on Diseases of Children," *American Journal of Obstetrics and Diseases of Women and Children* 70 (1914): 503–5.

13 The lone dissenter appears to have been Thomas Morgan Rotch, the Harvard pediatrician whose interest in scientific (and artificial) infant feeding was discussed in Chapter 5. Rotch, according to Voorhees, continued to favor the mixture prepared in the milk laboratory. Voorhees, "Care of Premature Babies in Incubators," p. 338. Rotch's successor at Harvard, John Lovett Morse, stated unequivocally that it was important for "premature babies to have breast milk." John Lovett Morse, *Diseases of Children Presented in Two Hundred Case Histories of Actual Patients . . . ,* 3d ed. (Boston: W. M. Leonard, 1920), p. 64.

14 Henry Dwight Chapin, "Discussion," *Archives of Pediatrics* 38 (1921): 40.

15 On colostrum see, for example, Benjamin Knox Rachford, *Diseases of Children: A Practical Treatise on Diagnosis and Treatment for the Use of Students and Practitioners of Medicine* (New York: D. Appleton, 1912), p. 67. On insufficient milk see, for example, Emelyn Lincoln Coolidge, *The Home Care of Sick Children: A Guide for Mothers in the Care of Sick Children* (New York: D. Appleton, 1916), p. 86.

constantly being sent to us by other hospitals in the hope that our wet-nurse feeding may save them, and many apparently hopeless cases are saved in this way."[16] The hospital also served, on occasion, as a resource for private families. In 1897, W. T. Bonner, treasurer of the New England Oil Company, arranged to have his infant sent to the Massachusetts Infant Asylum to be wet-nursed. Most likely, he had been unable to find a woman willing to work in his home. The Bonner baby remained for nearly two and a half months; the family paid five dollars a week for the privilege. Apparently well satisfied, the Bonner family admitted another infant in 1903.[17] Other families and physicians made indirect use of institutional wet nurses, arranging to purchase or otherwise obtain their milk. Thus, the directors of the Massachusetts Babies Hospital reported that resident wet nurses sometimes supplied local physicians with small quantities of milk until alternative arrangements could be made.[18]

The path to commodification began with the perception of human milk as a therapeutic agent. The second critical development was the creation of new systems for its procurement. Some doctors, as just noted, turned to local institutions housing wet nurses to get the vital fluid needed by their patients. Others simply sought out nursing mothers willing to sell or share their excess breast milk. St. Louis physician John Zahorsky, for instance, recalled in his autobiography purchasing milk for premature infants from needy women in the local community. Another doctor, Owen W. Wilson, reported to his colleagues in 1917 that he too had tried this method.[19] Although neither Zahorsky nor Wilson established a formal mechanism for buying human milk, they, along with the other practitioners who made individual efforts to buy milk, helped establish the concept of breast milk as a commodity.

As both physicians and families gradually became aware that the infant's need for human milk could be satisfied through means other than a wet nurse, they also learned the limits of these alternatives. The purchasing of milk, much like the hiring of a wet nurse, put the doctor in the business of seeking individual suppliers, hoping to find a source of milk before the infant's condition grew worse. Moreover, the disorganization that charac-terized the wet nurse marketplace in the nineteenth century also typified the twentieth-century marketplace for human milk. Under the circumstances, doctors called for the creation of organized wet nurse bureaus and agencies that could organize the sale of breast milk. One practitioner expressed hope

16 Massachusetts Babies Hospital, *Forty-sixth Annual Report* (Boston, 1913), p. 15.
17 Case records, Massachusetts Infant Asylum, 1897, p. 11; and case records, Massachusetts Infant Asylum, 1903, p. 1. HLUMB.
18 Massachusetts Babies Hospital, *Forty-six Annual Report*, p. 22.
19 John Zahorsky, *From the Hills: An Autobiography of a Pediatrician* (St. Louis: Mosby, 1949), p. 167; and Owen W. Wilson, "Discussion," *Journal of the American Medical Association* 69 (1917): 426.

that "with the growing appreciation of the importance of breast milk for young infants, systematized organizations for the supply of properly certified wet-nurses will soon supersede the haphazard method of selection now in vogue."[20] Another doctor, J. Ross Snyder of Birmingham, Alabama, recommended a breast-milk commission that would, among other activities, create a corps of wet nurses and establish depots selling human milk. Anticipating objections to his proposition, he argued resolutely that it was neither "*bizarre* or impossible."[21]

Snyder's proposal clearly encapsulated a new understanding of breast milk: He saw human milk as a product to be regulated by local authorities in much the same manner as cow's milk was regulated, and he also sought, as others had, to make wet nursing a profession controlled by the medical establishment.

One institution, the Boston Wet Nurse Directory, answered these demands. The experiences of this organization illustrate both the slow shift from hiring wet nurses to buying human milk and the growing perception of breast milk as a commodity. Founded in 1910, the Directory attempted to graft the Progressive Era ideal of efficiency on to a historically informal profession. At the same time, imbued with the legacy of moral reform that governed many of the institutions housing wet nurses, the Directory also endeavored to "save" the women who it placed in service. Such broad aspirations ultimately exceeded the Directory's narrow fiscal grasp; after fifteen years of service, it closed its doors. During its brief existence, the Directory "solved" the supposed problems of wet nursing by providing medical oversight for the wet nurse placement process, sharing managerial control of the wet nurse in the home, and ending the outplacement of the wet nurse's infant. The Directory's demise, therefore, serves as a coda to the history of private-duty wet nursing.

The Directory's founder, Fritz Bradley Talbot, a graduate of Harvard Medical School, served on the Harvard Medical School faculty as professor of pediatrics and was for twenty-one years chief of children's services at the prestigious Massachusetts General Hospital.[22] Talbot created the organization after he conducted a grueling three-day search for a wet nurse. During this search he observed that, had it been an emergency, "the baby

20 Alfred Cleveland Cotton, *The Medical Diseases of Infancy and Childhood* (Philadelphia: J. B. Lippincott, 1906), p. 108.
21 J. Ross Snyder, "The Breast Milk Problem," *Journal of the American Medical Association* 51 (1908): 1214.
22 *Medical Directory of Greater Boston* 3d ed. rev. (Boston: Boston Medical Publishing Co., 1911), p. 467; George C. Shattuck, [obituary of Fritz B. Talbot], *Harvard Medical Alumni Bulletin*, 39 (1965): 41; W. G. P., "Fritz B. Talbot, M.D. [obituary]," *New England Journal of Medicine* 272 (1965): 50.

Human milk in the twentieth century 185

might have died before the milk was obtained."[23] Like other physicians at the time, Talbot recognized the value of human milk and the need to make it available on short notice. He was also soon aware that others shared his interest.

Talbot carefully surveyed the needs of other practitioners, questioning eighty doctors. Eight reported having no use for wet nurses; seventy-one declared using 6 or more annually; and one, evidently a true believer in human milk, claimed to have placed 25 or more. Their collective demand amounted to 450 wet nurses annually, a substantial number that would justify the creation of a wet nurse bureau.[24]

Difficulties in juggling supply and demand had stymied an earlier effort to help doctors find wet nurses, the wet nurse registry begun in 1909 at the Boston Medical Library. The service had quickly failed because would-be wet nurses lacked shelter in the interim between their discharge from the hospital and the time that they obtained work.[25] Talbot solved this problem with a combination of personal connections and personal largess: He rented a house near the Massachusetts Infant Asylum, where he served as visiting physician and arranged for the women to suckle the Asylum babies there until they found other work. The average wait for a job was about two weeks. With the housing problem solved, Talbot proudly announced the Directory's opening with a mass mailing of eight thousand postcards to physicians throughout New England.[26]

The Directory positioned itself initially as a medical resource, promising to share medical and managerial oversight with private physicians representing the employers. By its own account, doctors from Maine to Connecticut made use of its residents. Each woman entered service after having been examined by a doctor at the Directory as well as by the family physician. Once ensconced in a private home she continued to be monitored. The employers received a postcard questionnaire asking a host of questions, among them: "Is the wet nurse neat? Willing and cheerful? Does she take correction well? Is she fond of her own baby? How much did your baby gain on her milk?" The family physician was also queried, being asked whether the wet nurse did well with the sick baby and well by her

23 Fritz B. Talbot, "An Organization for Supplying Human Milk," *New England Journal of Medicine* 199 (1928): 610. On the difficulty of finding wet nurses, see James H. McKee and William H. Wells, *Practical Pediatrics: A Modern Clinical Guide in the Diseases of Infants and Children for the Family Physician*, vol. 1, (Philadelphia: P. Blakiston's Sons, 1914) pp. 115–16. A more detailed description of Talbot's search was provided in 1937 by a colleague. See James A. Tobey, "The Newest Foster Mother," *Good Housekeeping* 104 (1937): 77.
24 Fritz B. Talbot, "The Wetnurse Problem," *Boston Medical and Surgical Journal* 169 (1913): 760–2.
25 Fritz B. Talbot, "A Directory for Wet-Nurses: Its Experiences for Twelve Months," *Journal of the American Medical Association* 56 (1911): 1715.
26 Talbot, "The Wetnurse Problem," pp. 760–2.

own child, and whether the doctor would recommend her again.[27] The questions reflected the fact that the wet nursing relationship remained fundamentally one of personal service in which friction between a wet nurse and her employer could upset a delicate arrangement. With this in mind apparently, Talbot's colleague, Harvard pediatrician John Lovett Morse, felt compelled to remind physicians that whereas the Directory could attest to the health of the wet nurse and the quality of her milk, it could not guarantee her character, habits, or disposition.[28]

Breaking with past medical orthodoxy, the Directory required that wet nurses keep their infants with them while in service. This practice melded social-welfare ideology with medical necessity. As noted previously, maternity homes began to stress the need for single mothers to remain with their babies in order for the women to be morally redeemed.[29] The Directory adopted the same practice, hoping to "save" the women it sent into service. The organization could also invoke a medical rationale; presumably, many of the babies being wet-nursed were premature infants who were too weak to suck and typically received milk by dropper. To keep up their milk supply, the women had to continue to feed their own babies.[30]

A new paradigm for interpreting domestic discord developed as a result of the changing clientele for wet nurses. Families now became the bad actors in the nursery drama. Medical accounts described how doctors struggled with reluctant families to win a place for the wet nurse's offspring. One practitioner declared, "Often it takes considerable persuasive power on the part of both physician and nurse" to convince the family that the wet nurse should bring her baby.[31] A second remarked, "It demands courage few physicians possess to place the available wet nurse and her child in the average household."[32] To gain support for their arguments, doctors developed additional justifications. One doctor alleged that keeping her own baby with her contributed to the wet nurse's "peace of mind."[33] Previously, it had been the employer's composure that most mattered.

27 Talbot, "A Directory for Wet-Nurses," pp. 1716–17.
28 John Lovett Morse, "Directory for Wet Nurses," *Boston Medical and Surgical Journal* 179 (1918): 218.
29 The policies of maternity homes are discussed in Chapter 3. The effect of this policy was noted by Isaac Abt, who reported that maternity homes were glad to secure positions in hospitals for their inmates because they had a policy of not separating mother and baby. Isaac A. Abt, "Technic of Wet Nurse Management in Institutions," *Journal of the American Medical Association* 69 (1917): 188.
30 Coolidge, *The Home Care of Sick Children*, p. 86; Rowland Godfrey Freeman, *Elements of Pediatrics for Medical Students* (New York: MacMillan, 1917), p. 214; Hess, *Premature and Congenitally Diseased Infants*, pp. 118–19; and LaFetra, "Hospital Care of Premature Infants," p. 28.
31 Carl G. Leo-Wolf, *Nursing in Diseases of Children* (St. Louis: Mosby, 1918), p. 106.
32 William Palmer Lucas, *The Modern Practice of Pediatrics* (New York: MacMillan, 1927), p. 132.
33 Hess, *Premature and Congenitally Diseased Infants*, pp. 118–19.

Now doctors depicted employers as stubborn and as ill-educated in matters of medicine, unwilling to follow the advice of professionals.

Physicians, in turn, may have seemed close minded to the employers, who had their own reasons for rejecting their blandishments. Although the medical writings were silent on the matter, the historical record was full of reports of families unhappy about having to house two infants or simply reluctant to sanction single motherhood by hiring wet nurses.

Even though the medical rationale for using wet nurses may have been bolstered by the new focus on assisting premature infants, the population of wet nurses remained relatively unchanged from that of previous decades. Evidence from the Boston Wet Nurse Directory strongly suggests that women who became wet nurses in the twentieth century closely resembled their nineteenth-century counterparts: they were young, single mothers. Of the 147 women who applied for admission to the Directory between 1910 and 1913, doctors rejected 12 (5 for an insufficient milk supply, 4 because of syphilis, 2 with tuberculosis, and 1 with gonorrhea). Of the 135 successful applicants, 125 (85 percent) were single, the vast majority were primiparae, and almost all were between the ages of eighteen and thirty. Work as wet nurses earned them eight dollars a week, still a relatively high salary, and most saved a significant portion of their pay.

At times the Directory's interest in aiding the wet nurses seemed to outstrip its goal of assisting physicians. Talbot's publications increasingly boasted of the work done by the organization on behalf of the wet nurses. The Directory made vigorous efforts to polish the women's tarnished reputations and to assist them in gaining economic independence. Talbot was an early supporter of medical social work and had initiated a cooperative arrangement between the Children's Medical Department and the Social Service Department of the Massachusetts General Hospital.[34] Not unexpectedly, he brought case workers into the Directory. There, they endeavored to teach the women "the love and responsibility of motherhood."[35] In Talbot's words, the Directory tried to make "Annie" a "much better woman," "Louise" a "good mother," and see that "Mary" was "making every effort to improve herself."[36] In addition to restoring the women morally, the social workers took concrete steps to help them

34 The program at the Massachusetts General Hospital was, according to Talbot, the first such venture in the United States. Fritz B. Talbot, "Early History of the Children's Medical Department, Massachusetts General Hospital, 1903–1922," in Nathaniel W. Faxon, ed., *The Massachusetts General Hospital, 1935–1955* (Cambridge: Harvard University Press, 1959), p. 267. Talbot's attitude toward wet nurses may have been influenced by Ida M. Cannon, chief of social services at the Massachusetts General Hospital, who believed that "unwed mothers were especially suitable for social service." Ida M. Cannon, *Social Work in Hospitals: A Contribution to Progressive Medicine*, rev. ed. (New York, Russell Sage Foundation, 1923), p. 54.
35 Massachusetts Babies Hospital, *Annual Report* (Boston, 1913), p. 13.
36 Talbot, "The Wetnurse Problem," pp. 761–2.

financially. One case worker persuaded a young man of seventeen to pay three dollars a week in child support. Another hauled a more recalcitrant father into court to be charged under the Bastardy Law; the father was forced to settle the suit for three hundred dollars. Other men chose a different solution. Talbot reported that five wet nurses were wed during the first three years of the Directory's operations, although he did not make clear whether love, honor, or fear of the law had brought the couples to the altar.[37] For most of the wet nurses, however, neither matrimony nor a financial settlement offered a viable solution to the problem of supporting their children. The social workers therefore assisted them in finding places to live and work after they finished their service.[38] Talbot described how one twenty-four-year-old single mother came to the Directory planning to give up her child for adoption and left with her baby in her arms. While employed, she saved two hundred dollars and learned to care for her own child. When her wet nursing days ended, the social worker arranged for her to board her baby, work in a factory, and study dressmaking in the evening. Other women too ended their wet nursing careers with a nice amount of savings. Talbot reported that some of the women managed to put aside between fifty and three hundred dollars, a substantial stake toward a new life.[39]

In its early years, the Directory placed between three and five women in service each month; by 1915 the number had risen to approximately fifteen per month.[40] The numbers mocked the argument that scientific infant feeding had made wet nursing obsolete but did little to suggest that wet nursing directories would soon blossom in other cities. For one thing, the supply of workers appeared to be ebbing along with the demand. John Lovett Morse argued that the Directory already attracted a "considerable proportion of the women who wish to be wet nurses."[41] In earlier decades, more women would have been going into service, many directly after their confinements.

Although physicians and families relied on the Directory, the organization foundered, apparently because of the high costs of its social-welfare program. Its attempts to aid wet nurses situated it in the world of reform rather than medicine and left its books in the red. Financial difficulties necessitated periodic increases in the fee schedule and ultimately spurred efforts to generate revenue by selling bottled breast milk. In 1910 employers paid ten dollars to hire a wet nurse from the Directory; the fee doubled

37 Ibid.
38 Fritz B. Talbot, "The Educational Work by Boston Hospitals for the Health of Children under 2 Years," pp. 3–4. Unpublished paper. Fritz B. Talbot Papers. FACLM.
39 Talbot, "The Wetnurse Problem," pp. 760–1.
40 George R. Bedinger, "The Wet Nurse Directory of Boston," *Transactions of the American Association for Study and Prevention of Infant Mortality* 6 (1915): 252–4.
41 John Lovett Morse, *Clinical Pediatrics* (Philadelphia: W. B. Saunders, 1926), p. 141.

in 1913. That same year the Directory began selling milk, earning four hundred eighty dollars from the sixty quarts it sold for twenty-five cents an ounce.[42] In 1915 fees rose again. The wet nurses received fifteen dollars a week and in turn paid the Directory seven dollars. In cases where the wet nurse was indispensable and the family unable to afford the total cost, a smaller fee was negotiated, with the difference subtracted from the Directory's share. Families with sufficient means had another alternative. For twenty-one dollars per week they could arrange for the delivery of bottled breast milk, sparing themselves the inconvenience of housing a wet nurse and her baby.[43] Those who chose to purchase the milk paid a high price; in 1918 the cost increased to thirty dollars per week.[44]

Ultimately, the medical and social controls exercised by the Directory were mere scaffolding erected to support a crumbling structure. The problems of wet nursing inhered in its role as a private service that placed poor women in the nurseries of rich families. In the end, it could not overcome the competition from bottled breast milk.

Despite frequent price increases, the Directory's income never equaled its expenses. Faced with high costs and low revenues, the institution survived because of Talbot's generosity – much of it anonymous. In addition to renting the house in which the wet nurses lived, he supplied the bulk of the Directory's operating funds.[45] The organization was, in effect, a private philanthropy and one that could not be maintained indefinitely. Capitulating to fiscal and practical realities, the Boston Wet Nurse Directory closed its doors in 1925. Having brought order to the structural arrangements of wet nursing by remaking relations among wet nurses, their infants, employers, and physicians, the Directory fell victim to its own expansive aims. Remaking the lives of poor, single mothers was an undertaking too costly to be supported only by the fees earned from wet nurse placement.

The shift from referring wet nurses to supplying bottled breast milk that occurred within the Boston Wet Nurse Directory was paralleled by changing practices within hospitals. The managerial difficulties posed by ward wet nurses were pale but still visible reflections of those encoun-

42 Talbot, "The Wetnurse Problem," p. 761.
43 Bedinger, "The Wet Nurse Directory," p. 253; and Talbot, "The Wetnurse Problem," pp. 760–1.
44 Morse, "Directory for Wet Nurses," p. 218.
45 In 1912, for example, the Boston Wet Nurse Directory received donations totaling $1,231.91; Talbot's portion was $1,091.91, the second-largest contribution was $50. Talbot never acknowledged these gifts. In one article he suggested that the difference between operating expenses and earnings was made up by the Ladies' Board of the Directory. Talbot was the scion of a prosperous family. He accepted no salary during his tenure as chief of pediatrics at the Massachusetts General Hospital and donated the salaries of his several assistants. See Talbot Papers. FACLM. Talbot is revealed as the renter of the house in Hazel M. Keene, "Maternal Milk Collection," *Public Health Nursing* 26 (1934): 649.

tered in private homes – problems of character and control. Although they made constant efforts to solve these problems in the hospitals, doctors also looked for alternatives, including new systems for collecting, bottling, and distributing breast milk. Slowly, a cadre of nursing mothers who sold their excess breast milk began to replace the wet nurses who lived and worked on incubator wards.

Writing to a colleague in 1914, the pediatrician John Price Crozer Griffith explained that maintaining wet nurses in "incubator wards" was the "trend in all children's hospitals in this country and in Europe."[46] Among the American institutions that did so were the St. Louis Children's Hospital and two children's hospitals in Chicago – Sarah Morris and Children's Memorial.[47] Other facilities adopted somewhat different arrangements. The New York Foundling Hospital, which had employed wet nurses since its founding, ceased using the women to suckle the babies and instead required them to pump the milk from their breasts.[48] And at least one institution, the University of Minnesota Hospital, eschewed wet nurses entirely, arranging instead for mothers to send in breast milk for their own babies.[49]

Both mothers and wet nurses produced milk for premature babies by manual expression or by using a pump. In some instances, the wet nurse would feed her own infant on one breast in order to stimulate the expression of milk from the other.[50] The premature babies received the milk via either specially designed feeding devices or the more old-fashioned droppers. With venereal disease a major cause of prematurity, feeding by device had the additional benefit of protecting the wet nurse from infection.

Hospitals recruited wet nurses from the same sources as private physicians. One doctor recalled that they came from "homes for unmarried mothers, such as the Florence Crittendon Missions."[51] The Children's Memorial Hospital in Chicago, for example, obtained them from the local Salvation Army.[52] Other facilities looked to their own patients when they needed to obtain milk for use on the wards. Griffith wrote to a colleague about a woman who refused to "give milk to save another baby's life,"

46 Letters of John Price Crozer Griffith, vol. 1, 1914–15, p. 97. CPP.
47 Bessie Ingersoll Cutler, *Pediatric Nursing, Its Principles and Practice* (New York: MacMillan, 1923), p. 144; F. S. Churchill, "The Wet Nurse in Hospital Practice," *American Journal of Obstetrics* 70 (1914): 499; and Isaac A. Abt, "Technic of Wet Nurse Management in Hospitals," *Journal of the American Medical Association* 69 (1917): 418–20.
48 Lewis A. Scheuer and Jessie E. Duncan, "A Method of Preserving Breast Milk," *American Journal of Diseases of Children* 51 (1936): 249–54.
49 Rodd Taylor, "Treatment of Prematurity," *Journal of the American Medical Association* 71 (1918): 1123.
50 Henry Dwight Chapin and Godfrey Roger Pisek, *Diseases of Infants and Children* (New York: William Wood, 1909), p. 4.
51 John C. Baldwin, *Pediatrics for Nurses* (New York: D. Appleton, 1924), p. 51.
52 Churchill, "The Wet Nurse in Hospital Practice," p. 499.

warning that she would lose "the special privilege of going to the Hospital out of ordinary times."[53]

On the wards, wet nurses functioned as suppliers of milk, yet they continued to be judged and managed according to traditional interpretations of their role and character. In the article "Technic of Wet Nurse Management in Institutions," pediatrician Isaac Abt described how wet nurses at Chicago's Sarah Morris Children's Hospital performed light work including room care and did their own laundry. Functioning in the dual role of housekeeping staff and providers of milk, the women earned eight dollars per week, the same as the private-duty wet nurses dispatched by the Boston Wet Nurse Directory.[54] Julius H. Hess, Abt's successor at Sarah Morris, created a Premature Infant Station and instituted more rigorous controls. Wet nurses ate "under the eye of a nurse," remained in the hospital at night, and bathed regularly.[55] The regime in the hospital mimicked that of the private home, as doctors attempted to compensate for the presumed duplicity of the wet nurses with strict regulation. Hess's efforts to achieve order were the most extreme. He designed two uniforms for the women to wear so as to "overcome the slovenly appearance of the wet nurse as she is seen wandering about the wards of an infants' hospital."[56] On a practical level, the uniforms permitted easy access to the breast; on a symbolic level, they brought the wet nurse into conformity with hospital practice in which clothing marked a worker's status and role.

The wet nurse's uniform masked her condition as a social outsider, as a woman who was judged not only by her ability to obey ward routines and produce good milk but also according to her background. In this regard, twentieth-century hospital-based wet nurses resembled the women employed in nineteenth-century private homes. The latter were carefully scrutinized by employers and physicians who were anxious to assure themselves that the women could control their emotions, follow the household routine, and refrain from polluting the child or the workplace. In the hospital setting, issues of obedience and order were more easily solved, but the question of character remained, although in an altered guise. Physicians no longer spoke about morals; they did, however, pay careful attention to race and ethnicity and to their presumed links to milk quality. Hess argued, for example, that women with "phlegmatic temperaments as seen in women from Northern and Central Europe of Teutonic and Slavic descent" offered the "ideal material," whereas "Italians and Southern negroes, when removed from their home environment . . . secrete a milk poor in

53 Letters of John Price Crozer Griffith, vol. 1, 1914–15, p. 46. CPP.
54 Abt, "Technic of Wet Nurse Management," p. 419.
55 Hess, *Premature and Congenitally Diseased Infants*, p. 129. See also Julius H. Hess, George J. Mohr and Phyllis F. Bartelme, *The Physical and Mental Growth of Prematurely Born Children* (Chicago: University of Chicago Press, 1934), pp. 7–9.
56 Julius H. Hess, "Uniform for the Wet Nurse," *Modern Hospital* 6 (1916): 265–6.

quality."[57] Others agreed with his findings – that there was a link between ethnicity and milk quality – but disagreed with his premise that women from Southern Europe supplied an inferior product. At a meeting of the American Medical Association's Section on Diseases of Children in 1917, in a session discussing human milk, one New York physician commended the Italian and Jewish women who voluntarily offered breast milk to needy neighbors.[58] The implication was that they also supplied "good" milk.

The race question also elicited conflicting judgments, seemingly based on physicians' personal experiences. At the same session, two Southern physicians, one from Charlotte, North Carolina, the other from Knoxville, Tennessee, disagreed about whether African-American women could make good wet nurses.[59] Neither made clear if the issue dividing them was race per se or the personal characteristics of African-American women.

The emerging interest in the race issue suggests that because the pool of private-duty wet nurses had shrunk, both private families and hospitals were now facing the question of whether they should hire African-American women, whom they had previously rejected for the job. One physician noted, in 1920, that families sometimes drew the line at "engaging of a woman other than white."[60] Another, the author of a nursing textbook, suggested that "colored wet nurses will usually be found easier to get along with than white ones," adding later that "their milk is equally good and usually more abundant."[61] His arguments were clearly mustered in defense of an unpopular opinion.

The topics of the debate – race and ethnicity – indicated that physicians and families persisted in seeing milk as a complex substance containing, in some form, the characteristics of its producers. Yet, the tenor of discussion in the twentieth century seems to have been far more sober than it had in the nineteenth. With the doctors in firm command of both the wet nursing and human milk business, talk of milkborne heredity and emotion-poisoned milk subsided. The ongoing process of commodification slowly transformed human milk from a substance produced by women to a therapy dispensed by doctors.

Commodities, Igor Kopytoff and other anthropologists argue, have cultural biographies, that is, identities conditioned by systems of exchange, by cultural rules, and by the tendency to separate people from things.[62]

---

57 Hess, *Premature and Congenitally Diseased Infants,* p. 114.
58 Jacob Sobel, "Discussion," *Journal of the American Medical Association* 69 (1917): 425–6.
59 Isaac W. Faison, "Discussion on Human Milk," *Journal of the American Medical Association* 69 (1917): 428; and Oliver Hill, "Discussion on Human Milk," *Journal of the American Medical Association* 69 (1917): 428.
60 John Price Crozer Griffith, *Diseases of Infants and Children* (Philadelphia: Saunders, 1921), p. 90.
61 Baldwin, *Pediatrics for Nurses,* p. 54.
62 Kopytoff, "The Cultural Biography of Things," pp. 64–91.

The creation of bottled breast milk illustrates each of these phenomena. In wet nursing, the labor process – feeding a baby – was indistinguishable from the labor product – breast milk. Women were paid to do both – to produce milk and to feed a baby. In milk selling, product and producer were distinct, and only the product was sold. Essentially, selling breast milk and wet nursing were distinguished by the separation of the woman and the milk, and by the inauguration of a new system of exchange – the payment of cash per ounce of milk rather than the provision of room, board, and a weekly wage to a wet nurse.

Yet, even if milk selling was, explicitly, not wet nursing, it was still fundamentally shaped by the cultural rules of wet nursing. Consequently, the perception of human milk remained ambiguous; human milk could never be appraised simply in terms of its cost or its chemical attributes, and it could not be bought from just anyone. Doctors, therefore, imported in modified form their wet nurse management techniques into the organizations they created to collect and process human milk. Furthermore, they searched for ways to purge human milk of its human history. Ultimately they would achieve both aims – tight control over milk sellers and the "purification" of their milk – through the creation of the modern milk bank.

A crucial stage in the commodification process involved the construction of a scientific system for collecting and distributing breast milk in a bottle. The effort to do so succeeded in widening the physical and psychological distance between the makers and the users of human milk. This led to the gradual shift in focus away from the producers of milk – the wet nurses – toward the consumers – the babies. Before this could occur, however, breast milk had to be cleansed of its individual characteristics, and the judgments made about milk sellers had to be based not on their economic status, housekeeping skills, character, race, or ethnicity, but on the quantity and quality of the product they produced and sold. The milk bank met both these challenges.

Milk banking, defined simply as the institutional collection, storage, and distribution of breast milk, evolved simultaneously with hospital-based wet nursing, and often the two schemes operated in tandem. Both depended upon medical oversight, both involved day-to-day management by nurses, and both had the same goal: obtaining the milk needed by frail and premature babies. Their differences lay largely in their organization of labor and in their respective work forces. Hospital wet nursing was a round-the-clock residential job, employing, for the most part, single mothers, whereas milk selling engaged married, working-class women for a brief period each day.

The first milk bank opened in Boston in 1910. In an article published in the *Boston Medical and Surgical Journal*, Fritz Bradley Talbot, the founder of the Boston Wet Nurse Directory, credited his colleague Francis Parkman Denny with inspiring the milk bank's creation, although Talbot himself was largely responsible for its development.[63]

Denny, a Harvard-trained bacteriologist and public-health physician, served for a time as visiting physician to the Massachusetts Infant Asylum, where he became familiar with the institutional use of wet nurses.[64] He developed a scheme for breast-milk collection after having arranged for four women to supply breast milk to a sick baby. Denny later calculated that in five weeks he had obtained twelve quarts of milk and that two quarts would have been sufficient for the infant's needs. The remaining, he recognized, could have been used to "save the lives of other sick babies."[65] Having developed a successful method for collecting human milk, Denny first employed it in an inconclusive medical experiment he conducted involving adult typhoid patients.[66] According to Talbot, Denny's milk-collection program laid the groundwork for the breast-milk collection service that he later began at the Boston Floating Hospital.

So named because it operated on a ship that sailed around Boston harbor each summer, the Floating Hospital purchased approximately four quarts of milk each day during its summer operating season in 1910.[67] Subsequently, both the amount collected and the numbers of infants served grew substantially. In 1911 the hospital used over two hundred quarts of milk, and by 1915 it collected and distributed a total of 368.5 quarts in one eighty-day period.[68] The Floating Hospital's crew of milk sellers consisted

63 Fritz B. Talbot, "Two Methods of Obtaining Human Milk for Hospital Use," *Boston Medical and Surgical Journal* 164 (1911): 305–6. Much of the following discussion is drawn from Janet Golden, "From Wet Nurse Directory to Milk Bank: The Delivery of Human Milk in Boston, 1909–1927," *Bulletin of the History of Medicine* 62 (1988): 589–605.

64 *Medical Directory of Greater Boston* (Boston: Boston Medical Publishing Co., 1906), p. 84; *Medical Directory of Greater Boston* (1911), p. 125; "Francis Parkman Denny [obituary]," *Journal of the American Medical Association* 138 (1948): 982; Harvard College Class of 1891, *Twenty-fifth Anniversary Report* (privately printed), p. 85; Harvard College Class of 1891, *Fiftieth Anniversary Report* (privately printed), p. 60.

65 Francis P. Denny, "Value of Small Quantities of Human Milk in the Treatment of Infantile Atrophy and the Infections of Infants," *Journal of the American Medical Association* 47 (1906): 1907.

66 Francis P. Denny, "The Use of Human Milk in Typhoid Fever to Increase the Bacteriolytic Power of the Blood," *Boston Medical and Surgical Journal* 158 (1908): 625–30.

67 On the Boston Floating Hospital, see *The Boston Floating Hospital: A Gangway to Health* (Boston, 1935); Paul Beaven, ed., "A History of the Boston Floating Hospital," *Pediatrics* 19 (1957): 629–38; G. Loring Briggs, "The Floating Hospital," *Transactions of the American Association for Study and Prevention of Infant Mortality* 5 (1914): 303–4; and John Lovett Morse, "The History of Pediatrics in Massachusetts," *New England Journal of Medicine* 205 (1931): 174. On the milk collection at the hospital, see Talbot, "Two Methods," pp. 305–6.

68 "Close of the Boston Floating Hospital Season," *Boston Medical and Surgical Journal* 165 (1911): 459; and Paul W. Emerson, "The Collection and Preservation of Human Milk," *Journal of the American Medical Association* 78 (1922): 642.

of married women living in the neighborhood. They earned approximately
$4.20 per week if they provided the one quart daily that was typical of
women selling milk – a wage approximately half that received by live-in
wet nurses but, nonetheless, a significant contribution to the family
economy.

Several other hospitals initiated milk-bank programs in the 1910s and
1920s, typically as a means of replacing staffs of resident wet nurses. The
Manhattan Maternity and Dispensary and the Boston Children's Hospital
began using drawn breast milk sent into their nurseries.[69] In 1911, the
Clinic for Infant Feeding in Grand Rapids, Michigan, substituted a milk-
collection service for its system of carrying sick babies to the homes of wet
nurses.[70] In a retrospective analysis of its work, the clinic's director would
attribute the city's low infant-mortality rate to the work of the breast-
milk service.

In some instances, hospitals looked to their patients, developing strate-
gies for collecting human milk from women in the maternity ward or
served by the outdoor delivery department.[71] Bellevue Hospital inaugurated a well-documented milk-collection service under the direction of
physician B. Raymond Hoobler.[72] Employees of the Social Service Department identified potential milk sellers from among their clients, and if the
women had an ample supply of milk, they were asked to sell their excess.
Those who agreed underwent a medical examination and, if approved,
made daily visits to the hospital to express their milk. Initially, nurses
instructed them in the use of the breast pump; after their first visit, resident
wet nurses supervised their work. The women earned fifty cents for each
hospital visit, and the hospital collected approximately thirty-one quarts of
milk each month.[73]

Several years later, Hoobler began a much more extensive milk-
collection and -distribution service at the Detroit Women's Hospital and
Infants' Home. At this juncture, he turned both to single mothers giving
birth at the hospital and to women recruited through local dispensaries and
by advertisements in the newspaper. In some cases the women became
private-duty wet nurses rather than milk sellers, a further indication that

69 Walter Lester Carr, "A Clinical Report of Simple Methods in the Care of Premature
   Babies," *Archives of Pediatrics* 38 (1921): 402; Letters of John Price Crozer Griffith, vol. 1,
   1914–15, p. 97. CPP.
70 Blanche H. DeKoning, "A Twenty-two-year-old Breast Milk Service Reaps Its Reward,"
   Public Health Nursing 25 (1933): 569–70.
71 J. Clarence Chambers, Jr., "Mothers' Milk Bank in a Large Municipal Hospital," *Hospitals*
   16 (1942): 79–81. Junior League of Evanston, Illinois, "Premature Babies Milk Bank," in
   Clement A. Smith papers (copies in author's possession).
72 LaFetra, "Hospital Care of Premature Infants," p. 27; and Letters of John Price Crozer
   Griffith, vol. 1, 1914–15, p. 97. CPP.
73 B. Raymond Hoobler, "An Experiment in the Collection of Human Milk for Hospital
   and Dispensary Uses," *Archives of Pediatrics* 31 (1914): 171–3.

milk banks did not completely eradicate demand for private help in the home. However, most of the work of the Detroit Bureau of Wet Nurses, as the service was named, consisted of collecting and distributing breast milk from nursing mothers who came to the hospital two or three times a day to express their milk.[74] In 1917 the Bureau supplied 79 babies with 16,400 ounces of milk and placed twenty-seven wet nurses. A decade later, 323 babies received 41,395 ounces of milk, and no wet nurses went out to service.[75]

The women selling their milk in the opening decades of the twentieth century resembled those who took in babies to suckle half a century earlier. They had homes of their own, for the most part, but also needed to contribute to the family economy. In a 1925 article, Hoobler observed that one mother came to the Detroit Bureau of Wet Nurses during three "lactating periods," earning over thirty-five hundred dollars (approximately eight dollars per day) during one fourteen-month stretch. When the Bureau began refusing to buy her milk, Hoobler believed that she "deliberately became pregnant that she might again be a producing mother." Her income, he reported, enabled her to buy her own home.[76] A similar account of an extraordinarily lucrative arrangement came from New York City, where Henry Dwight Chapin reported in 1926 that one Italian-American woman earned almost one thousand dollars during a single year of selling milk to the Children's Welfare Federation.[77] More typical were the women selling their milk to the Directory for Mothers' Milk in Boston who received seven cents an ounce and earned approximately twenty-five dollars a month and in some cases much more.[78] According to public-health nurses working in the various milk banks around the country, payments ranged from twenty-five to one hundred dollars a month.[79] At the Registry for Mother's Milk in Pittsburgh, women earned five cents per ounce; the California Babies Hospital in Los Angeles paid seven cents; and the Chil-

74 B. Raymond Hoobler, "Problems Connected with the Collection and Production of Human Milk," *Journal of the American Medical Association* 69 (1917): 421–5; and idem, "Human Milk: Its Commercial Production and Distribution," *Journal of the American Medical Association* 84 (1925): 165–6.
75 Katherine Jones, "The Mothers Milk Bureau of Detroit," *Public Health Nurse* 20 (1928): 142.
76 Hoobler, "Human Milk: Its Commercial Production," p. 166. By 1928 the women were earning twelve cents an ounce. Jones, "Mothers Milk Bureau," p. 142.
77 Henry Dwight Chapin, "The Production and Handling of Human Milk," *Journal of the American Medical Association* 87 (1926): 1364. On the milk collection by the Children's Welfare Federation, see also Mary D. Blankenhorn, "A Breast Milk Dairy," *Hygeia* 11 (1933): 412.
78 Helene Walker, "Maternal Milk Collection," *Public Health Nurse* 20 (1928): 23–4; and Clement A. Smith papers (copies in author's possession).
79 "Maternal Milk Collection," *Public Health Nurse* 20 (1928): 384. For comparative statistics on prices and other aspects of milk banking, see Dorothy Deming, "The Wet Nurse Past and Present," *Public Health Nurse* 20 (1928): 87–90.

dren's Welfare Federation in New York City paid carfare as well as thirteen cents an ounce.[80]

The specter of charity hung over the job of milk selling, even though women were paid by the ounce for their milk. This reflected, in part, the fact that the hospitals recruited from among their own clinic patients. During his term at Bellevue, Hoobler explicitly termed the hospital's purchase of milk an act of "charity," believing that the needy mothers selling their milk would otherwise have had to receive assistance from "some organization."[81] Whether the women considered themselves to be workers or aid recipients remains unclear, although there is good evidence that the job provided at least some of them with an enviable income.

In addition to acknowledging their high-volume producers, doctors freely elaborated on the cases in which women were caught trying to exploit the system. Some women succumbed to the temptation to cheat and tried to boost their earnings by adding cow's milk or water to the collection bottle. According to the Children's Welfare Federation in New York City, so many attempted this deception that they had to change their procedures. Instead of the Federation's picking up the milk at the women's homes, it required them to express their milk at the local health station.[82]

Other evidence makes clear that the motives of milk sellers ranged from greed to altruism. Whereas some mothers poured water into the collection bottle, others refused payment and confided their emotional attachment to the unseen recipients of their milk. Public-health nurses reported that many of the "contributing mothers" asked about the progress and weight of the babies they were feeding.[83] One woman told the Boston Floating Hospital she preferred a letter of thanks to twenty-five dollars, and another claimed she always stayed in town on Sundays so she could make her "little contribution."[84] Undoubtedly, these women saw providing milk as a means of expressing their gratitude toward the hospital that treated them and their children without charge. Just as nineteenth-century wet nurses ranged from the noble to the venial, so too did the twentieth-century mothers who pumped their breasts in order to earn a few dollars a week.

Milk banks carefully selected and managed their staffs of lactating women. At the Boston Floating Hospital, for example, physicians evaluated the potential contributors, eliminating those they believed to be suffering from tuberculosis, syphilis, and other contagious diseases. The candi-

---

80 In a more old-fashioned arrangement, the Ingleside Home in Buffalo provided the wet nurses with a place to live in addition to four cents per ounce for their milk. Helen F. Leighty, "Preserving Human Milk," *Trained Nurse and Hospital Review* 103 (1939): 228.
81 Hoobler, "Experiment in the Collection of Human Milk for Hospital and Dispensary Uses," pp. 172–3.
82 Chapin, "Operation of a Breast Milk Dairy," p. 152.
83 "Maternal Milk Collection," p. 384.
84 Talbot, "Two Methods," p. 305.

dates also submitted to an examination by their own physicians, who attested to whether or not they had sufficient milk to supply their own babies as well as the hospital's. At this point, the nurse took charge, visiting each potential milk seller and excluding from participation any woman judged "dirty." Approved candidates received instructions in hygiene and milk-collection procedures, learned how to make ice boxes, and were taught to use the breast pumps supplied by the hospital.[85]

In milk banking, tasks were carefully apportioned among staff members, reflecting the division of labor within the hospital and the need to achieve maximum efficiency. Nurses handled the day-to-day responsibilities of collecting and processing the milk; physicians provided more distant oversight. A 1922 account described the rounds of a nurse who visited nursing mothers to collect their milk and stopped periodically at "a convenient drug store, where the clerk obligingly places [the milk] on ice." When she finished gathering the milk, she returned with it to the hospital, where it was mixed, pasteurized, and refrigerated.[86]

Once the milk reached the milk station little thought was given to its producers. Pooling milk from a number of women served to eradicate the characteristics of its individual producers. Pasteurization eliminated the potential for passing on disease. Concern shifted to maintaining milk freshness and to seeing to its prompt and safe distribution. These latter tasks made human milk analogous to cow's milk, and many technologies developed at the dairy found applications at the milk bank. Among them were efforts to move beyond refrigeration and develop new methods for long-term storage. Experiments begun at the Boston Floating Hospital in 1920 led to a method of drying the milk.[87] Research conducted at the Directory for Mothers' Milk in conjunction with the Borden Company led to development of a freezing process.[88] By the early 1930s, scientists at Cornell

85 Emerson, "Collection and Preservation of Human Milk," pp. 641–2; and Talbot, "Two Methods," p. 305.
86 Emerson, "Collection and Preservation of Human Milk," p. 642.
87 Ibid., pp. 641–2; idem, "Dried Human Milk," *American Journal of Diseases of Children* 30 (1925): 769–73; Paul W. Emerson and Lawrence W. Smith, "Dried Human Milk," *American Journal of Diseases of Children* 31 (1926): 1–21; Paul W. Emerson, "The Preservation of Human Milk," *New England Journal of Medicine* 209 (1933): 893–905; Lawrence Weld Smith, "The Experimental Feeding of Dried Breast Milk," *Journal of Biological Chemistry* 61 (1924): 625–31; and Lawrence Weld Smith and Paul W. Emerson, "Notes on the Experimental Production of Dried Breast Milk," *Boston Medical and Surgical Journal* 191 (1924): 938–40.
  The New York Foundling Hospital used a heating, sealing, and refrigeration technique for storing human milk. Scheuer and Duncan, "A Method of Preserving Breast Milk," pp. 249–54; and Jean Broadhurst and Jessie E. Duncan, "Preserving Mother's Milk," *American Journal of Nursing* 33 (1933): 453.
88 Paul Emerson and Washington Platt, "The Preservation of Human Milk: A Preliminary Note on the Freezing Process," *Journal of Pediatrics* 2 (1933) 472–7; Smith and Emerson, "Experimental Production of Dried Breast Milk," pp. 938–40.
  The Borden Company owned the patent on the process for freezing breast milk and

University had developed a means of canning breast milk that allowed it to be stored for up to two years.[89] With each step, the distance between producer and consumer expanded, and, ironically, human milk in its new packaging came to resemble the artificial foods meant to replace it.

The closing of the Boston Wet Nurse Directory in 1925 and the opening two years later of the Directory for Mothers' Milk demonstrate the evolution of milk banking. The home in which wet nurses once lived became a milk laboratory, and the goal of the organization moved from helping needy young women to assisting medically needy infants.[90] In a 1928 radio talk Talbot told listeners how each day three public-health nurses set out from the Directory in their Chevrolet coupe with an ice chest in the back seat. After making their rounds of lactating mothers, the nurses brought the milk back to the laboratory to be weighed, inspected, pooled, strained, pasteurized, and bottled for distribution.[91] Where Talbot once boasted about the moral reclamation of wet nurses, he now remained silent on the subject of who sold milk to the new organization, which, unlike its predecessor, remained in business for several decades. In 1930 the Directory for Mothers' Milk became affiliated with the Boston Lying-In Hospital, where it remained in service until 1962.[92]

The high cost of breast-milk collection meant that few milk banks broke even and that breast milk was an expensive product.[93] To make up the difference between income and expenses, many milk banks turned to charitable donations. The Directory for Mothers' Milk enjoyed the personal patronage of its founder, Talbot; other milk banks located institutional

offered the rights to the American Academy of Pediatrics in 1936. The academy rejected the offer because of the administrative expenses involved. "Report of the Committee on Clinical Investigation and Scientific Research on the Offer of the Borden Company to give to the American Academy of Pediatrics Directions for the Use of the Rights of the Patent of the Borden Company for Freezing Milk"; and "Meeting Between Dr. James A. Tobey of the Borden Company, Dr. Paul Emerson and Dr. F. B. Talbot, Wednesday, May 27, 1936." Talbot Papers. FACLM.

89 "Mother's Milk: Babies Now to Get Nature's Food in Cans," *Newsweek* 4 (November 10, 1934): 37.

90 Emerson, "Collection and Preservation of Human Milk," p. 205. On Talbot's continuing involvement with the Directory, see Talbot Papers. FACLM; and Clement A. Smith papers (copies in author's possession).

91 Fritz B. Talbot, "Radio Talk for the Directory for Mother's Milk Incorporated," Talbot Papers. FACLM.

92 Letter from Clement A. Smith to Mrs. William W. Carson, November 29, 1962. Smith papers (copies in author's possession). Smith, a leading neonatologist and director of pediatrics at the Boston Lying-In Hospital, served for twenty years as consultant and research director for the Directory for Mothers' Milk.

93 Both the Detroit and Boston milk banks had a sliding fee scale. In Detroit, private patients paid between ten and thirty cents an ounce, whereas institutions paid eight cents – lower than the purchase price. Hoobler, "Human Milk," pp. 165–6. In Boston, private patients spent between twelve and thirty cents an ounce for milk; private hospitals paid twelve cents an ounce and semiprivate hospitals fifteen cents. Walker, "Maternal Milk Collection," pp. 23–4; and Smith papers (copies in author's possession).

backers as well. The Visiting Nurse Association of Hartford, Connecticut, ran a milk bank supported by the local Junior League; the Kansas City Milk Bank depended upon the sponsorship of the Women's City Club; and the Clinic for Infant Feeding in Grand Rapids received funding from the Community Chest.[94]

In less than two decades milk banks evolved from relatively simple efforts to collect breast milk for hospitalized infants to sophisticated medical organizations producing processed human milk for distribution or sale. By 1929 at least twenty cities had milk banks in operation; in some cases they were run by child-welfare organizations, in other instances, by hospitals.[95] Meanwhile, physicians in cities without milk banks sometimes struggled to provide for their patients and called for milk banks to be established. A "Hospital and Health Survey" conducted in Philadelphia noted, for example, that the supply of human milk was "sporadic" and that there was a need for a central milk bureau.[96] Clearly, access to human milk was considered a basic (if sometimes unmet) need by health-care professionals.

When human milk became a commodity, wet nursing largely ceased to exist. A door of opportunity closed to poor single mothers who a generation earlier might have found work in private homes or on hospital wards. At the same time, milk selling was an occupation in which working-class women could earn small, and in a few instances, large, sums of money. Milk's commodification rested on the creation of technical, bureaucratic, and structural systems that allowed for the procurement, processing, and distribution of this new product. And the perception of newness was a critical element as well. Commodification was a cognitive step; human milk had taken on the guise of therapeutic merchandise and thus had been transformed. Once this had occurred, interest in breast milk shifted from the characteristics of its producers, lactating women, to those of its consumers, frail infants. And once infants became the focus, new questions arose. Should a woman sell or should she donate a commodity that could keep an infant alive?

94 Deming, "Wet Nurse Past and Present," p. 87; Mary Katherine Herwick, "A Mother's Milk Station," *American Journal of Nursing* 33 (1933): 455; and Blanche H. DeKoning, "A Twenty-two-year-old Breast Milk Service Reaps Its Reward," p. 570.
95 Tobey, "New Foster-Mother," p. 110.
96 Philadelphia Health and Hospital Survey Committee, *Philadelphia Hospital and Health Survey* (Philadelphia: Philadelphia Health and Hospital Survey, 1930), pp. 262, 280–1.

From commodity to gift

Bottled breast milk remains to this day a vital product for a small number of infants. However, it is collected and distributed far differently than it was early in the twentieth century. It is no longer a commodity sold by working-class women, but has become, instead, a gift. And it is given not in the expectation of reciprocity, but as part of a "moral transaction" encompassing late twentieth-century perceptions of infancy, mothering, economy, and society.[1] The idea that an infant might die because its family lacks the means to purchase breast milk has become morally repugnant, just as has the notion that a woman might earn a living by selling her milk.[2]

The transformed meaning of breast milk production is illustrated by an article in the December 1982 Boston Globe describing the meeting between Lacie Lynette Smith of Oklahoma and the women whose milk had kept her alive. Born with a rare allergic condition, Lacie could ingest nothing but breast milk. Her mother, unable to feed her because she was on medication, drained "every milk bank we could find." On the verge of running out of milk, she contacted the milk bank of Worcester, Massachusetts – one of thirty operating milk banks in the United States, and one with 275 donors. The Worcester milk bank started sending Lacie the milk she needed, and at the age of nineteen months Lacie traveled to New England to meet her unseen benefactors. One hundred and twenty women gathered at the airport to greet her arrival. A reporter asked one about her thoughts. "I prayed for this baby," she replied, "I just can't wait to meet her."[3] We can envision the airport tableau – the assembly of donating women surrounding the infant protagonist and her mother – and see a phenomenon transformed, but marked by the legacy of wet nursing. Social

1 This analysis of human milk as gift is drawn from Richard Titmuss's classic study of blood donation. Richard M. Titmuss, *The Gift Relationship: From Human Blood to Social Policy* (New York: Pantheon, 1971).
2 Thus the horrified reaction of a colleague who reports that a friend in Moscow is selling breast milk in order to have the money to buy meat.
3 "Okla. couple visit Mass. mothers who are keeping their baby alive," *Boston Globe*, 7 December 1982.

class, medical authority, and the cultural construction of motherhood are all elements in the modern history of breast milk.

Milk selling proved, in fact, to be a rather brief career opportunity for women, lasting perhaps sixty years – from the opening of the first milk-collection service in 1910 to the 1970s, when milk banks grew in number and became places where women could go to donate milk. As early as the 1930s, however, questions began to be raised about the appropriateness of selling breast milk, first because of the cost, especially when the milk was needed by poor infants, and second, as will be discussed shortly, in the context of World War II blood-donation drives and patriotism.

The birth of the Dionne quintuplets in May 1934 proved to be a pivotal event in the public's perception of breast milk. Their birth proclaimed a medical miracle. The story of the survival of the five tiny baby girls born in the backwoods of Canada's Ontario Province quickly attracted a Depression-era audience fascinated by what appeared to be a dramatic struggle between nature and science. As the babies clung to life, the local physician looking after them, Allan Roy Dafoe, emerged from obscurity to become an international hero.[4] Ironically, although the quintuplets grew up to become celebrities whose faces graced advertisements for Carnation Milk, in the early months of their lives they survived exclusively on donated human milk.

Initially, milk for the quintuplets came from the family's "lactating neighbors"; by the fourth day, however, it was arriving in regular rail shipments from the Toronto Hospital for Sick Children.[5] Like many of the other supplies needed by the babies, the milk was sent without charge. The Dionne family, although prosperous by local standards, had no money to spend on the medical personnel, equipment, and breast milk needed to keep their youngest children alive. Before becoming bottle babies, the quintuplets consumed over five hundred gallons of breast milk in a five-month period.

4 For popular accounts of the birth and subsequent development of the quintuplets, see *Time* 23 (June 11, 1934): 40; ibid. 23 (July 23, 1934): 31; ibid. 23 (September 3, 1934): 35; *Newsweek* 4 (June 9, 1934): 20; ibid. 4 (August 18, 1934): 20–1.
5 The milk was collected from nursing mothers by members of the Toronto Junior League who took the milk to the hospital where it was boiled, bottled, refrigerated, and shipped by train to Callander, Ontario. Pierre Berton, *The Dionne Years* (New York: W. W. Norton, 1977) p. 63. Berton states that the quintuplets received over eight thousand ounces of milk and that 120 shipments were made from Toronto. Dafoe, who became a well-paid spokesman for Carnation milk, had relatively little to say about the importance of the milk in his descriptions of the quintuplets. His brother wrote two articles on their care. See Allan Roy Dafoe, "The Survival of the Dionne Quints," *American Journal of Obstetrics and Gynecology* 39 (1940): 162; and idem, "Further History of the Care and Feeding of the Dionne Quints," *Canadian Medical Association Journal* 34 (1936): 31. Louise De Kiriline, one of the babies' nurses, offers more detail about how they were fed, but says very little about the milk shipments. Louise De Kiriline, *The Quintuplets' First Year; The Survival of the Famous Five Dionne Babies and Its Significance for All Mothers* (Toronto: MacMillan, 1936).

Americans as well as Canadians rushed forward with offers to aid the quintuplets. Immediately after learning of their birth, James A. Tobey, a physician affiliated with the Directory for Mothers' Milk in Boston, wired Dafoe to offer him frozen breast milk. His generosity came too late; the Toronto Hospital had already begun its shipments. Perhaps eager to steal a little of the limelight for his own work, Tobey explained to the readers of *Good Housekeeping* that bottled breast milk was neither a new product nor one that was exclusively available in Canada. With a nod to his own institution, Tobey proudly announced that the Kasper quadruplets of New Jersey received frozen mother's milk sent daily by plane from Boston.[6] Popular magazine articles about the Dionne quintuplets brought the work of milk banks before the public, shedding light on what had been an obscure medical phenomenon. *Newsweek* ran a brief article describing a milk bank in New York City, where "healthy, young Italian mothers" (who reportedly had the most and the best milk) earned an average of $13.65 a week selling their excess milk. The milk, the author reported, had been collected under strict control and had aided 333 babies.[7]

Although breast milk remained a commodity, the attention given to the Dionne quintuplets raised the question of whether such a vital fluid was best governed by the rules of commerce. Articles about milk banks made clear that the infants receiving bottled breast milk were those in the most precarious health. It was also evident from the press accounts that hospitals and milk banks met the infants' needs regardless of their parents' ability to pay. Yet, the propriety of women selling something that babies needed for their survival began to be challenged during World War II, when blood donation started to be touted as a patriotic duty. In one case, the media drew simplistic parallels between milk donation and blood donation. An article in *Parent's Magazine* in November 1943 reminded readers that "Over two million American blood donors have answered the call to help save our fighting men." The author then inquired: "Is it too much to ask that American mothers give milk to save American babies?"[8]

The analogy between blood and milk had little practical meaning. Whereas blood had no substitute and was in constant and great demand, only a few infants actually required human milk for their survival. As a leading pediatrician, William McKim Marriott pointed out in his 1930 textbook on infant feeding, "Most infants deprived of mother's milk may be fed artificially with as great success as with collected breast milk."[9] Thus milk banks remained on the periphery of medical practice, quietly engaged

6 James A. Tobey, "The Newest Foster Mother," *Good Housekeeping* 104 (1937): 76.
7 "Mother's Milk: Babies Now to Get Nature's Food in Cans," *Newsweek* 4 (November 10, 1934): 36–7.
8 Pearl P. Puckett, "Milk Banks for Babies," *Parent's Magazine* 18 (1943): 20.
9 William McKim Marriott, *Infant Nutrition* (St. Louis: C. V. Mosby, 1930), p. 113.

in the business of buying and distributing mother's milk. Their numbers appear to have grown during the Depression, reflecting perhaps their ability to attract women suddenly in need of income support. In 1939 Harlem Hospital in New York City opened a milk bank, as did the Chicago Board of Health. Philadelphia's first milk bank opened at the Pennsylvania Hospital in 1940.[10] During the war years and after, as new employment opportunities opened for women, the number of milk banks began to shrink. By 1955, only seven remained in operation.[11]

The Directory for Mothers' Milk in Boston, one of the last survivors, closed its doors in 1962. In its waning years, however, the Directory pointed the way to what would become the late twentieth-century pattern of human milk collection: it purchased milk not from low-income women but from middle-class mothers. An article in the *Boston Globe* reported that "mostly college grads" were "selling mother's milk" and that the women were using the money to "help put papa through graduate school."[12] The denouement of the wet nursing story thus had an ironic twist. Wet nursing was an occupation in which poor women served the babies of the rich. Milk selling, an occupation spawned in part by the poisoned class relations among mothers, doctors, and wet nurses in the contested terrain of the private nursery, became a job for the middle class. Because discussions of wet nursing often turned on whether the infant imbibed the characteristics of its wet nurse, the reference to college graduates could be a veiled hint that they were selling "smart milk."

More significantly, as the economic backgrounds of Boston's milk sellers imply, maternal nursing was gradually becoming more popular among middle-class women. The founding in 1956 of the La Leche League, an organization dedicated to "the womanly art of breast feeding," and the resurgence of maternal nursing in the "baby bust" years that soon followed, suggest that a fundamental reconception of middle-class maternity was underway.[13] According to the National Center for Health Statistics, the number of American women nursing their babies immediately after birth rose from 24.7 percent in 1971 to 55.3 percent in 1981.[14] In many cases the duration of nursing proved very brief. Even so, the figures seem to indicate that women believed they should make an effort to breast-feed.

10 J. Clarence Chambers, Jr., "Mothers' Milk Bank in a Large Municipal Hospital," *Hospitals* 16 (1942): 79–81; "Philadelphia's First Human Milk 'Bank' Saves Lives of Frail Babies," *Philadelphia Evening Bulletin*, 22 February 1940; and "Saving Lives with Mothers' Milk," *Hygeia* 18 (1940): 424–8.
11 E. Robbins Kimball et al., "The Breast Milk Bank as Community Project," *Pediatrics* 16 (1955): 264–7.
12 "Mostly College Grads Selling Mothers' Milk," *Boston Daily Globe*, 21 January 1961, p. 3.
13 Lynn Y. Weiner, "Reconstructing Motherhood: The La Leche League in Postwar America," *Journal of American History* 80 (1994): 1357–81.
14 Rima D. Apple, *Mothers and Medicine; A Social History of Infant Feeding* (Madison: University of Wisconsin Press, 1987), p. 197.

In 1982 maternal breast-feeding rates peaked at 61.9 percent, although by six months of age only 27.1 percent of babies were still being breast-fed. The latter figure was, nevertheless, five times higher than it had been in 1971, when the rate was only 5.4 percent.[15]

The reasons for the recrudescence of maternal nursing are numerous and to some degree contradictory. They include a feminist and countercultural rejection of medical authoritarianism (also evident in the embrace of the natural-childbirth movement) and at the same time reflect the continuing influence of the earlier "baby boom" generation, which constructed motherhood as a vocation.[16] Yet, motherhood was not women's only vocation in the 1970s. The growth in maternal nursing paralleled an increase in the labor force participation rate of women with young children.[17] this points to another critical factor: growing rates of maternal nursing were not universal, but were class based. Middle-class mothers embraced breast-feeding at a time when low-income women continued the practice of bottle-feeding. The use of mothering style as a demarcation of class – evident in the nineteenth century when well-to-do women saw breast-feeding by lower-class women as animallike – obviously continued in the late twentieth century.

Maternal nursing today remains highly regarded but not wholly unproblematic, again for reasons that appear familiar. In the highly sexualized society of the late twentieth century, female breasts are seen largely as sexual objects rather than in their role in lactation. One result is that lactation is expected to continue for only a brief time. Another is that when sexuality and lactation converge or threaten to do so women's behavior is called into question. In 1992 Denise Perrigo inquired at a volunteer center about being sexually aroused while nursing her child, setting off a chain of investigation that led to her being jailed, charged with sexual abuse and neglect, and separated from her baby for a year. According to the *Chicago Tribune* this was not the only case in which extended nursing was used against a woman in court, nor was it the first time that lactation was a

---

15 Alan S. Ryan, David Rush, Fritz W. Krieger, and Gregory E. Lewandowski, "Recent Declines in Breast-Feeding in the United States, 1984 Through 1989," *Pediatrics* 88 (1991): 719–27.

16 Elaine Tyler May, *Homeward Bound: American Families in the Cold War Era* (New York: Basic Books, 1988).

17 On sexuality after World War II, see John D'Emilio and Estelle B. Freedman, *Intimate Matters: A History of Sexuality in America* (New York: Harper & Row, 1988), pp. 301–43.
    The percentage of married women in the labor force with children aged six to seventeen grew from 28.3 percent in 1950 to 49.2 percent by 1970; the percentage of married women in the labor force with children under six grew from 11.9 percent in 1950 to 30.3 percent in 1970. Lynn Y. Weiner, *From Working Girl to Working Mother: The Female Labor Force in the United States, 1820–1980* (Chapel Hill: University of North Carolina Press, 1985), p. 5, Table 7, "Percentage of Married Women in the Labor Force, by Presence and Age of Children, 1948–1970."

subject for adjudication.[18] Lactation consultants sometimes testify in custody trials, as expert witnesses who can support a woman's argument that she should not be separated from her nursing child.[19]

Breast milk, like breast-feeding, also provokes ambivalence. In the late twentieth century, human milk is a symbol of purity, albeit one sometimes sullied by pollution. Anti-war activists of the 1960s decried the presence of the radioactive element strontium 90 in mother's milk; environmental activists of the 1980s rued the discovery that human milk contained dioxin. Now, of course, doctors debate whether breast-feeding should be forbidden to women infected with the human immunodeficiency virus.[20] Strontium 90, dioxin, and human immunodeficiency virus can be found in other parts of the body, but it is their presence in mother's milk that sends the loudest message. For, just as nineteenth-century Americans argued about character, heredity, and the environment by posing questions about the foreign-born wet nurse, so too do twentieth-century Americans express their deepest anxieties in their questions about the purity of human milk.

The fact that we voice public concerns by referencing the breast and the baby speaks to the enduring cultural resonance of actions performed in the nursery. The end of the wet nurse has not, as some nineteenth-century critics had hoped, left us free to chose between what mothers can provide and what science can create. Rather, it has left us as a culture still struggling to frame the social and biological definitions of motherhood and the shifting ideologies upon which they rest.

18 *Chicago Tribune*, 9 February 1992, p. 17. Perrigo called a community volunteer center to find the number of the La Leche League, mentioning that nursing her two-year-old child caused her to sometimes become sexually aroused. The volunteer center gave her the number of a rape crisis center, and the rape crisis center in turn called a child abuse hot line.

19 Ann Suhler, Priscilla G. Bornmann, and JoAnne W. Scott, "The Lactation Consultant as Expert Witness," *Journal of Human Lactation* 7 (1991): 129–35; and "Review of Cases Related to Breastfeeding and Custody Cases," *Journal of Human Lactation* 7 (1991): 140.

20 Margaret J. Oxtoby, "Human immunodeficiency virus and other viruses in human milk: placing the issues in broader perspective," *Pediatric Infectious Diseases* 7 (1988): 825–35.

INDEX

A. M. B. [magazine correspondent], 169,
171
abandoned babies, 102
abortion, 24
Abt, Isaac, M.D., 77, 136, 146, 186(n29),
191
Adams, Abigail, 34
advertisements
for infant foods, 134, 167
for wet nurses, 26–7, 67–73, 74–6, 95,
108–9
Advice to Mothers (Buchan), 16
African-Americans
as domestics, 73, 112
as wet nurses, 25–7, 30, 32, 34, 72, 73,
108, 112, 192
alcohol, 156
wet nurses' use of, 150–1, 155
Alcott, Louisa May, 75
Alcott, William, 52
Aldrich, F. L. S., M.D., 140
Allen, Mary Wood, 175–6
Allen, Nathan, 137
amenorrhea, during breast-feeding, 23–4
*The American Domestick Medicine; or, Medical
Admonisher* (Gates), 51
American Journal of Diseases of Children, 155
*American Journal of Obstetrics and Diseases of
Children*, 144
American Medical Association, 139, 154,
166, 172, 192
American Medical Monthly, 55
American Revolution, 39
Anchorage, 87
The Angel of Bethesda (Mather), 11
Anglo-Saxon race and traits, 153, 157
antebellum period, wet nursing during, 70,
73
Apple, Rima D., 156
Archives of Pediatrics, 140, 154
artificial formulas and feeding, 9, 17, 96,
131, 139, 157, 165

bacterial contamination of, 17
commercial, 164, 165, 167
development of, 135–6
effect on wet nursing, 156, 160
history of, 1(n2), 116, 134
problems with, 158
promotion by physicians, 5, 135, 168–
169
Ashbrooke, Mrs. [wet nurse], 17
Astor, John Jacob, 61

*Baby: A Monthly Magazine Devoted to the
Care of Babies and Children: Medical, Men-
tal and Physical*, 167
Baby Doctor (Abt), 77
baby farmers, 101, 113, 175
Babyhood, 141, 150, 159, 160
as forum for scientific mothers and wet
nursing, 165, 166–7, 168, 169, 170–1,
174, 176
bacteriology, 132–3
Badger, Mary, 36
Bakewell, J. (Mrs.), 48
Ballard, Martha, 18, 20
Baltimore Board of Supervision of City
Charities, 144
Baltimore Sun, 71, 72
Barrett, Kate Waller, 86
Bastardy Law, 188
Beach, Wooster, M.D., 51–2
Beecher, Catherine, 49, 50
beer, perceived lactogenic affect of, 150
Bellevue Hospital (New York), 181, 195,
197
Bellevue Hospital Medical College (New
York), 166
benevolent institutions, effect on wet nurse
marketplace, 87, 92
birthrate, changes in, 137–8, 158
Blackberry Winter (Mead), 1
Blackwell's Island Almshouse, 113–14
Blanton, Wyndham, 25

Bok, Edward, 167
Bonner, W. T., 183
The Borden Company, 198
Boston
    foundling hospitals in, 119, 120
    single-mother shelters in, 86, 88, 89
    wet nursing in, 22, 31, 78, 79, 95, 105–7,
        119
Boston Board of Health, 119
Boston Children's Hospital, 195
Boston City Temporary Home, 78, 79, 80,
    81, 95, 98, 99, 100, 101, 102, 105, 106,
    108, 109, 126
Boston Evening Transcript, 68, 69, 71, 72, 75
Boston Floating Hospital, 194–5, 197, 198
Boston Globe, 201, 204
Boston Lying-In Hospital, 76, 88, 89, 102,
    104, 110, 199
Boston Medical and Surgical Journal, 194
Boston Medical Library, 185
Boston Wet Nurse Directory, 184, 187, 188,
    191, 194, 199
bottle-feeding, 9, 16, 17, 95
    breast-feeding compared to, 123–4, 139
    of institutionalized babies, 117
    replacement of breast-feeding by, 132, 134
Brace, Charles Loring, 113
Bradlee, John Tisdale, 80
breast-feeding
    amenorrhea during, 23–4
    among well-to-do women, 138–9, 205
    bottle-feeding as choice over, 1, 139
    current notions of sexuality and, 205
    current revival of, 204–5
    maternal rejection of, 45, 138–9
    as means of birth limitation, 24, 33
    perceived as confining, 138
    physical demands of, 148–9
    problems associated with, 19–20
    in public, 138
breast milk
    artificial expression of, 190, 195, 196
    bottled, 9, 193, 201, 203
    commodification of, 179–200
    examination of, 129
    as gift, 201–6
    pollutants in, 206
    preservation methods for, 198–9
    price of, 195, 196–7, 199(n93), 203
    use for premature babies, 179, 180–1, 182,
        186, 187
Bridgwater Almshouse, 78
Brieux, Eugene, 147
Buchan, William, M.D., 16–17, 50
Buckingham, Charles E., 164
Burns, Doris [wet nurse], 99
Burns, John, M.D., 55(n61)

Busey, Samuel, M.D., 98
Butler, Elisa, 60

Cabot, Elizabeth, 43
Cabot, Stephen Perkins, 143
Cadogan, William, M.D., 15
California Babies Hospital (Los Angeles),
    196
caloric system, for scientific infant formulas,
    135
Calvinism, 41
Canada, as wet-nurse birthplace, 108, 109,
    110
*Care and Feeding of Children: A Catechism for
    the Use of Mothers and Children's Nurses*
    (Holt), 135
Carnation Milk, 202
Carnrick's Soluble Food, 167
Carpenter, James, 158
Carpenter, Julia, 158
Carter, Alice P. [magazine correspondent],
    160
Carter, Landon, 25, 26
Carter, Robert, III, 26
Catholicism, 109, 114
chancre, 143
Chapin, Henry Dwight, M.D., 182, 196
Charles Street Temporary Home (Boston),
    126
Charleston Courier, 73
Chicago, single-mother shelters in, 87
Chicago Board of Health, 204
Chicago Tribune, 205
Child, Lydia Maria, 52, 57
child and infant welfare, 113, 115
childbirth, maternal mortality from, 18, 44–
    5
child rearing, 38, 64, 156, 167
children, value of, 130
Children's Aid Society, 85
Children's Bureau, 132, 181
children's hospitals, 130
Children's Memorial Hospital (Chicago),
    190
Children's Welfare Federation (New York),
    196–7
cholera infantum, 34
Christian Home (Philadelphia), 83, 84, 87
Churchill, Frank S., M.D., 155
Civil War, 39, 44, 47, 107, 136
clergymen, early views on wet nursing, 11–
    13
Clinic for Infant Feeding (Grand Rapids),
    195, 200
Clinton, Elizabeth, 13
Codman, William C. (Mrs.), 90
colic, 149, 150, 176

Colles's law, 145
colonial America, wet nursing in, 8, 11–37
colostrum, 128, 182
Colson, Victoria [wet nurse], 103
Combe, Andrew, 50
Community Chest (Grand Rapids), 200
condensed milk, use in infant feeding, 158
Condie, D. Francis, M.D., 56, 58
congenital debility and malformations, as infant death causes, 124
Consumptives Home (Boston), 143
contamination, of milk and water supplies, 124
contraceptive effects, of breast-feeding, 23–4, 25, 33, 35
convulsions, in babies, 151, 170
Coolidge, David H., 103
Cornell University, 198–9
Cott, Nancy, 41
cottage industry, wet nursing as, 22–3
Cotton, Alfred Cleveland, M.D., 139
The Countesse of Lincolnes Nursery (Clinton), 13
country areas, outplacement of infants to, 56
Courtney, Jane [wet nurse], 59
cow's milk
    adulteration and contamination of, 132–3, 136, 143
    certification of, 133, 141
    modified, for infant feeding, 134
    pasteurization of, 132
    raw, 133–4
    use in early infant feeding, 1, 9, 132–3, 158, 171
Crane, Sophie [wet nurse], 132
crippled children's homes, 130
Crosby, Darius, 81
cross-racial wet nursing, 26, 73, 74, 153
cult of domesticity, 41
Cummings, William H., 55

Dafoe, Allan Roy, M.D., 202, 203
Damaged Goods (Brieux), 147
Dana, Richard Henry, Jr., 60
"dangerous poor," 83
Daughter's of Charity of St. Vincent De Paul, 119
Davenport, Bridget [wet nurse], 21
Davis, Effa V., M.D., 97, 177
death of mother. *See* maternal mortality
death rate. *See* infant mortality; maternal mortality
Deland, Margaret, 86
Dennis, Vinnie [wet nurse], 107–8, 112
Denny, Francis D., 80
Denny, Francis Parkman, M.D., 194

Depression era, 204
desertion, as factor for wet nurses, 107–8
Detroit Bureau of Wet Nurses, 196
Detroit Women's Hospital and Infants' Home, 195
Devine, Hugh, 59
Dewees, William Potts, M.D., 38–9, 52, 54, 57, 62
Dionne quintuplets, breast-milk donations for, 202–3
dioxin, in breast milk, 206
diphtheria, 132
Directory for Mothers' Milk (Boston), 196, 198, 199, 203, 204
diseases
    among institutionalized foundlings, 123
    of wet nurses, 16, 54, 140, 143–6, 167–8, 187
domestic feminism, 156
Domestic Medicine (Buchan), 16, 50
domestic service
    single mothers in, 83
    wet nursing as path to, 60–2, 174–5
    as women's occupation, 42–3
"Dr. Holt's Bible," 135
Drake, George, B., 143
Drinker, Ann, 33
Drinker, Benjamin, 33
Drinker, Charles, 35
Drinker, Elizabeth Sandwith, 32–7, 38, 43, 46
Drinker, George, 33
Drinker, Henry Sandwith, 34
Driscoll, Catherine [wet nurse], 99
drugs, wet nurses' use of, 150, 155
Du Bois, Mary Delafield, 84, 91, 93

E. B. L. [magazine correspondent], 175
Earle, Charles Warrington, 140
Eberle, John, M.D., 52, 53, 57
eighteenth century, wet nursing in, 8, 11–37
Elizabeth in Her Holy Retirement (Mather), 11
Ellington, George [pseudonym], 76
Elmira (New York), 87
Ely, Will, M.D., 172
Emile (Rousseau), 13
emotions, supposed effect on lactation, 65–6, 151–2, 153, 170
England
    as wet-nurse birthplace, 108, 109, 110
    wet nursing in, 13, 16–17, 115
Ennis, Mary, 91
Erring Women's Refuge, 87
An Essay upon Nursing, and the Management of Children (Cadogan), 15
Esther Waters (Moore), 97
ethinc origin, of wet nurses, 108, 191–2, 196, 203

Europe
  foundling hospitals in, 114
  wet nursing in, 2–3, 8, 13, 14, 190
Eve's Daughters (Harland), 138, 166
Ewell, James, M.D., 50
Excell, Hannah [wet nurse], 28

Fairchild's Peptogenic Powder, 165
family size
  limitation after colonial period, 39–40
  limitation by lactation, 23
Fanny [motherless baby], 172–4
farming-out system. *See* outplacement
fertility, limitation in nineteenth century,
  39–40
*The First Baby: His Trials and the Trials of His
  Parents* (Walker), 64–6, 141
Fischer, Louis, M.D., 128, 129
Fisher, Betsy Rhoads, 20
Fithian, Philip Vickers, 26
Flanigan, Eva [wet nurse], 107
Flint, Ann [wet nurse], 30
Florence Crittendon Missions, 86, 190
Foster, Alfred S., 108
Foundling Hospital (Ackworth, Yorkshire),
  16
Foundling Hospital of the Sisters of Charity
  (New York), 117(n54), 119, 120
foundling hospitals and infant asylums, 83,
  84, 90, 102–27, 129, 130, 174
  history of, 114
  wet nursing in, 13, 77, 84, 112, 118,
  179
foundlings, in early America, 113
France, wet nursing in, 8, 13, 14, 114, 115
Frankford (Philadelphia), 33, 34
Franklin, Benjamin, 14
Freeman, Rowland Godfrey, 162
frontier residents, early medical treatise for,
  51
Fullerton, Anna M., 167

gastrointestinal diseases, among infants, 123,
  124, 125
General Federation of Women's Clubs, 157
Georgia Gazette, 27
Germany
  American domestic servants from, 43, 72
  as wet-nurse birthplace, 108, 109, 110,
  137, 165
  wet nursing in, 13
germ theory, 129, 132, 157
Getchell, F. H., M.D., 148, 151
Gibbs, Robert, 28
Gilman, Charlotte Perkins, 149
Girard, Stephen, 31–2

goat's milk, use in infant feeding, 1, 9, 51
Godey's Lady's Book, 56
gonorrhea, 187
Good Housekeeping, 167, 203
Goodwife Taylor [wet nurse], 28
Gouge, William, 24
Green, Louise [wet nurse], 103
Griffith, John Price Crozer, M.D., 148, 153,
  190
Grimes, Charles, 105
Grimes, Wallace Theodore, 105
Guardians of the Poor (Philadelphia), 30,
  59
Gunn, John, M.D., 51
Gwyn, Charles L., M.D., 140

Hale, Annie, M.D., 151
hand-feeding, 9, 12
Harland, Marion. *See* Terhune, Mary
Harlem Hospital, 204
Harper, Alice, 31
Harper's Weekly, 91
Hartshorne (Prof.), 167
Harvard Medical School, 132, 155, 184
health concerns, maternal feeding and, 23
Hearth and Home, 134
Helen Brent, M.D., 143
heredity, lactational, 152–3, 170
Hess, Julius H., M.D., 182, 191
Hill, Richard, M.D., 23
Hints for the Nursery (Hopkinson), 58
Hirst, Mary, 22
Hitchcock, Enos, 12
Hoffert, Sylvia, 44
Holt, Luther Emmett, M.D., 97, 135, 141,
  161
home, concept of, in nineteenth century,
  40–1
Home Comfort, 138
Hoobler, B. Raymond, M.D., 195, 197
Hopkinson, C. A. (Mrs.), 58
"Hospital and Health Survey" (Philadel-
  phia), 200
hospitals, as wet-nurse sources, 97–127
Hough [police captain], 81
Household News, 167
House of Reception (New York Infant Asy-
  lum), 118
How Women Can Make Money, 141
human immunodeficiency virus, in breast
  milk, 206
human milk. *See* breast milk
hypoprolactinemia, 19

Ideaal Married Life (Allen), 175
infant asylums. *See* foundling hospitals and
  infant asylums

Infant Feeding: In its Relation to Health and Disease (Fischer), 128
Infant Hospital (New York), 117
infanticide, 101, 114
infant mortality
  comparison among breast-fed and bottle-fed babies, 123–4
  feeding decisions affecting, 2
  of foundlings, 116, 117, 118, 119, 120, 121, 122
  rates of, 157–8, 180, 195
  wet nursing and increase of, 13, 97, 116, 117
infant nourishment
  artificial formulas as. *See* formulas and feeding
  comparison among breast-fed and bottle-fed babies, 123–4
  medical management of, 52, 53, 131, 135
  mother's milk as. *See* breast-feeding
  science of, 9
  wet nursing for. *See* wet nurses; wet nursing
infants, abandoned, 29
intelligence offices, for female domestics, 75, 83–4, 95
Interested Reader [magazine correspondent], 165, 171
Ireland
  as source of American domestic servants, 43, 61, 108, 112(n34)
  as wet-nurse birthplace, 108–10, 137, 152, 153, 162, 163, 175
Irish Marys [wet nurses], 162, 163, 175
Italy
  immigrants from, 112
  as wet nurse birthplace, 152, 203

Jacobi, Abraham, M.D., 94, 126, 137
Jameson, Horatio Gates, M.D., 51
Jenny [wet nurse], 172
Jewish immigrants, 112
Journal of the American Medical Association, 144, 145
Junior League (Hartford), 200
Just's Food, 165

K. H. [magazine correspondent], 170, 172
Kansas City Milk Bank, 200
Kasper quadruplets, breast-milk donations for, 203
Katzman, David, 67
Kilmer, Theron, 148
Kinney, Anna, 90
Kopytoff, Igor, 192

lactation. *See* breast-feeding
lactational heredity, 152–3, 170

Ladies Home Journal, 137, 167
LaFetra, Linnaeus, M.D., 181
La Leche League, 204
Larkey, Betty [wet nurse], 35, 36
laudanum, use to pacify infants, 57, 150
Lawrence Fire Insurance Company, 80
Lebsock, Suzanne, 41
Leibig's infant food, 134
let-down reflex, interference with, 19
Letters to Married Women on the Nursing and Management of Children (Smith), 16, 24
Logan, George, M.D., 74
London Foundling Hospital, 15, 115
Loomis, Elizabeth [wet nurse], 99
Louise J. [magazine correspondent], 165
Love, I. N., M.D., 154, 155
lying-in hospitals, as wet nurse source, 87, 89–95, 129

M. M. [magazine correspondent], 174–5
M. S. [magazine correspondent], 176
McCall, Katie [wet nurse], 103
McDernish, Grace [wet nurse], 59
McFarlaine, Betsy, 78
McIntosh, Maria, 48
McLean, Maggie [wet nurse], 104
McMillen, Sally, 44
malaria, 18, 19
male heirs, wet nursing and desire for, 13–14
Malthus, Thomas, 115
"mammy," African-American woman as, 74
The Management of Infancy (Combe), 50
Manhattan Maternity and Dispensary, 195
Maria [wet nurse], 61–2
Marion-Sims College of Medicine (St. Louis), 154
married women
  as milk sellers, 198, 204
  as wet nurses, 99, 103, 105, 107
Marriott, William McKim, 203
Maryland Lying-In Asylum, 71
Massachusetts, wet-nurse regulation in, 101
Massachusetts Babies Hospital, 182, 183
Massachusetts General Hospital, 184, 187, 189(n45)
Massachusetts Infant Asylum, 95, 102–3, 104, 105, 107, 108, 110, 111, 120–21, 122, 123, 143, 182, 183, 185, 194
Massachusetts Infant Hospital, 122
mastitis, 20
Materfamilias [magazine correspondent], 170, 171
Mater [magazine correspondent], 169
maternal morbidity, wet nursing during, 19–20, 34, 45
maternal mortality, wet nursing after, 17–18, 19, 32

The Maternal Physician, 38
maternity homes, as source of wet nurses, 75, 76
Mather, Cotton, 11, 12, 38
Mead, Margaret, 1, 2
Meckel, Richard, 131
medical practice
    effects and views on infant feeding, 15–16, 52
    effects and views on wet nursing, 3–4, 5, 7, 14, 16, 42, 50, 127–55, 186–7
medical social work, 187
Mellin's Food, 164, 165, 17
Memoirs of the Bloomsgrove Family (Hitchcock), 12
middle class
    breast-feeding among, 205
    effects on wet nursing, 42, 62
    motherhood values of, 47–8, 156–8
milk. *See* breast milk; condensed milk; cow's milk' goat's milk
milk banks, 193–200, 201, 202, 203–4
"milk punch," nursling affected by, 150
milk science, 134
Miss M. T. Finn's Select Registry for Wet Nurses and Female Help, 75, 76
Moore, Edward Mott, M.D., 172
Moore, George, 97
"moral lepers" and "moral monsters," wet nurses depicted as, 5, 10
moral motherhood, 41, 47
morals
    of single mothers, 85–6, 154, 168, 169, 191
    of wet nurses, 162, 166
Morris, Margaret Hill, 23, 31
Morse, John Lovett, M.D., 155, 186, 188
mortality
    of infants. *See* infant mortality
    of mothers. *See* maternal mortality
Moscow Foundling Home, 114
The Mother and Her Offspring (Tracey), 52
Motherhood, 141
motherhood
    medicalization of, 6–7, 8
    in postrevolutionary era, 38–63
    scientific, 5, 157
    social dichotomies of, 60
    social meaning of, 5
    as women's career, 156, 205
mother love, development of, 5(n12)
The Mother's Practical Guide (Bakewell), 48
multiple births, prematurity and, 180(n6)
Munn, Aristeen Pixley, 172–4

N. N. [magazine correspondent], 168–9, 170, 171, 172

Nanny Harper [wet nurse], 33–4, 36
Nanny Oats [wet nurse], 34–5, 35
Nantucket, maternal mortality in, 18–19
Napheys, George, 151
National Center for Health Statistics, 204
National Congress of Mothers, 157
Native Americans, as wet nurses, 226
neighbors, as wet nurses, 20, 35, 36–7, 39, 43, 202
neurasthenia, 137
New England
    maternal mortality in, 18
    motherhood concepts in, 41
    wet nursing in, 18–19, 20, 21, 22–3, 28, 31, 36
New England Hospital for Women and Children, 89, 90, 102, 103, 104, 110
New England Oil Company, 183
New Orleans, wet nurses in, 72
New Orleans Daily Picayune, 73
Newsweek, 203
New York City Alms-House, 117
New York Female Asylum for Lying-In Women, 88, 89
New York Foundling Hospital, 190
New York Herald, 65
New York Infant Asylum, 94, 117(n54), 118–19, 121
New York Nursery and Child's Hospital, 102, 117(n54)
New York State, foundling hospital system in, 117(n54)
New York Times, 170
nineteenth century, wet nursing in, 44–5, 77–8, 128–55, 156
Northern United States, wet nursing in, 25, 26, 28, 30, 73, 74
Norton, Mary Beth, 25
Norwood, Laura Lenoir, 54
nursery, domestic help in, 160–1
Nursery and Child's Hospital (New York), 93–4, 95, 108, 117(n54), 125, 126
Nursery for the Children of Poor Woman (New York), 90–1, 92, 93
nursery maids, 160, 161
nurses
    trained. *See* trained nurses
    wet. *See* wet nurses
    work day of, 161(n14)

O'Connor, Mary [wet nurse], 105
opium tincture. *See* laudanum
Orphan Society of Philadelphia, 58, 59
outplacement, of infants for wet nursing, 56, 58, 114, 115, 117, 120
Overseers of the Poor of Philadelphia, 29, 30

Pacific Fur Company, 61
pap boat, 9, 17
paregoric, use to pacify infants, 150
Parent's Magazine, 203
Parkman, Ebenezer, 20, 21(n45)
Parkman, Hannah, 20, 21(n45)
pasteurization, of breast milk, 198
Peckham, Grace, 141
pediatrics, as medical specialty, 9, 14(n14), 52, 53, 74, 97, 129, 130-1
Penniston, Clara, 141
Pennsylvania Hospital (Philadelphia), 31, 204
percentage system, for scientific infant formulas, 135
Perrigo, Denise, 205
pewter, in early pap boats, 17
Phelps, Almira, 56
Philadelphia Home for Infants, 84, 102, 107, 123, 125
Philadelphia Orphan Asylum, 59
Philadelphia Public Ledger, 68, 71, 72
Philadelphia Temporary Home, 84
Philadelphia, wet nursing in early, 27, 29, 30-1, 32-7, 58, 83, 84
physicians. *See also* medical practice
  views and effects on wet nursing, 7, 16, 26, 42, 50, 53, 54, 55, 128-55, 160
The Planter's and Mariner's Medical Companion (Ewell), 50-1
Pool, Nancy [wet nurse], 35
post-Civil War period, wet nursing in, 8-9
postpartum fever, 20
A Practical Treatise on the Diseases of Children (Stewart), 52
Premature and Congenitally Diseased Infants, 182
premature infants, 124, 146, 178
  breast milk use for, 179, 180-1, 182, 186, 187
  medical care of, 180-2
Pridham, N. C., 73
Protestant Home of Philadelphia, 83, 84-5, 87
puerperal fever, 61, 88
Puritans, wet nurse use by, 22
Pynchon, John, 28

Quakers, wet nurse use by, 27, 33, 34

race, maternal feeding and, 23
race suicide, 137
Randall's Island Infant Hospital, 116-17, 119, 122
raw milk, 133
Registry for Mother's Milk (Pittsburgh), 196

republican motherhood, 41
rescue homes, 83
respiratory diseases, among infants, 123, 124
Reynell, John, 27
Richmond, Sarah A., 118
Riis, Jacob, 119
Rockdale (Pennsylvania), wet nursing study of, 45-7
Rodale, Ellen [wet nurse], 103
Rosell, M. D., 72
Rosenberg, Charles, 52
Rotch, Thomas Morgan, M.D., 135, 136, 149
Rousel Law [France], 115
Rousseau, Jean-Jacques, 13
Royal Pennsylvania Gazette, 27
Rush, Benjamin, M.D., 16, 36
Russia, wet nursing in, 114-15

St. Louis Children's Hospital, 190
St. Mary's Infant Asylum and Lying-In Hospital (Boston), 119
St. Petersburg, wet nursing in, 114-15
Salvation Army, 86, 87, 190
Sarah Morris Children's Hospital (Chicago), 190, 191
Scandinavia
  diseased wet-nurse case in, 54
  as source of American domestic servants, 43, 112(n34)
  as wet-nurse birthplace, 108, 110
scarlet fever, 132
The Science of Motherhood (Smith), 157
scientific infant foods and feedings, 178
  artificial formulas for, 9-10
scientific mothers and motherhood, 5, 156-8, 166, 167
Scott, Elizabeth [wet nurse], 35-6
Scovil, Elisabeth Robinson, 167
scrofula, 143
septic sore throat, 132
Sewall, Hannah, 21, 22
Sewall, Henry, 22
Sewall, Judith, 21
Sewall, Mary, 22
Sewall, Samuel, 21, 22, 23
sexual activity, supposed effect on lactation, 65-6, 151, 152
sexual double standard, 82, 83
sexuality
  attitudes toward, 147
  maternal feeding and, 23, 45, 205
sexual relations, during nursing, 13, 24, 151
Sheppard-Towner Act (1921), 132, 181
Sigourney, Lydia, 41
Sinclair, Upton, 147

single mothers
  lying-in homes and shelters for, 64–5, 83,
    86, 88–90, 104
  rehabilitation of, 187–8
  as wet nurses, 6, 63, 76, 77–8, 103, 104–5,
    154–5, 166, 168, 170, 173–4, 187, 188
slaves, as wet nurses, 25–7, 32, 34, 73
Smith, Clementina, 46–7
Smith, Hannah Whitall, 157
Smith, Harriet, 46, 59, 164
Smith, Hugh, M.D., 15–16, 24
Smith, J. Lewis, M.D., 113, 118, 151
Smith, Laci Lynette, 201
Smith, Lanta Wilson, 170
Snyder, J. Ross, M.D., 184
social welfare, in nineteenth century, 81
social work, medical. *See* medical social
    work
Society for the Prevention of Cruelty to Chil-
    dren, 101, 119
Society for the Relief and Employment of
    the Poor (Philadelphia), 98
South Carolina Gazette, 14–15
Southern United States
  motherhood concepts in, 41
  wet nursing in, 17, 18, 25–7, 29, 44, 72,
    73, 153
Spencer, Charles, 177
spoons, use for infant feeding, 17
Spruill, Julia Cherry, 25
Stanton, Elizabeth Cady, 50
Stedman, Charles H., M.D., 60
Stewart, James, M.D., 52
Stiles, Ezra, 18
stillbirths, 19
Stowe, Charles Edwards, 49
Stowe, Harriet Beecher, 49–50
strontium 90, in breast milk, 206
Stuart, Emma Elizabeth Sullivan, 60–1
Sweden, as wet-nurse birthplace, 72
swill milk, 132
syphilis, 70, 143, 144–7, 161, 187, 197

Talbot, Fritz Bradley, M.D., 184–5, 186,
    187, 188, 189(n45), 194, 199
Taylor, William H., M.D., 180
Terhune, Mary [pseud. Marion Harland],
    138, 152, 166–7
Tewksbury State Almshouse (Massachu-
    setts), 78, 104–5, 120
Thorne, Matilda, 59, 60
Ticknor, Caleb, M.D., 52
tobacco, as payment for wet nursing, 29
Tobey, James A., M.D., 203
Toronto Hospital for Sick Children, 202
Tower, Esther [wet nurse], 107

Tracey, Stephen, 52
Trained Motherhood, 164, 167, 170
trained nurses, 142, 160–2
*A Treatise on the Diseases and Physical Educa-
    tion of Children* (Eberle), 52
Treatise on the Domestic Economy (Beecher),
    49
*Treatise on the Physical and Mental Treatment
    of Children* (Dewees), 52
tuberculosis, 132, 143, 161, 187, 197
Turner, Arthur, 17–18
twentieth century, breast milk commodifi-
    cation in, 179–200
twins, wet nursing of, 152–3, 177
Two Lives; or To Seem To Be (McIntosh), 48
Tyler, Mary Palmer, 38, 48–9
typhoid fever, 132, 194
"tyranny of the household," 62

Underwood, Michael, M.D., 15
University of Minnesota Hospital, 190
University of Pennsylvania, 39
urban areas, wet-nurse marketplace in, 64–
    96
urban growth rate, 42(n15)

Vannater, Lydia, 59, 60
venereal disease
  as prematurity cause, 190
  in wet nurses, 54–5, 143, 144–6, 187
"vicious poor," wet nurses as members of,
    154
violence, supposed effect on lactation, 151
Visiting Nurse Association (Hartford), 200
Vogel, Morris, 76

Wadsworth, Benjamin, 12
Walker, Jerome, M.D., 64, 112, 141
Walters, Jane [wet nurse], 99
Warner, Amos, 116
Wassermann test, 144, 146
Waters, Ethel, 126
weaning, from wet nurses, 21–2, 33, 36
The Well-Ordered Family; Or, Relative Duties
    (Wadsworth), 12
well-to-do women
  breast-feeding among, 138–9, 205
  child rearing by, 160
wet nurses
  age of, 102–3
  bonds with nurslings, 62, 100, 159
  bureaus and agencies for, 183–5, 186
  clothes purchases for, 141–2
  defenders of, 172–6
  diet of, 149–50, 162, 163, 164
  difficult working conditions for, 177–8

wet nurses (*Continued*)
  as disease carriers, 16, 54, 140, 143–6,
    167–8, 187
  domestic-labor experiences of, 110, 177
  domestic servants compared to, 154, 177
  effects on nursling's health, 152
  employers of, 9, 28, 80–1
  ethnic origin of, 108, 191–2, 196, 203
  gratitude toward, 172–4, 175
  household power of, 155–78
  infants of, 57, 91, 97–127, 142, 163, 164,
    186
  as instinctive entrepreneurs, 58, 60
  as instinctive mothers, 58–60
  institutional, 183, 194
  live-in, 3–4, 35, 45–7, 58–9, 99, 100, 102,
    121–2, 177
  loss of own babies by, 70, 127, 142, 143
  managerial problems of, 147–8
  marketplace for, 6, 9, 28, 31, 64–96, 183
  medical profession and. *See under* medical
    practice; individual physicians
  milk examination of, 142, 143
  monitoring of, 185–6
  morals of, 162, 166
  neighbors as, 20, 35, 36–7, 39, 43, 202
  nurslings' disease transmission to, 144,
    145
  personalistic accounts of, 168
  physicians as intermediaries for, 128–55,
    158–9, 172, 186
  poverty of, 103
  previous occupation of, 111
  problems with, 46, 67, 139–40, 162–6,
    167, 188–9
  relationships with employers, 5, 28, 33–7,
    47, 60, 62, 147–8, 172–3
  selection criteria for, 142
  separation from own babies, 82, 124–7
  single mothers as. *See under* single
    mothers
  uniforms for, 191
  wages for, 80, 91–2, 140–2, 162, 176, 187,
    188–9
wet nursing
  after maternal death, 17–18
  in America, 3, 8
  in colonial America, 8, 11–37
  decline of, 2, 6, 9, 139, 156, 200, 206

  as domestic service,
    in eighteenth century, 8, 11–37
    in Europe, 2–3, 8, 13
  history of, 4, 6–7
  as livelihood for women, 6, 7, 10, 17, 21,
    27, 29, 58, 98, 99, 200
  Margaret Mead and, 1, 2
  medicalization of, 128–55
  middle-class views of, 42
  moral complexities of, 129, 153(n111),
    155
  in nineteenth century, 44–5, 77–8, 128–55
  outplacement of infants for, 56, 58, 98
  as social custom, 32
  statisitcs on, 44
  as temporary employment, 21(n44)
  in twentieth century, 179–200
  in Western societies, 3(n7)
White [wet nurse's husband], 172, 173
White, Deborah Gray, 73
Wiggin, Oliver C., M.D., 127, 140
Wilson, E., M.D., 70
Wilson, Owen W., M.D., 183
Winters, Joseph Edcil, 138, 152–3
"woman of leisure," wet nursing and, 5
women
  as breast-milk sellers, 193, 194–5, 196
  as domestic servants, 42–3
  inability to breast-feed, 136–7
*The Women of New York or the Under-World
  of the Great City* (Ellington), 76
Women's Christian Association, 87
Women's Christian Temperance Union, 86,
  87, 156
Women's City Club (Kansas City), 200
women's magazines, infant food ads in, 134
work, concept of, in nineteenth century, 40–
  1
Work (Alcott), 75
Workman, Fanny Bullock, 141, 159–60,
  162–6, 171, 175, 178
World's Columbian Exhibition [Chicago,
  1893], 121

Yale, Leroy M., 166, 171
yellow fever, 31, 32

Zahorsky, John, M.D., 183
Zelizer, Viviana, 130

Continued from the front of the book

The science of woman: Gynecology and gender in England, 1800–1929
ORNELLA MOSCUCCI
Quality and quantity: The quest for biological regeneration in twentieth-century France WILLIAM H. SCHNEIDER
Bilharzia: A history of imperial tropical medicine JOHN FARLEY
Preserve your love for science: Life of William A. Hammond, American neurologist BONNIE E. BLUSTEIN
Patients, power, and the poor in eighteenth-century Bristol MARY E. FISSELL
AIDS and contemporary society EDITED BY VIRGINIA BERRIDGE AND PHILIP STRONG
Science and empire: East Coast fever in Rhodesia and the Transvaal PAUL F. CRANEFIELD
The colonial disease: A social history of sleeping sickness in Northern Zaire, 1900–1940 MARYINEZ LYONS
Mission and method: The early nineteenth-century French public health movement ANN F. LABERGE
Meanings of sex differences in the Middle Ages: Medicine, science, and culture JOAN CADDEN
Public health in British India: Anglo-Indian preventive medicine, 1859-1914 MARK HARRISON
Medicine before the Plague: Practitioners and their patients in the Crown of Aragon, 1285–1345 MICHAEL R. MCVAUGH
The physical and the moral: Anthropology, physiology, and philosophical medicine in France, 1750-1850. ELIZABETH A. WILLIAMS

For EU product safety concerns, contact us at Calle de José Abascal, 56–1°,
28003 Madrid, Spain or eugpsr@cambridge.org.

www.ingramcontent.com/pod-product-compliance
Ingram Content Group UK Ltd.
Pitfield, Milton Keynes, MK11 3LW, UK
UKHW042133130625

459647UK00003B/21